CONSTRUCTIVE THERAPIES
Volume 2

CONSTRUCTIVE THERAPIES
Volume 2

Edited by

Michael F. Hoyt

THE GUILFORD PRESS
New York   London

© 1996 The Guilford Press
A Division of Guilford Publications, Inc.
72 Spring Street, New York, NY 10012

Printed in the United States of America

This book is printed on acid-free paper.

Last digit is print number: 9 8 7 6 5 4 3 2 1

Library of Congress Cataloging-in-Publication Data

Constructive therapies / Michael F. Hoyt, editor.
    p. cm.
   Includes bibliographical references and index.
   ISBN 0-89862-094-5 (Vol. 1)   ISBN 1-57230-096-5 (Vol. 2)
   1. Brief psychotherapy.   2. Solution-focused therapy.
I. Hoyt, Michael F.
   [DNLM: 1. Psychotherapy, Brief.   WM 420 C758 1994]
RC480.55.C66 1994
616.89—dc20
DNLM/DLC
for Library of Congress   94-14220
                                     CIP

To Alexander
who said, at age six,
"Dad, there's a nation in my head.
It's called imagination!"

Information is news of the difference.
—GREGORY BATESON

I hate and renounce as a coward any person
who consents to being born and does not choose
to re-create himself.
—ANTONIN ARTAUD

From the conception the increase.
From the increase the swelling.
From the swelling the thought.
From the thought the remembrance.
From the remembrance the desire.
—MAORI SONG (NEW ZEALAND)

Time comes into it.
Say it. Say it.

The universe is made of stories,
not of atoms.
—MURIEL RUKEYSER

Rabbi Moshe Hayyim Efraim, the Baal Shem's
grandson, told: "I heard this from my grandfather:
Once a fiddler played so sweetly that all who heard
him began to dance, and whoever came near enough
to hear, joined in the dance. Then a deaf man, who
knew nothing of music, happened along, and to him
all he saw seemed the action of madmen—senseless
and in bad taste."
—MARTIN BUBER

Be a lamp to yourself. Be your own confidence. Hold
to the truth within yourself, as to the only truth.
—THE BUDDHA

Contributors

CONNIRAE ANDREAS, PhD, NLP Comprehensive, Boulder, Colorado

TAMARA ANDREAS, MM, NLP Comprehensive, Boulder, Colorado

GENE COMBS, MD, Evanston Family Therapy Center, Evanston, Illinois; Chicago Center for Family Health, Chicago, Illinois

VICTOR CORSIGLIA, PhD, private practice, San Jose, California

STEVE DE SHAZER, MSW, Brief Family Therapy Center, Milwaukee, Wisconsin

JOHN DYCKMAN, PhD, Kaiser Permanente Medical Center, Vallejo, California; California Institute of Integral Studies, San Francisco, California

DAVID EPSTON, MA, Family Therapy Centre, Sandringham, Auckland, New Zealand

KENNETH GERGEN, PhD, Swarthmore College, Swarthmore, Pennsylvania

STEPHEN G. GILLIGAN, PhD, private practice, Encinitas, California

JOSEPH A. GOLDFIELD, MSW, private practice, New York, New York

JEFFREY GOLDMAN, MSW, Peaceful Alternatives in the Home, Denver, Colorado

MICHAEL F. HOYT, PhD, Kaiser Permanente Medical Center, Hayward, California; University of California School of Medicine, San Francisco, California

CHARLES E. JOHNSON, MSW, The Solution Group, Lakewood, Colorado

BRADFORD P. KEENEY, PhD, University of St. Thomas, St. Paul, Minnesota

CLIFFORD LEVIN, PhD, private practice, Palo Alto, California; Mental Research Institute, Palo Alto, California; EMDR Research Center, Palo Alto, California

DONALD MEICHENBAUM, PhD, University of Waterloo, Waterloo, Ontario, Canada

DAVID NYLUND, LCSW, Kaiser Permanente Medical Center, Stockton, California

WILLIAM HUDSON O'HANLON, MS, Possibilities, Omaha, Nebraska

HAIM OMER, PhD, Tel-Aviv University, Tel-Aviv, Israel

WENDEL A. RAY, PhD, Mental Research Institute, Palo Alto, California; Northeast Louisiana University, Monroe, Louisiana

ROBERT ROSENBAUM, PhD, Kaiser Permanente Medical Center, Hayward, California; California Institute of Integral Studies, San Francisco, California

SALLYANN ROTH, MSW, Family Institute of Cambridge, Watertown, Massachusetts; Harvard Medical School at Cambridge Hospital, Cambridge, Massachusetts

FRANCINE SHAPIRO, PhD, Mental Research Institute, Palo Alto, California; EMDR Institute, Pacific Grove, California; EMDR Humanitarian Assistance Programs, El Granada, California.

JOHN H. WEAKLAND (deceased), ChE, MFCC, Brief Therapy Center, Mental Research Institute, Palo Alto, California

MICHAEL WHITE, MSW, Dulwich Centre, Adelaide, South Australia, Australia

Acknowledgments

An editor is blessed to have colleagues as fine as the contributors to this volume. I thank each and every one of them for their skill and friendship.

Thanks also to Seymour Weingarten, Editor-in-Chief at The Guilford Press, and to his fine staff, especially Senior Production Editor Anna Brackett; to Kaiser Permanente, for its continuing support; and to Sherran Boll, my secretary.

My special gratitude to Jennifer and Alex, for much more than words can express.

Finally (for now), I would like to acknowledge the passing of Carl Whitaker and John Weakland, both of whom died during the preparation of this book. Long ago Carl helped light my light, and more recently John provided clarity and encouragement. Like so many others, I am richer for having known them.

Contents

CHAPTER 1

Introduction
Some Stories Are Better Than Others

MICHAEL F. HOYT

The doors of therapeutic perception and possibility have been opened wide by the recognition that we are actively constructing our mental realities rather than simply uncovering or coping with an objective "truth." What makes us most human is not our opposable thumbs nor our use of tools but, rather, our capacity to conceive a future, recall a past, construct meaning, and make choices. How we choose to conceive and pattern the present, the past, and the future profoundly influences our course. This is a book about ways of enhancing such choices within the context of psychotherapy.

We conceive our "reality," creating "his-story" and "her-story" and "our-story" and "your-story," which in turn helps to create us, round and round.[1] Self-recursive autopoiesis. We can speculate regarding the origins of this narrative function, as does the novelist John Barth (1995, p. 96):

> [One can] wonder whether people reflexively think of their lives as stories because from birth to death they are exposed to so many narratives of every sort, or whether, contrariwise, our notion of what a "story" is, in every age and culture, reflects an innately dramatistic sense of life: a feature of the biological evolution of the human brain and of human consciousness, which appears to be essentially of a scenario-making character.

Whatever the source, organizing our world through the telling of stories is fundamental (Bruner, 1986; Omer & Strenger, 1992; Parry, 1991;

---

[1]Modern mass media make this feedback loop all the quicker. A recent article in *Newsweek* (Cowley & Springen, 1995) was entitled "Rewriting Life Stories." It not only heralded the narrative therapy approach, but also directed public consciousness toward a different way of thinking, with large type declaring "Instead of looking for flaws in people's psyches, 'narrative therapy' works at nurturing their forgotten strengths." This is part of the "technology of saturation" described by Gergen (1991).

Sarbin, 1986). As Engel (1995, p. 14; see also Singer & Salovey, 1993) describes it:

> Whether a particular story is remembered or not, the act of telling a story is always important to the developing child, because in the telling the child is both practicing telling stories and building up an inventory of stories that contribute to a life story and a self-representation. Who knows how she will use, save, savor, and blend these stories in the future. What does that matter? Because to a great extent we are the stories we tell, and our memories of personal experiences are what give us a history and a sense of who we are—past, present, and future.

Mary Catherine Bateson (1994, p. 11) elaborates:

> Wherever a story comes from, whether it is a familiar myth or a private memory, the retelling exemplifies the making of a connection from one pattern to another: a potential translation in which narrative becomes parable and the once upon a time comes to stand for some renascent truth. . . . Our species thinks in metaphors and learns through stories.
>
> Many tales have more than one meaning. It is important not to reduce understanding to some narrow focus, sacrificing multiplicity to what might be called the rhetoric of merely: merely a dead sheep, only an atavistic ritual, nothing but a metaphor. Openness to peripheral vision depends on rejecting such reductionism and rejecting with it the belief that questions of meaning have unitary answers.

MAKING A DIFFERENCE

What makes some stories better than others? Ultimately, of course, the answer must come from each individual freely, lest we impose our own values or beliefs. In general terms, stories involve a plot in which characters have experiences and employ imagination to resolve problems over time (Gergen & Gergen, 1986; also see Bruner, 1986; Berg, 1995; Yeung, 1995; Held, 1995, pp. 202–206). Our focus is on the therapeutic, making a difference, and the *sine qua non* must be the ultimate effect or change in the patient's or client's[2] life. Most of us would prefer images of "self" and "other" organized into a "narrative" that promotes a sense of autonomy, that "empowers" and allows a reasonably successful pursuit

---

[2]The terms *client* and *patient* are both used throughout this volume, at the discretion of respective authors. Each term may carry certain implications about the nature of the therapeutic relationship and the very reason for professional contact. *Client* may emphasize the egalitarian and minimize the implication of pathology, whereas *patient* may connote both a medical model (sickness and doctor–patient hierarchy) and the idea of the problem having to do with the alleviation of suffering (Hoyt, 1979, 1985). Whatever one calls the participants and the process (*therapy? treatment? intervention? consultation?*) helps to establish a meaning context and influences their work together.

of health and happiness—however one understands such concepts. Most people who become psychotherapy patients or clients are construing a different kind of story, however, and getting a different result.[3] Within this framework, the therapeutic endeavor can be understood as an attempt to construct and live within a more salutary reality. As Anderson and Goolishian (1988, p. 372) have written:

> Meaning and understanding are socially and intersubjectively constructed. By intersubjective, we refer to an evolving state of affairs in which two or more people agree (understand) that they are experiencing the same event in the same way. . . . Therapy is a linguistic event that takes place in what we call a therapeutic conversation. The therapeutic conversation is a mutual search and exploration through dialogue, a two-way exchange, a crisscrossing of ideas in which new meanings are continually evolving toward the "dis-solving" of problems and, thus, the dissolving of the therapy system and, hence, the *problem-organizing, problem-dis-solving system. Change is the evolution of new meaning through dialogue.* (emphasis in original)

Sometimes only a small (albeit significant) pattern change is wanted or needed; a client may revise some "viewing and doing" (O'Hanlon & Weiner-Davis, 1989), but is only looking for some simple problem solving and does not have life-encompassing problems that require an "identity overhaul" (O'Hanlon, 1994, p. 28; White, 1989b). Other times, however, for a client to achieve his/her/their goal one may need to engage the narrating function more fully, broadening the scope to assist in a "reauthoring" or "restorying" or "retelling" of a life (White, 1995; White & Epston, 1990; Freeman, 1993; Goulding & Goulding, 1979; Parry & Doan, 1994; Schafer, 1992; Spence, 1982; Polster, 1987; Steiner, 1974; Hudson & O'Hanlon, 1991).[4]

---

[3]Serving as a kind of Linnaeus of tormented tales as well as a cartographer of routes to less twisted territories, Gustafson (1992, 1995a, 1995b; see also Sluzki, 1992; McGoldrick, 1995; Omer, 1994; Roberts, 1994) presents numerous interesting nosologies. He situates the main stories of helping within the first world of objectivity, the second world of subjectivity, and the third world of narrative; he then categorizes (with many variations and nuances) the main stories of persons on fields of power into those having to do with subservience, bureaucratic delay, and overpowering. I particularly like his description (1992, p. 76) of the themes of marital conflict: "The first dilemma is whether to be in or out. The second is whether to be top or bottom. The third is whether to be near or far." To which I might add: "A fourth is whether to be hot or cold."

[4]Clinical practices in this realm are marked by terms such as *solution-oriented, solution-focused, possibility, narrative, postmodern, cooperative, competency-based*, and *constructivist*. An extensive bibliography is available in the first volume of *Constructive Therapies* (Hoyt, 1994a), and excellent overviews are available in *Therapy as Social Construction* (McNamee & Gergen, 1992), *The New Language of Change* (Friedman, 1993), *Therapeutic Conversations* (Gilligan & Price, 1993), *Constructing Realities* (Rosen & Kuelhwein, 1996), *The Reflecting Team in Action* (Friedman, 1995), *Constructivism in Psychotherapy* (Neimeyer & Mahoney, 1995), and *Narrative Therapy* (Freedman & Combs, 1996). For a critical analysis, see also *Back to Reality* (Held, 1995).

Life is not just lived "in the head," however, so intrapsychic modification is seldom sufficient. For the clinical endeavor to be therapeutic, change must become manifest in the world. "It takes two to speak the truth—one to speak and another to hear," said Henry David Thoreau (1854/1975). Hoffman (1993b, 1995) refers to "collaborative knowing"; de Shazer (1991, p. 50) succinctly says, "Between, not inside." While Lax (1992, p. 69) notes, "Psychotherapy is the process of shifting the client's 'problematic' discourse to another discourse that is more fluid and allows for a broader range of possible interactions," it is important that some of the "possible interactions" be realized. "Reality" may be a socially mediated construction, but, as Anderson and Goolishian (1988, p. 377, emphasis added) say, "*We live and take action* in a world that we define through our descriptive language in social intercourse with others." We "perform" (Omer, 1993) or "enact" (Sluzki, 1992) our narratives in the world. As discussed with Michael White and Gene Combs in Chapter 2, this is "taking steps on the path" and the "little sacraments of daily existence," with the recognition that alternative discourses "will have different real effects on the shape of the therapeutic interaction, different real effects on the lives of the people who consult us, and different real effects on our lives as well" (p. 34).

A radical constructivist position may hold that we are always part of the equation, that there is no knowing without the knower; but there are also other, extralinguistic forces to be reckoned with. One who ignores context, circumstances, consequences, events, objects, and various social structures and systems risks ignoring a lot (see Speed, 1984, 1991; Held, 1995). As discussed in the conversation with Bill O'Hanlon in Chapter 4, someone unmindful of traffic can still be run over! We may be making meaning and only be able to know approximately what's "out there" (we always more or less "misread," to use Steve de Shazer's [1991; de Shazer & Berg, 1992] term), but, as discussed with de Shazer in Chapter 3, there is a *there* there. The one is constituted in relation to the many and can only show stasis or change when situated socially. Hence, we ask: What (where, who, when) difference will therapy make, and how will we know it?

TO INTERVENE OR TO INTERVENE: *HOW* IS THE QUESTION

We cannot *not* communicate (Ruesch & Bateson, 1951; Watzlawick, Beavin, & Jackson, 1967). As John Weakland (1993, p. 143, emphasis in original) has written about strategic intervention:

> Just as one cannot *not* communicate, one cannot *not* influence. Influence is inherent in all human interaction. We are bound to influence our clients, and they are bound to influence us. The only choice is between doing so without reflection, or even with attempted denial, and doing so deliberately

and responsibly. Clients come seeking change which they could not achieve on their own; expertise in influencing them to change usefully seems to us the essence of the therapist's job. Therefore, we give much thought—guided, of course, by what a client does and says—to almost every aspect of treatment: To whom we will see in any given session, to the timing of sessions, to what suggestions we will offer as to new thoughts and actions, to responses we make to clients' reports of progress or difficulties encountered, and especially not just to the content of what we say, but to how we will phrase it. This strategic emphasis, however, does not mean that we propose or favor any arrangement in which a therapist has all the power, knowledge, control, and activity, while the patient is just a passive object of therapeutic actions—if indeed this were possible, which is very doubtful.

TAKING/MAKING HISTORY

All questions are leading questions (Epston, 1995; Madigan, 1993; Tomm, 1988; White & Epston, 1990), inviting (Freedman & Combs, 1993) us to focus our attention and consciousness here rather than there, suggesting or giving "privilege" to certain "knowledges" (patternings of awareness and conduct) rather than others. "Reality," therapeutic or not, is co-created in relationships, a social weaving of meaning (Watzlawick, 1976, 1984, 1992). Consequently, hermeneutics (Frank, 1987; Fine & Turner, 1995) rather than engineering, and poetics rather than physics, are the fields of study that examine the warp and weft of human life.[5]

Consider the observation of St. Augustine in his *Confessions* (quoted in Boscolo & Bertrando, 1993, p. 34):

> What is by now evident and clear is that neither future nor past exists, and it is inexact language to speak of three times—past, present, and future. Perhaps it would be exact to say: there are three times, a present of things past, a present of things present, a present of things to come. In the soul there are these three aspects of time, and I do not see them anywhere else. The present considering the past is the memory, the present considering the future is expectation.

Memory is active and constructive. As autobiographer Mary Helen Ponce (1993, p. ix) writes: "The memory is a mysterious—and powerful—thing. It forgets what we want most to remember, and retains what we often wish to forget. We take from it what we need." Mary Catherine Bateson (1994) refers to "peripheral visions: learning along the way." Along similar lines, Milton Erickson (1980, p. 27) spoke of the "uncon-

---

[5]Hence, my protoconstructivist *bubbe* (grandmother) was on to something when she asked, "A PhD? So what kind of disease is philosophy that it needs a doctor?" (Hoyt, 1994b, p. 77).

scious" as a "storehouse" and a "reservoir of learning," and commented, "any knowledge acquired by your unconscious mind is knowledge that you can use at any appropriate time. But you need not necessarily be aware that you have that knowledge until the moment comes to use it" (quoted in R. A. Havens, 1989, p. 69). As Shakespeare (1623/1974) asked in *The Tempest* (Act I, Scene ii, lines 48–50):

> . . . But how is it
> That this lives in thy mind? What seest thou else
> In the dark backward and abysm of time?[6]

With this awareness, one can assist a client in "looking back" to elicit histories that will support an alternative present and future (White, 1993; Madanes, Keim, Lentine, & Keim, 1990). A "history of the present recovery" may be more salutary than the conventional psychiatric "history of the present complaint." One can also assist clients to imagine future times (in a kind of "forward to the present" rather than "back to the future"), which will then give better meanings to current life as it is lived (Furman & Ahola, 1992; Penn, 1985).[7] As Thoreau advised in *Walden* (1854/1975, pp. 562–563):

> If one advances confidently in the direction of his dreams, and endeavors to live the life which he has imagined, he will meet with a success unexpected in common hours. . . . If you have built castles in the air, your work need not be lost; that is where they should be. Now put the foundations under them.

As we will see, there are many ways to look, and how we look determines what we see. Events may happen, but what meaning will be given? The ancient Greek philosopher Epicritus (quoted in Watzlawick,

---

[6]Henry Miller (quoted in Brassai, 1995, p. 144) notes: "Autobiography is the purest romance. . . . What can possibly be more fictive than the story of one's life?" Novelist Vladimir Nabokov (quoted in McGoldrick, 1995, p. 58) also reminds us that the stories we hear are subject to various influences: "Remember, what you are told is really threefold: Shaped by the teller, reshaped by the listener, and concealed from them both by the deadman of the tale." Aesop's fable of the three blind men examining the elephant, Faulkner's *The Sound and the Fury*, and the classic Japanese film *Rashomon* all illustrate the profound influence of perspective.

[7]There is no time but the present; or, as C. S. Lewis described it in *The Screwtape Letters* (1941/1982, pp. 80–81), the present is where time and eternity meet. Eric Berne, the originator of transactional analysis, observed many people organizing their life story in terms of an approach to time: "Winning or losing, the script is a way to structure the time between the first Hello at mother's breast and the last Good-by at the grave. This life time is emptied and filled by not doing and doing; by never doing, always doing, not doing before, not doing after, doing over and over, and doing until there is nothing left to do. This gives rise to 'Never' and 'Always,' 'Until' and 'After,' 'Over and Over,' and 'Open-Ended' scripts" (Berne, 1972, p. 205). For other perspectives on time and therapy, see Boscolo and Bertrando (1993), Hoyt (1990), Melges (1982), and Ricoeur (1983).

1992, p. 61) made this recognition when he wrote, "It is not the things that bother us, but the opinions that we have about these things." In this century, Albert Einstein (quoted by Watzlawick, 1994) noted: "Theories do not come from observations; rather, observations come from theories." Along related lines, Alfred Adler (1931/1958, p. 4, emphasis in original; see also Ellis, 1990; Kelly, 1955) recognized:

> Human beings live in the realm of *meanings*. . . . We experience reality always through the meaning we give it; not in itself, but as something interpreted. It will be natural to suppose, therefore, that this meaning is always more or less unfinished, incomplete; and even that is never altogether right. The realm of meanings is the realm of mistakes.

As James Hillman (Goulding & Hillman, 1995) has commented: "Your countertransference is there long before the transference begins." For better or worse, the beliefs that result from the processes of attribution (Jones et al., 1972; Collins & Hoyt, 1972; Furman & Ahola, 1989) can have great influence.

Behold the constructive power in statements such as these:

> I discovered I had no resentment toward my mother, as I had believed, and could remember her with the goodwill that neither of us was able to express while she was alive. I no longer had to invent a [mother] that suited my needs, and anyway, we shape our own past and build memories of many fantasies. (Isabel Allende, *The Infinite Plan,* 1993, p. 347)

> She had indeed stepped from the road which seemed to have been chosen for her and cut herself a brand-new path. . . . Each of us has the right and the responsibility to assess the roads which lie ahead, and those over which we have traveled, and if the future road looms ominous or unpromising, and the roads back uninviting, then we need to gather our resolve and, carrying only the necessary baggage, step off that road into another direction. If the new choice is also unpalatable, without embarrassment, we must be ready to change that as well. (Maya Angelou, *Wouldn't Take Nothing for My Journey Now,* 1993, p. 24)

> "A warrior is aware that the world will change as soon as he stops talking to himself," he said, "and he must be prepared for that monumental jolt."
> "What do you mean, Don Juan?"
> "The world is such-and-such and so-and-so only because we tell ourselves that that is the way it is. If we stop telling ourselves that the world is so-and-so, the world will stop being so-and-so. At this moment I don't think you're ready for such a momentous blow, therefore, you must start slowly to undo the world." (Carlos Castaneda, *A Separate Reality,* 1971, p. 264)

> Black Elk, a very famous Sioux Medicine Man, was asked, "Are these stories true?" He answered, "Well, I don't know if they happened exactly that way,

but if you listen to them long enough, you will hear how they are true."
(Susan Strauss, *Coyote Stories for Children*, 1991, n.p.)

When you play songs, you can bring back people's memories of when they
fell in love. That's where the power is. (Johnny Mercer, songwriter of "Moon
River," etc.; quoted in John Berendt, *Midnight in the Garden of Good and Evil*,
1994, p. 90)

Happiness lies in the endowment with value of all of the things you
have.—Dad. (Milton H. Erickson, birthday card message to his daughter-in-
law, Kathy Erickson, March 19, 1980; personal communication from Kathy
Erickson)

PERSONS VERSUS PROBLEMS

Constructivist approaches are based on the construction that we are
constructive—that we are engaged in a process of actively building
our reality or world view, instead of there being an "objective" world
that can be known independent of the knower. Emphasizing how
language shapes and is shaped by human relationships, Gergen
(1993, p. x) writes:

> The various accounts brought to therapy by the client—tales of misery,
> oppression, failures, and the like—serve not as approximations to the truth,
> perhaps biased by desires or cognitive incapacities, but as life constructions,
> made up of narratives, metaphors, cultural logics, and the like. They are
> more like musical or poetic accompaniments than mirrors or maps. And
> their major significance lies not in their relative validity, but in their social
> utility. In this context a major aim of therapy becomes one of freeing the
> client from a particular kind of account and opening the way to alternatives
> of greater promise.

A gateway into this perspective was neatly opened in the statement
by Milton Erickson: "Not everything you see is the way you see it is"
(quoted by Carl Hammerschlag in the videotape by Haley & Richeport,
1993). Creating uncertainty opens the door. Hence, McGoldrick (1995,
p. 56) suggests "jostling" your view of your family. Writing within the
context of architecture, Papadakis, Cooke, and Benjamin (1989, flyleaf)
say: "Deconstruction is characterized by an essential distrust of the
authenticity of apparent meaning and form and the traditional distinction between the two."[8] According to Goolishian (quoted in de Shazer,
1991, p. 50), "to deconstruct means to take apart the interpretive

---

[8]Art criticism and literary criticism have yielded fertile ground for variegated development of this concept. As Bennington (1989, p. 84) expands:
   1. Deconstruction is not what you think.

assumptions of the system of meaning that you are examining, to challenge the interpretive system in such a manner that you reveal the assumptions on which the model is based. At the same time, as these are revealed, you open the space for alternative understanding." As Hoffman (1993a, p. 104) notes:

> Postmodern and poststructural thinking has allowed us to look afresh at all prized or sacred writings and to "deconstruct" them. The purpose behind deconstructing a text is basically one of political emancipation: by laying bare the relations of domination and submission embedded in the text, one (hopefully) weakens its power to oppress.

Michael White (1991/1993, pp. 34–36) elaborates the implications of *deconstruction* for psychotherapy:

> According to my rather loose definition, deconstruction has to do with procedures that subvert taken-for-granted realities and practices: those so-called "truths" that are split off from the conditions and the context of their production; those disembodied ways of speaking that hide their biases and prejudices; and those familiar practices of self and of relationship that are subjugating of persons' lives. Many of the methods of deconstruction render strange these familiar and everyday taken-for-granted realities and practices by objectifying them. In this sense, the methods of deconstruction are methods that 'exoticize the domestic.' . . . Deconstruction is premised on what is generally referred to as a 'critical constructivist' or, as I would prefer, a 'constitutionalist' perspective on the world. From this perspective, it is proposed that persons' lives are shaped by the meaning that they ascribe to their experience, by their situation in social structures, and by the language practices and cultural practices of self and of relationship that these lives are recruited into. . . . This constructionalist perspective is at variance with the dominant structuralist (behavior reflects the structure of the mind) and functionalist (behavior serves a purpose for the system) perspectives of the world of psychotherapy.

Inherent in this view is the narrative therapy motto, "It is not the person who is . . . the problem. Rather, it is the problem that is the problem" (White, 1989b, p. 6; see also O'Hanlon, 1994). Redekop (1995,

---

[. . .]
1.3   Deconstruction is not what you think. If what you think is a content, present to mind, in "the mind's presence-room" (Locke). But that you think might already be Deconstruction.
2.   Deconstruction is not (what you think if you think it is) essentially to do with language.
2.1   Nothing more common than to hear Deconstruction described as depending on "an extension of the linguistic paradigm." "There is nothing outside the text" (Derrida): proves it, obviously.
2.1.1   Everybody also knows this is not quite right. "Text" is not quite an extension of a familiar concept, but a displacement or reinscription of it. Text in general is any system of marks, traces, referrals (don't say reference, have a little more sense than that). Perception is a text. [etc.]

p. 317, emphasis added; see also Madigan, 1992) quotes Michel Foucault (1988) as saying: "*Problematization* is the 'totality of discursive and non-discursive practices that introduces something into the play of the true and false and constitute[s] it as an object for thought (whether in the form of moral reflection, scientific knowledge, political analysis, etc.).' "[9] The consequent practices of *externalizing the problem* are steps toward reclaiming autonomy:

> "Externalizing" is an approach to therapy that encourages persons to objectify, and at times, to personify, the problems that they experience as oppressive. In this process, the problem becomes a separate entity and thus external to the person who was, or the relationship that was, ascribed the problem. Those problems that are considered to be inherent, and those relatively fixed qualities that are attributed to persons and to relationship, are rendered less fixed and less restricting. (White, 1989b, p. 5)

As White (1991/1993, p. 39) elaborates:

> These externalizing conversations "exoticize the domestic" in that they encourage persons to identify the private stories and the cultural knowledges that they live by; those stories and knowledges that guide their lives and that speak to them of their identity. These externalizing conversations assist persons to unravel, across time, the constitution of their self and of their relationships. Externalizing conversations are initiated by encouraging persons to provide an account of the effects of the problem on their lives. This can include its effects on their emotional states, familial and peer relationships, social and work spheres, etc., and with a special emphasis on how it has affected their "view" of themselves and of their relationships. Then, persons are invited to map the influence that these views or perceptions have on their lives, including on their interactions with others. This is often followed by some investigation of how persons have been recruited into these views.
>
> As persons become engaged in these externalizing conversations, their private stories cease to speak to them of their identity and of the truth of their relationships—these private stories are no longer transfixing of their

---

[9]Constructive therapists truly respect their clients' own capacities. Hence, Anderson and Goolishian (1992) write of "the client as expert"; Lipchik (1994) describes solution focus as a basic attitude or orientation rather than a set of techniques; and Michael White (Wylie, 1994) is noted for his "congruence" rather than harboring a privately disrespectful view that would put down clients while elevating therapist authority. Similarly, Gergen (1995b) and Tomm (1990) reveal some of the many ways therapists have developed a clinical language that reinforces and disseminates deficit; and de Shazer and Weakland (quoted in Hoyt, 1994c, p. 20) comment that the activity of many professionals is "not a mental health industry; it's a mental illness industry." (For an antipathologizing exercise, see Dickerson & Zimmerman, 1995.) A fundamentally healthy attitude was expressed by Carl Rogers (quoted in Satir, 1993, p. 75) when he declared: "What I am is good enough if I would only be it openly."

lives. Persons experience a separation from, and an alienation in relation to, these stories. In the space established by this separation, persons are free to explore alternative and preferred knowledges of who they might be; alternative and preferred knowledges into which they might enter their lives.

Following White's description (see also O'Hanlon, 1994; Redekop, 1995; Freedman & Combs, 1996; and Roth & Epston, in press, plus Roth & Epston's training exercise in Chapter 6), externalizing in narrative therapy typically involves separating the person from the problem by naming the problem and exploring the person's relationship to the problem, including ways the problem may achieve influence over him or her and ways he or she sometimes resists the problem's attempts. There are also methods drawn from other theoretical approaches that can be seen, through the narrative lens, as forms of externalization. For example, Miller (1994; see also Bateson, 1972a) notes the externalizing function of substance "addiction" models; Hoyt (1994d) calls attention to the externalizing function of Gestalt therapy two-chair work ("Put your guilt in that chair and tell it how you feel"); and L. L. Havens (1986, p. 6) describes Harry Stack Sullivan as sometimes sitting next to a patient so that they could look out together at the problem that was troubling the person. Aspects of psychodrama, mindfulness meditation, mask and play therapy, and various "alternative" healing practices could be added to the list. Unlike classic psychodynamic theory, which construes externalization as a "defense mechanism" that "distorts reality" by the disowning of personal responsibility, narrative therapy construes the process as the externalizing of the problem and the internalizing of personal agency (Tomm, 1989).

Although not all cases require exposition of mystified sociocultural power/knowledge factors (Laing, 1967; Foucault, 1980; White, 1989b), clinicians need to be careful that they do not simply adjust clients to more of the same rather than assisting them toward "exceptions" (de Shazer, 1985), "new directions" (O'Hanlon & Weiner-Davis, 1989), or "unique outcomes" (White & Epston, 1990). There is the risk—as Lerner (1995) has passionately argued—that health care policies may in effect seal off awareness of such factors if therapists are restricted to managing immediate symptomatology and are enjoined from looking at antecedent or systemic issues. " 'History' is written by the winners," as they say, with the dominant culture's voice (or discourse) given privilege and recognition over others'. The caution sounded by Marshall McLuhan (quoted in Karrass, 1992, p. 78) is worth noting: "For any medium has the power of imposing its own assumptions on the unwary. But the greatest aid is simply in knowing that the spell can occur immediately upon contact, as in the first bars of a melody." With this understanding, "resistance" can be seen quite differently from the conventional psychiatric pejorative.

Not identifying and honoring the client's treatment goals may make it necessary for the client to "resist" (de Shazer, 1984). Clients who are described as "noncompliant" or "resistant" may be in a power-politics struggle (see Tomm, 1993), engaged in counteroppressive practices to refuse being psychologically colonized or bent in directions they don't wish to go. In such cases, *vive la résistance!*

A meta-view of some of the broader pragmatic implications of a constructivist or postmodern perspective for psychotherapeutic prac-tice—in which (following Neimeyer, 1995) therapy may be conceived as a form of personal science, selfhood development, narrative reconstruc-tion, or conversational elaboration—is presented in Table 1.1.

RESPONSIBILITIES

At its finest, a constructivist approach increases our sense of empower-ment and participation, and reminds us that the essence of being human is that we are "meaning makers" and that no one can remain neutral in the "art of experience" (Hoffman, 1990; Rosenbaum & Bohart, 1994; White, 1995).[10] There are, however, numerous perils potentially lurking when one forgoes the safety of the positivist/objectivist shore. Beware pitfalls. One can slide into an antiscientism or lack of standards of knowledge or critical thinking (Gergen, 1994; Held, 1995; Lincoln, 1990; Smith, 1994). The application of logic and rationality to shared meanings is important, lest chaos reign if we imitate the mind-boggling March Hare and Mad Hatter in Lewis Carroll's *Alice in Wonderland* as they redefine terms willy-nilly. Even if more prosaic or straightforward,

> There are circumstances in which people are just wrong about what they are doing and how they are doing it. It is not that they lie . . . but that they confabulate; they fill in the gaps, guess, speculate, mistake theoretizing for observing. The relation between what they say and whatever it is that drives them to say what they say could hardly be more obscure. . . . [They] are

[10]We are always part of the equation, even if, as Bruner (1986, p. 155) comments, "there is no end to belief in meaning and reality. We thirst after them. We are natural ontologists but relevant epistemologists." Lyddon and Bradford (1995) note how trainees' personal philosophical beliefs influence their preferences for different therapy approaches. In a recent *American Psychologist* article, Madigan, Johnson, and Linton (1995) also note that how we are trained to tell the story (i.e., the forms we learn to follow in professional writing) teaches us how to think and thus inculcates a particular viewpoint, which in turn shapes what we see and report, and so on. Lest we think that "scientific" writing is exempt from subjective influences, Gould (1987, p. 85) cautions: "Scientific papers are polite or self-serving fictions in their statements about doing science; they are, at best, logical reconstructions after the fact, written under the conceit that fact and argument shape conclusions by their own inexorable demands of reasons. Levels of interacting complex-ity, contradictory motives, thoughts that lie too deep for either tears or even self-recog-nition—all combine to shape this most complex style of human knowledge."

TABLE 1.1. Selected Strategic and Technical Preferences of Constructivist Therapies

Area	Strategic preferences	Representative interventions
Assessment focus	Exploration of personal narratives, autobiography, personal and family construct systems and hierarchies	Identification of central metaphors, life review, repertory grids, laddering techniques
Goal of therapy	Creative rather than corrective; promotion of meaning-making and personal development	Fixed-role therapy, stream-of-consciousness technique, facilitation of meaningful accounts
Interpretation of emotion	Treatment of negative emotion as integral to constructive change; to be respected rather than controlled	Reprocessing of emotional schemata, systematic evocative unfolding, psychodramatic exploration
Level of intervention	Attention to selfhood processes, core role structures, family constructs or premises	Movieola technique, enactment of deep role relationship, circular questions, ritual prescription
Style of therapy	Personal rather than authoritative; empathic grasping of client's outlook as basis of negotiation	Credulous approach, adoption of "not-knowing approach, elaboration of metaphor or story
Approach to resistance	To understand as a legitimate attempt to protect core-ordering processes; modulate pace of change	"Allowing" resistance, externalizing of the problem, identification of unique outcomes

Note. From Neimeyer (1995, p. 17). Copyright 1995 by the American Psychological Association. Reprinted by permission.

unwitting creators of fictions, but to say that they are unwitting is to grant that what they say is, or can be, an account of exactly how it seems to them. (Dennett, 1991, quoted in Fancher, 1995, p. 1)

Others worry that we may overlook the inevitability of our influence, as well as the miserable circumstances of some individuals and families, especially amongst the poor and disadvantaged. Thus, while acknowledging "the richness that the constructivist movement contributes to our understanding of language, stories, and co-construction" (p. 10), Minuchin (1992; see also Held, 1995) argues:

> I am extremely concerned about the preservation of strengths that, I think, are vitiated by the constructivist framing. [p. 5] . . . When the constructivists equate expertise with power . . . and develop a new technology of interventions that avoid control, they are only creating a different use of power. Control does not disappear from family therapy when it is renamed "cocreation." All that happens is that the influence of the therapist on the family is made invisible. Safely underground, it may remain unexamined. Therapy is a temporary arrangement. Hierarchies are mutually organized for a period of time and for a "more or less" specific purpose. Temporary as it is, this arrangement would be a sham if the therapist were not an expert—that is, a person of informed uncertainty—on the human condition, the variety of family systems, family and individual development, processes of change, and the handling of dialogues, metaphors, and stories. . . . The bottom line is that the constructivist approach, by bracketing the idiosyncratic story, obscures the social fabric that also constructs it. [pp. 7–8] . . . Constructivist practice, with some exceptions, binds the therapist to the procrustean bed of talking and meaning, robbing the therapist of human complexity. [p. 10]

Especially because meaning is so fluid, there are risks of (perhaps unknowingly) imposing one's own values; Mahoney (1995) cautions that the psychological demands of being a constructive psychotherapist are many and that a great degree of openness to self-examination and ambiguity is required. There is also the danger of those who are deliberately misleading or nefarious, including actual perpetrators as well as persons who knowingly ignore or dismiss claims of individual or societal abuse (e.g., incest, the Holocaust). Hence, Frank Pittman decries those who hide behind "It's all in your mind" or "That's just how *you* look at it" to justify an irresponsible "It's not my fault":

> Postmodernism entered family therapy in the form of constructivism, espousing that reality is in the eye of the beholder, and that it doesn't matter what people do, only what story they tell about it. What a breakthrough! People don't have to change what they do! They can just use different words instead! Constructivism is fun intellectual masturbation, until we notice that the world constructivism is defining away is a cruel, unsafe, unfair place that hurts real people. (Pittman, 1992, p. 58)

In addition, there is the perhaps more subtle but also pernicious practice of reducing experience to explanation (Hillman, 1975), with a resultant loss of purposefulness, passion, and soul. Theorizing and categorizing experience can produce "petrification" (Polster, 1992, p. 144; see also Whitaker, 1976). Moreover, empathy and human relatedness can get short shrift if attention is too centered on the technologies of adjusting the calculus of cognition. As West (1993, p. 22) comments:

Nihilism is to be understood here not as a philosophical doctrine that there are no rational grounds for legitimate standards or authority; it is, far more, the lived experience of coping with a life of horrifying meaninglessness, hopelessness, and (most important) lovelessness. The frightening result is a numbing detachment from others and a self-destructive disposition toward the world. Life without meaning, hope, and love breeds a cold-hearted, mean-spirited outlook that destroys both the individual and others.

The Jungian analyst Robert Moore (1994, p. 9) counsels us to take the high road:

Is there an understandable reason why contemporary Western culture seems to be deconstructing itself into nihilism and anarchy? Careful reflection . . . can help us to understand some of the primary reasons for our deep—and contagious—disease. The culture of modernism with its attendant secularization and de-emphasis on the role of ritual in human adaptation has been dominated by the archetype of the magician and its shadow or dysfunctional forms. One might say that our culture is 'possessed' by the immature shadow-magician. When human beings use their magical potentials in the service of healing and community, the deconstructive and sociopathic energies of the immature magician—the trickster—are transformed into a mature, shamanic form that heals both self and the larger community.[11]

WHAT'S AHEAD

The psychotherapy practitioners and theorists who have contributed to this volume (and its predecessor, Hoyt, 1994a) have provided a veritable cornucopia of creative concepts, specific techniques, and fascinating case examples to illustrate ways of working respectfully, collaboratively, and successfully with people who have a broad range of problems. In addition to an explicit emphasis on how the client constructs "reality," of course, with its attendant and intrinsic awareness of language, the authors repeatedly highlight the value of the alliance relationship, respect for the client's own strengths and capacities, the power of imagina-

---

[11]Halifax (1993, p. 148) also describes the "deep interconnectedness" of traditional peoples as a corrective to the dualistic view of reality often dominant in contemporaneous constructions: "The wisdom of the peoples of elder cultures can make an important contribution to the postmodern world, one that we must begin to accept as the crisis of self, society, and the environment deepens. This wisdom cannot be told, but it is to be found by each of us in the direct experience of silence, stillness, solitude, simplicity, ceremony, and vision." But how "real" is "real"? How "natural" is "nature" (Pollan, 1991)? Is it ersatz if media mediate? In *The Age of Missing Information*, McKibben (1992) reports an interesting experiment in which he compares what is experienced over 24 hours sitting in nature with what is experienced over the same 24 hours in front of a television.

tion to go beyond or expand the present, and the importance of making a positive and practical difference in the person's life. While no single chapter (or book) can fully teach a method of psychotherapy, the hope is that readers will, through transcripts and commentaries, get a sense of what actually happens and what characterizes particular approaches. This is a "how to" book, a user's guide, intended to promote skills in various forms of constructive therapy.

Chapter 2, "On Ethics and the Spiritualities of the Surface: A Conversation with Michael White," goes right to the heart of the matter. White's many works, of course, include his recent *Re-Authoring Lives: Interviews and Essays* (1995) and *Selected Papers* (1989a), as well as (with David Epston) the signal *Narrative Means to Therapeutic Ends* (White & Epston, 1990) and *Experience, Contradiction, Narrative and Imagination* (Epston & White, 1992). Joining me as an interviewer was Gene Combs, who is well known for having co-authored both *Symbol, Story, and Ceremony* (Combs & Freedman, 1990) and *Narrative Therapy: The Social Construction of Preferred Realities* (Freedman & Combs, 1996). A complicated interview schedule had been prepared about many of the theoretical and technical features of the narrative approach, but, in the moment, we instead focused on the spirit that informs the work. Our ensuing discussion about the values of caring, compassion, and service—the importance of constructing a path with love—took us to the far shore. An exercise is included to help readers recognize and resist ways in which their conscious purpose and commitment to psychotherapeutic work may be undermined by common pathologizing discourses.

Chapter 3, "Solution Building and Language Games: A Conversation with Steve de Shazer," explores some of the history and minimalist elegance of the solution-focused approach that de Shazer has described in works such as *Keys to Solution in Brief Therapy* (1985), *Clues* (1988), *Putting Difference to Work* (1991), and *Words Were Originally Magic* (1994). Special attention is paid to the way language is used to construct reality and therapeutic solutions. As a bonus, at the end of the conversation Insoo Kim Berg joins us and provides some perspective on her perspective.

Chapter 4, "Welcome to PossibilityLand: A Conversation with Bill O'Hanlon," elaborates ways of using brief therapy and solution-oriented therapy methods to help clients expand their perceived options and to move safely into more desirable ways of being, with a special focus on assisting persons suffering aftereffects from sexual abuse and other trauma. The coauthor of many books, including *In Search of Solutions* (O'Hanlon & Weiner-Davis, 1989), *A Field Guide to PossibilityLand* (O'Hanlon & Beadle, 1994), and *Love Is a Verb* (O'Hanlon & Hudson, 1995), O'Hanlon emphasizes the importance of acknowledgment and validation as a first and essential (and often overlooked) part of (brief) therapy. The discussion of the *narrative* and the *experiential* senses of self is particularly fascinating within the context of current controversies regarding "true" and "false" recall of abuse.

Chapter 5, "Cognitive-Behavioral Treatment of Posttraumatic Stress Disorder from a Narrative Constructivist Perspective: A Conversation with Donald Meichenbaum," also addresses issues in the treatment of persons who have been abused. Like the other interviewees, Meichenbaum is extraordinarily articulate and informed, drawing on an extensive clinical and research background. His many publications include the classic *Cognitive-Behavior Modification* (1977) and the recent *A Clinical Handbook/Practical Therapist Manual for Treating PTSD* (1994). In our discussion, he, too, focuses on the importance of the therapeutic relationship being collaborative and the need for careful attention to language, and addresses ways (including some cultural nuances) of helping clients to get "unstuck" by continuing their telling of the story until they construct a narrative that allows them to move forward beyond the trauma.

Chapter 6, "Consulting the Problem about the Problematic Relationship: An Exercise for Experiencing a Relationship with an Externalized Problem," is by Sallyann Roth and David Epston. Roth's previous contributions include an excellent chapter on narrative couples therapy (Roth & Chasin, 1994) in the first volume of *Constructive Therapies,* as well as her work in the Public Conversations Project (Roth, 1993; Roth, Chasin, Chasin, Becker, & Herzig, 1992). Epston, of course, is one of the originators and leaders of the narrative therapy movement. In addition to his well-known books with Michael White, *Narrative Means to Therapeutic Ends* (White & Epston, 1990) and *Experience, Contradiction, Narrative and Imagination* (Epston & White, 1992), a fine volume of his *Collected Papers* (1989) has also been published. Here Roth and Epston present a powerful exercise to engage participants actively in the externalizing process. Their chapter makes especially clear how the construction of metaphoric relationships to "the problem" helps free the client from the language trap of "disease–cure" and opens a plenitude of possibilities.

Chapter 7, "From Deficits to Special Abilities: Working Narratively with Children Labeled 'ADHD,'" is by David Nylund, coeditor of *Narrative Therapy with Children and Adolescents* (Nylund & Smith, in press), and Victor Corsiglia. They suggest that the medical/psychiatric model may, in various ways, impose a disempowering and demoralizing view upon children, parents, and treating professionals. Instead, they offer and illustrate with case examples ways in which the diagnosis of ADHD (attention-deficit/hyperactivity disorder) can be understood (deconstructed) in cultural context and everyone's energies can be directed to supporting an appreciation of the child's abilities, especially as they are applied to coping with (externalized) disturbing symptoms. The authors emphasize that a narrative approach provides a useful alternative and that the choice is not either/or; conventional psychiatric treatment (medication) and the more constructive therapeutic approach they advocate can coexist and even work synergistically.[12]

Chapter 8, "A Solution-Focused Approach to Safety in Cases of Domestic Violence," is by Charles E. Johnson and Jeffrey Goldman. Using several case illustrations, they describe ways of joining with and empowering clients. Rather than exploring family-of-origin dynamics, detailing episodes of violence, or imposing psychoeducation, their approach places strong emphasis on a collaborative therapeutic relationship that actively builds on positive "differences that make a difference" (de Shazer, 1991) to help clients achieve their treatment goals. The authors also note that when clients' capacities for self-determination are supported, sometimes one or both members of a relationship may recognize that their goals will not be met within the relationship; in such instances, one partner may bring safety home by separating from the other.

Chapter 9, "When the Past Is Present: A Conversation about EMDR and the MRI Interactional Approach," is by Clifford Levin, Francine Shapiro, and John H. Weakland. Levin (1993) is the author of a *Family Therapy Networker* case study that used both eye movement desensitization and reprocessing (EMDR) and the Mental Research Institute (MRI) brief therapy model, and Shapiro is the originator of the rapidly emerging EMDR approach and the author of the highly informative 1995 book, *Eye Movement Desensitization and Reprocessing: Basic Principles, Protocols, and Procedures*. Weakland, of course, was long associated with MRI and the development of strategic brief therapy; his death during this project was a significant loss for the entire field. He was a coauthor of both the seminal *Change: Principles of Problem Formation and Problem Resolution* (Watzlawick, Weakland, & Fisch, 1974) and *The Tactics of Change: Doing Therapy Briefly* (Fisch, Weakland, & Segal, 1982), as well as *Counseling Elders and Their Families: Practical Techniques for Applied Gerontology* (Herr & Weakland, 1979). He also coedited *The Interactional View* (Watzlawick & Weakland, 1977) and *Propagations: Thirty Years of Influence from the Mental Research Institute* (Weakland & Ray, 1995). He was a participant

---

[12]*Restoring restorying* is the term I prefer to describe the use of medication to support clients' self-empowerment. Issues of informed consent are paramount, of course, with adults or children; Nylund and Corsiglia articulate well some of the ways in which children's own expertise and autonomy can be engaged and respected. Used appropriately and respectfully, psychiatric/medical intervention need not be construed negatively. While there is great room for abuse (mind control), there are also many patients for whom medication allows thinking to focus and mood to abate enough for them to get on with the "reauthoring" and living of their lives. For more on the importance of the *meaning* patients ascribe to their medication, see Meichenbaum (1994, pp. 299–301).

in many published conversations with Milton Erickson (Haley, 1985) and was also one of the coauthors of the original double-bind hypothesis (Bateson, Jackson, Haley, & Weakland, 1956). Typical of his wide interests and collaborative energy, he recently coauthored an article describing the consultative application of brief strategic therapy within the context of a psychodynamic treatment framework (Weakland, Johnson, & Morrissette, 1995), and in the present chapter was engaged in developing an interactional understanding of the EMDR process.

Chapter 10, "The Relational Self: The Expanding of Love beyond Desire," is by Stephen G. Gilligan. The author of *Therapeutic Trances: The Cooperation Principle in Ericksonian Hypnotherapy* (1987), and the coeditor of *Brief Therapy: Myths, Methods, and Metaphors* (Zeig & Gilligan, 1990) and *Therapeutic Conversations* (Gilligan & Price, 1993), here he distinguishes between two basic approaches to psychological experience—fundamentalism versus aesthetics—and then explicates ways in which the former leads to rigidity and violence, whereas the latter leads to openness and harmony. Conceptualizing self as consciousness, as relational field, and as relational differences, he describes detailed clinical procedures to suggest ways to help clients restore and expand their being and relatedness.[13]

Chapter 11, "No Self? No Problem! Actualizing Empty Self in Psychotherapy," by Robert Rosenbaum and John Dyckman, presents an entrancing discussion situated in the nexus of systemic epistemology and Buddhist theory/practice. They suggest that we tend to define or construct our sense of self by what we exclude or rule out, and that concepts of a reified "self" are literally small-minded and unnecessarily limited. Numerous examples are provided to help readers and clients engage in a freer and broader experience.

Chapter 12, "Core Transformation: A Brief Therapy Approach to Emotional and Spiritual Healing," is by Connirae Andreas and Tamara Andreas. The senior author, recognized as a major figure in the neurolinguistic programming (NLP) field through her trainings and coauthorship (with her husband, Steve) of such volumes as *Change Your Mind–and Keep the Change* (S. Andreas & Andreas, 1987) and *Heart of the Mind* (C. Andreas & Andreas, 1989), here joins with her sister to report some of the developments described at length in their book, *Core Transformation: Reaching the Wellspring Within* (C. Andreas & Andreas, 1994). They

---

[13]As Gregory Bateson (1972a, p. 331) wrote in discussing the cybernetics of "self": "The 'self' as ordinarily understood is only a small part of a much larger trial-and-error system which does the thinking, acting, and deciding. This system includes all the informational pathways which are relevant at any given moment to any given decision. The 'self' is a false reification of an improperly delimited part of this much larger field of interlocking processes." See also Bateson (1972b, 1980), de Shazer (1991) and White (1986) on the importance of using *difference* to open therapeutic possibilities.

present a theory of how problematic "parts" of one's self are formed and produce conflict, and illustrate through several case examples a powerful step-by-step process that incorporates "resistance" as it promotes a profound sense of wholeness and well-being. Readers may note links to other constructive approaches that emphasize respect for the client's experience; careful attention to language and the use of client-generated metaphor; and the belief that the client has, with skillful facilitation, the capacity for self-healing.

Chapter 13, "A Golfer's Guide to Brief Therapy (with Footnotes for Baseball Fans)," reports my effort to vivify ideas presented in *The First Session in Brief Therapy* (Budman, Hoyt, & Friedman, 1992), *Constructive Therapies* (Hoyt, 1994a), and *Brief Therapy and Managed Care: Readings for Contemporary Practice* (Hoyt, 1995). Using the format of a golf course, after a few warm-up swings, various stories are told as we traverse 18 holes and return to the clubhouse.

Chapter 14, "Three Styles of Constructive Therapy," is by Haim Omer. Known for his instructive *Critical Interventions in Psychotherapy* (1994), here Omer explores some of the different ways language is used to create therapeutic realities by different well-known practitioners. "It's in the telling of the story," said Erickson (quoted by Hammerschlag in the videotape by Haley & Richeport, 1993).[14] Omer reminds us that as we move away from positivism in psychotherapy, we must pay keen attention to the purpose and specifics of different intervention styles lest we wander into a morass of fuzzy and arbitrary justification.

Chapter 15, "Resource-Focused Therapy," is by Bradford F. Keeney and Wendel A. Ray. In addition to coauthoring their book of the same name, *Resource Focused Therapy* (Ray & Keeney, 1993), Ray is the coeditor of *Propagations: Thirty Years of Influence from the Mental Research Institute* (Weakland & Ray, 1995), and Keeney is the senior editor of *The Systemic Therapist* (Keeney, Nolan, & Madsen, 1990), as well as the author of *Aesthetics of Change* (1983), *Mind in Therapy* (Keeney & Ross, 1985), *Improvisational Therapy* (1990), and the extraordinary *Shaking Out the Spirits: A Psychotherapist's Entry into the Healing Mysteries of Global Shaman-*

---

[14]At another point on the same videotape, *Milton H. Erickson, M.D.: Explorer in Hypnosis and Therapy*, a dog barks in the background while a woman is recounting her experiences with Erickson. It seems incidental, until one recognizes the naturalistic style and human context of Erickson's approach. The work is done in life, as part of life. Along the same vein, writer/photographer Will Baker (1983, p. 262) remarks on his two attempted encounters with conventional psychiatry during times of despair: "Both times, and only those times, I had gone to see the shaman of my own culture, the psychiatrist. I learned, this past night [spent around the fire with Indian friends], what had been missing from those sessions—which I very soon abandoned—missing from those offices with their polished wood, filing cabinets, soft lighting and black leather. There was nothing to drink. There was no singing. There was no ring of honest old friends with a yen to talk. There were no small boys to occupy the lap, or to tickle the feet."

ism (1994). In their chapter here, Keeney and Ray focus on the overriding importance of context in generating resourcefulness in all participants in the therapeutic endeavor. A schematic clinical procedure and two cases are presented to illustrate ways of moving out of problem–solution contexts into resourceful contexts.

Chapter 16, "Postmodernism, the Relational Self, Constructive Therapies, and Beyond: A Conversation with Kenneth Gergen," addresses some of the evolving problems of living and doing therapy in these postmodern times, including issues of character and integrity, relational responsibility and conflict resolution between competing value systems, and the possibilities of relatedness and the limits of narrative. A major contributor to the social constructionist movement, whose numerous volumes include *The Saturated Self* (1991), *Therapy as Social Construction* (McNamee & Gergen, 1992), and *Realities and Relationships* (1995a), Gergen eloquently portrays both the potentials and challenges that lie ahead.

An appendix, "Songs for Constructive Therapists," containing the lyrics of four interesting and very different compositions, rounds out the volume. First, Bill O'Hanlon offers "Tranceplants," the loving ballad he wrote in 1982 for Milton H. Erickson (for whom Bill worked as a gardener while studying with the master). Next, Joseph Goldfield, an innovative therapist who specializes in working with adolescents (Goldfield, 1994), gives us "Rapnotic Induction No. 1," the song he wrote (Goldfield, 1993) and first performed at the 1993 Louisiana Association of Marriage and Family Therapists conference in honor of John Weakland (see Efron, 1993). Robert Rosenbaum, with a nod to Gilbert and Sullivan, then takes us through many of the schools of psychotherapy in "Modern Major Therapists." Finally, there is a set of haiku I wrote late one night while preparing for the First Pan-Pacific Brief Psychotherapy Conference, held in July 1995 in Fukuoka, Japan.

TWO IMAGES[15]

Some years ago it was my good fortune to visit the village of Don José Rios Matsuwa, the venerable Huichol shaman, high in the Mexican Sierra Madre mountains. While I was there, participating in the annual harvest festival, I became intrigued by the motif of a two-headed eagle with a special star-like figure in its breast that was repeated in many weavings (see Figure 1.1). I inquired and was told (in Spanish and

[15]"Imagine," as John Lennon (1971) said.

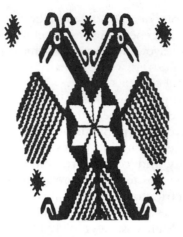

FIGURE 1.1. Soar like an eagle: Huichol representation of the two-headed eagle, *welika.*

Huichol) that the figure was called *welika* (see Berrin, 1978). When I asked "Why two heads?", I was informed, "When the heart opens, one can see the past and the other can see the future, at the same time. This is how we make our lives."

More recently, I was viewing a videotape of Insoo Kim Berg (1994; see Hoyt & Berg, in press) working with a married couple. On the tape, in her introduction to the session, she commented on the importance of attending to language and the value of using a "not-knowing" (Anderson & Goolishian, 1992) posture in which the clients' expertise is especially respected and supported. This combined in my mind with the idea that all questions are, in effect, leading questions (Epston, 1995; Tomm, 1988). Watching Insoo work, I suddenly had the image of the Compassionate Buddha (perhaps prefigured by her Asian countenance), who holds up his palm facing the viewer so as to reflect back whatever is offered. (As Levin, 1987, notes, such hand postures are called *mudras* in Buddist iconography and embody an overall attitude and way of being.) However, I had the idea that the therapist's hand, rather than simply "reflecting and clarifying" like a flat mirror *à la* Carl Rogers (1951),[16] was a special kind of mirror that could become convex or concave and swivel this way and that—expanding or shrinking the reflected image, opening parts of the story and closing others! Isn't this what (constructive) therapists do? Questions draw interest here or there, inviting one to focus attention and consciousness in (it may be hoped) more helpful ways. If a picture is worth a thousand words, this image suggests that with skillful inquiry parts of the picture can be elided or contracted into a mere mote, or perhaps can be expanded into the gateway to a new life story.[17]

R.S.V.P.

In the introduction (Hoyt, 1994e) to the first volume of *Constructive Therapies,* readers were invited to apply, adapt, cross-fertilize, follow up, and learn more than appeared on the printed pages. As the adage says, "The teacher can open the door, but the student must walk through." The authors contributing to *Constructive Therapies: Volume 2* have opened the door wide. The invitation is again extended.

REFERENCES

Adler, A. (1958). *What Life Should Mean to You.* New York: Capricorn Books. (Original work published 1931)

Allende, I. (1993). *The Infinite Plan.* New York: HarperCollins.

Anderson, H., & Goolishian, H. A. (1988). Human systems as linguistic systems: Preliminary and evolving ideas about the implications for clinical theory. *Family Process, 27,* 371–393.

Anderson, H., & Goolishian, H. A. (1992). The client is the expert: A not-knowing approach to therapy. In S. McNamee & K. J. Gergen (Eds.), *Therapy as Social Construction* (pp. 25–39). Newbury Park, CA: Sage.

Andreas, C., & Andreas, S. (1989). *Heart of the Mind.* Moab, UT: Real People Press.

Andreas, C., & Andreas, T. (1994). *Core Transformation: Reaching the Wellspring Within.* Moab, UT: Real People Press.

Andreas, S., & Andreas, C. (1987). *Change Your Mind–and Keep the Change.* Moab, UT: Real People Press.

---

[16]Even Rogers's "mirror" was not so flat: All therapists select (consciously or not) what to attend to, what to highlight (by inquiry, interpretation, reinforcement, etc.) or to ignore, what to "privilege" and what not (see Hare-Mustin, 1992, 1994; Rorty, 1979). Even if the therapist remained somehow "blank" or only gave grunts on a random schedule, the client would still be in the position of deciding what meanings to attribute to these events. And the therapist would concurrently and sequentially respond in kind, and so on and so on. Hence, the therapeutic reality is co-created; we cannot *not* communicate.

[17]One might speak of "panning for gold" (Wylie, 1994) and finding and expanding a "unique outcome" or "sparking moment" to enlarge a part of the "path" discussed with White and Combs in Chapter 2; or one might think of these gems as "exceptions" and "symptoms of solutions" (Miller, 1992) *à la* de Shazer's discussion in Chapter 3. Myriad images are possible, of course; for example, Furman and Ahola (1992) refer to "latent joy." Or perhaps we are photographic processors trying to bring forth a latent image with our special developing bath (Greenleaf, 1994, p. 253); if that metaphor is appealing, it is good to remember the words of Richard Avedon (1994, p. 9): "All photographs are accurate. None of them is the truth."

Angelou, M. (1993). *Wouldn't Take Nothing for My Journey Now.* New York: Random House.

Avedon, R. (1994). *Evidence 1944-1994.* New York: Random House/Eastman Kodak.

Baker, W. (1983). *Backward: An Essay on Indians, Time, and Photography.* Berkeley, CA: North Atlantic Books.

Barth, J. (1995, March). Stories of our lives. *Atlantic Monthly,* pp. 96-110.

Bateson, G. (1972a). The cybernetics of "self": A theory of alcoholism. In G. Bateson, *Steps to an Ecology of Being* (pp. 309-337). New York: Ballantine.

Bateson, G. (1972b). Form, substance, and difference. In G. Bateson, *Steps to an Ecology of Being* (pp. 448-466). New York: Ballantine.

Bateson, G. (1980). *Mind and Nature: A Necessary Unity.* New York: Bantam.

Bateson, G., Jackson, D. D., Haley, J., & Weakland, J. H. (1956). Toward a theory of schizophrenia. *Behavioral Science, 1,* 251-264.

Bateson, M. C. (1994). *Peripheral Visions: Learning Along the Way.* New York: HarperCollins.

Bennington, G. (1989). Deconstruction is not what you think. In A. Papadakis, C. Cooke, & A. Benjamin (Eds.), *Deconstruction: Omnibus Volume* (p. 84). New York: Rizzoli.

Berendt, J. (1994). *Midnight in the Garden of Good and Evil.* New York: Random House.

Berg, I. K. (1994). *Irreconcilable Differences: A Solution-Focused Approach to Marital Therapy* [Videotape]. New York: Norton.

Berg, I. K. (1995, July). *Beginning with the End: A New Therapeutic Conversation.* Paper presented at First Pan-Pacific Psychotherapy Conference, Fukuoka, Japan.

Berne, E. (1972). *What Do You Say After You Say Hello?* New York: Grove Press.

Berrin, K. (1978). *Art of the Huichol Indians.* New York: Abrams.

Boscolo, L., & Bertrando, P. (1993). *The Times of Time.* New York: Norton.

Brassai, G. (1995). *Henry Miller: The Paris Years.* New York: Arcade.

Bruner, J. (1986). *Actual Minds, Possible Worlds.* Cambridge, MA: Harvard University Press.

Budman, S. H., Hoyt, M. F., & Friedman, S. (Eds.). (1992). *The First Session in Brief Therapy.* New York: Guilford Press.

Castaneda, C. (1971). *A Separate Reality: Further Conversations with Don Juan.* New York: Simon & Schuster.

Collins, B. E., & Hoyt, M. F. (1972). Magnitude of inducement, consequences, and responsibility-choice: An integration and extension of the "forced compliance" literature. *Journal of Experimental Social Psychology, 8,* 558-593.

Combs, G., & Freedman, J. (1990). *Symbol, Story, and Ceremony: Using Metaphor in Individual and Family Therapy.* New York: Norton.

Cowley, G., & Springen, K. (1995, April 17). Rewriting life stories. *Newsweek,* pp. 70-74.

de Shazer, S. (1984). The death of resistance. *Family Process, 23,* 79-93.

de Shazer, S. (1985). *Keys to Solution in Brief Therapy.* New York: Norton.

de Shazer, S. (1988). *Clues: Investigating Solutions in Brief Therapy.* New York: Norton.

de Shazer, S. (1991). *Putting Difference to Work.* New York: Norton.

de Shazer, S. (1994). *Words Were Originally Magic.* New York: Norton.

de Shazer, S., & Berg, I. K. (1992). Doing therapy: A post-structural re-vision. *Journal of Marital and Family Therapy, 18,* 71–81.

Dennett, D. C. (1991). *Consciousness Explained.* Boston: Little, Brown.

Dickerson, V. C., & Zimmerman, J. L. (1995). A constructionist exercise in anti-pathologizing. *Journal of Systemic Therapies, 14*(1), 33–45.

Efron, D. (1993). Review and comments. Looking back, looking forward—the development of brief therapy: A workshop in honor of John Weakland. *Journal of Systemic Therapies, 12*(2), 86–88.

Ellis, A. (1990). Is rational–emotive therapy (RET) "rationalist" or "constructivist"? In W. Dryden (Ed.), *The Essential Albert Ellis* (pp. 114–141). New York: Springer.

Engel, S. (1995). *The Stories Children Tell: Making Sense of the Narratives of Childhood.* New York: Freeman.

Epston, D. (1989). *Collected Papers.* Adelaide: Dulwich Centre Publications.

Epston, D. (1995, February 13–14). *Toward a Child-Focused Family Therapy: Narrative, Play and Imagination.* Workshop held in San Rafael, CA.

Epston, D., & White, M. (1992). *Experience, Contradiction, Narrative and Imagination.* Adelaide: Dulwich Centre Publications.

Erickson, M. H. (1980). *The Collected Papers of Milton H. Erickson* (Vol. 3, E. L. Rossi, Ed.). New York: Irvington.

Fancher, R. T. (1995). *Cultures of Healing: Correcting the Image of American Health Care.* New York: Freeman.

Fine, M., & Turner, J. (1995). Hypotheses and hypothesizing: Following a thread through the weave. *Journal of Systemic Therapies, 14*(1), 61–68.

Fisch, R., Weakland, J. H., & Segal, L. (1982). *The Tactics of Change: Doing Therapy Briefly.* San Francisco: Jossey-Bass.

Foucault, M. (1980). *Power/Knowledge: Selected Interviews and Other Writings, 1972–1977.* New York: Pantheon.

Foucault, M. (1988). On power. In L. Kritzman (Ed.), *Michel Foucault: Politics, Philosophy: Interviews and Other Writings, 1977–1984* (pp. 96–109). New York: Routledge.

Frank, J. D. (1987). Psychotherapy, rhetoric, and hermeneutics: Implications for practice and research. *Psychotherapy, 24*(3), 293–302.

Freedman, J., & Combs, G. (1993). Invitations to new stories: Using questions to explore alternative possibilities. In S. G. Gilligan & R. Price (Eds.), *Therapeutic Conversations* (pp. 291–303). New York: Norton.

Freedman, J., & Combs, G. (1996). *Narrative Therapy: The Social Construction of Preferred Realities.* New York: Norton.

Freeman, M. (1993). *Rewriting the Self: History, Memory, Narrative.* New York: Routledge.

Friedman, S. (Ed.). (1993). *The New Language of Change: Constructive Collaboration in Psychotherapy.* New York: Guilford Press.

Friedman, S. (Ed.). (1995). *The Reflecting Team in Action: Collaborative Practice in Family Therapy.* New York: Guilford Press.

Furman, B., & Ahola, T. (1989). Adverse effects of psychotherapeutic beliefs. *Family Systems Medicine, 7*(2), 183–195. (Reprinted in B. Furman & T. Ahola, *Pickpockets on a Nudist Camp: The Systemic Revolution in Psychotherapy* [pp. 69–86]. Adelaide: Dulwich Centre Publications, 1992.)

Furman, B., & Ahola, T. (1992). *Solution Talk: Hosting Therapeutic Conversations.* New York: Norton.

Gergen, K. J. (1991). *The Saturated Self.* New York: Basic Books.

Gergen, K. J. (1993). Foreword. In S. Friedman (Ed.), *The New Language of Change: Constructive Collaboration in Psychotherapy* (pp. ix–xi). New York: Guilford Press.

Gergen, K. J. (1994). Exploring the postmodern: Perils or potentials? *American Psychologist, 49,* 412–416.

Gergen, K. J. (1995a). *Realities and Relationships: Soundings in Social Construction.* Cambridge, MA: Harvard University Press.

Gergen, K. J. (1995b). Therapeutic professions and the diffusion of deficit. In K. J. Gergen, *Realities and Relationships: Soundings in Social Construction.* Cambridge, MA: Harvard University Press.

Gergen, K. J., & Gergen, M. M. (1986). Narrative form and the construction of psychological science. In T. R. Sarbin (Ed.), *Narrative Psychology: The Storied Nature of Human Conduct* (pp. 22–44). New York: Praeger.

Gilligan, S. G. (1987). *Therapeutic Trances: The Cooperation Principle in Ericksonian Hypnotherapy.* New York: Brunner/Mazel.

Gilligan, S. G., & Price, R. (Eds.). (1993). *Therapeutic Conversations.* New York: Norton.

Goldfield, J. (1993). Rapnotic Induction No. 1. *Journal of Systemic Therapies, 12*(2), 89–91.

Goldfield, J. (1994). *A Utilization Approach for Working with Adolescents and Their Families.* Workshop held at the Sixth International Congress on Ericksonian Approaches to Hypnosis and Psychotherapy, Milton H. Erickson Foundation, Los Angeles.

Gould, S. J. (1987). The power of narrative. In *An Urchin in the Storm: Essays about Books and Ideas* (pp. 75–92). New York: Norton.

Goulding, M. M., & Goulding, R. L. (1979). *Changing Lives through Redecision Therapy.* New York: Grove Press.

Goulding, M. M., & Hillman, J. (1995, December). *Growth and Development of the Therapist.* Dialogue held at the Evolution of Psychotherapy conference, Milton H. Erickson Foundation, Las Vegas.

Greenleaf, E. (1994). Solving the unknown problem. In M. F. Hoyt (Ed.), *Constructive Therapies* (pp. 251–275). New York: Guilford Press.

Gustafson, J. P. (1992). *Self-Delight in a Harsh World: The Main Stories of Individual, Marital and Family Therapy.* New York: Norton.

Gustafson, J. P. (1995a). *The Dilemmas of Brief Psychotherapy, and Taking Care of the Patient.* New York: Plenum Press.

Gustafson, J. P. (1995b). *Brief versus Long Psychotherapy: When, Why, and How.* Northvale, NJ: Jason Aronson.

Haley, J. (Ed.). (1985). *Conversations with Milton H. Erickson, M.D.* (Vols. 1–3). New York: Triangle Press.

Haley, J., & Richeport, M. (1993). *Milton H. Erickson, M.D.: Explorer in Hypnosis and Therapy* [Videotape]. New York: Brunner/Mazel.

Halifax, J. (1993). *The Fruitful Darkness: Reconnecting with the Body of the Earth.* San Francisco: HarperCollins.

Hare-Mustin, R. T. (1992). Meanings in the mirrored room: On cats and dogs. *Journal of Marital and Family Therapy, 18,* 309–310.

Hare-Mustin, R. T. (1994). Discourses in the mirrored room: A postmodern analysis of therapy. *Family Process, 33,* 19–35.

Havens, L. L. (1986). *Making Contact: Uses of Language in Psychotherapy.* Cambridge, MA: Harvard University Press.

Havens, R. A. (Ed.). (1989). *The Wisdom of Milton H. Erickson: Vol. 2. Human Behavior and Psychotherapy.* New York: Irvington.

Held, B. S. (1995). *Back to Reality: A Critique of Postmodern Theory in Psychotherapy.* New York: Norton.

Herr, J. J., & Weakland, J. H. (1979). *Counseling Elders and Their Families: Practical Techniques for Applied Gerontology.* New York: Springer.

Hillman, J. (1975). *Re-Visioning Psychology.* New York: Harper & Row. (Excerpted in T. Moore [Ed.], *A Blue Fire: Selected Writings of James Hillman.* New York: HarperCollins, 1989.)

Hoffman, L. (1990). Constructing realities: An art of lenses. *Family Process, 29,* 1–12.

Hoffman, L. (1993a). Definitions for simple folk. In *Exchanging Voices: A Collaborative Approach to Family Therapy* (pp. 103–109). London: Karnac Books.

Hoffman, L. (1993b). *Exchanging Voices: A Collaborative Approach to Family Therapy.* London: Karnac Books.

Hoffman, L. (1995, December). *The Rise of Social Therapies.* Address at the Evolution of Psychotherapy conference, Milton H. Erickson Foundation, Las Vegas.

Hoyt, M. F. (1979). "Patient" or "client": What's in a name? *Psychotherapy: Theory, Research and Practice, 16,* 46–47. (Reprinted in M. F. Hoyt, *Brief Therapy and Managed Care: Readings for Contemporary Practice* [pp. 205–207]. San Francisco: Jossey-Bass, 1995.)

Hoyt, M. F. (1985). "Shrink" or "expander": An issue in forming a therapeutic alliance. *Psychotherapy, 22,* 813–814. (Reprinted in M. F. Hoyt, *Brief Therapy and Managed Care: Readings for Contemporary Practice* [pp. 209–211]. San Francisco: Jossey-Bass, 1995.)

Hoyt, M. F. (1990). On time in brief therapy. In R. A. Wells & V. J. Giannetti (Eds.), *Handbook of the Brief Psychotherapies* (pp. 115–143). New York: Plenum Press. (Reprinted in M. F. Hoyt, *Brief Therapy and Managed Care: Readings for Contemporary Practice* [pp. 69–104]. San Francisco: Jossey-Bass, 1995.)

Hoyt, M. F. (Ed.). (1994a). *Constructive Therapies.* New York: Guilford Press.

Hoyt, M. F. (1994b). The four questions of brief therapy. *Journal of Systemic Therapies, 13,* 77–78. (Reprinted in M. F. Hoyt, *Brief Therapy and Managed Care: Readings for Contemporary Practice* [pp. 217–218]. San Francisco: Jossey-Bass, 1995.)

Hoyt, M. F. (1994c). On the importance of keeping it simple and taking the patient seriously: A conversation with Steve de Shazer and John Weakland. In M. F. Hoyt (Ed.), *Constructive Therapies* (pp. 11–40). New York: Guilford Press.

Hoyt, M. F. (1994d). Single-session solutions. In M. F. Hoyt (Ed.), *Constructive Therapies* (pp. 140–159). New York: Guilford Press.

Hoyt, M. F. (1994e). Introduction: Competency-based future-oriented therapy. In M. F. Hoyt (Ed.), *Constructive Therapies* (pp. 1–10). New York: Guilford Press.

Hoyt, M. F. (1995). *Brief Therapy and Managed Care: Readings for Contemporary Practice.* San Francisco: Jossey-Bass.

Hoyt, M. F., & Berg, I. K. (in press). Solution-focused couple-therapy: Helping clients construct self-fulfilling realities. In F. M. Dattilio (Ed.), *Integrative Cases in Couples and Family Therapy*. New York: Guilford Press.

Hudson, P. O., & O'Hanlon, W. H. (1991). *Rewriting Love Stories: Brief Marital Therapy*. New York: Norton.

Jones, E. E., Kanouse, D. E., Kelley, H. H., Nisbett, R. E., Valins, S., Weiner, B. (Eds.). (1972). *Attribution: Perceiving the Causes of Behavior*. New York: General Learning Press.

Karrass, C. L. (1992). *The Negotiating Game* (rev. ed.). New York: HarperCollins.

Keeney, B. P. (1983). *Aesthetics of Change*. New York: Guilford Press.

Keeney, B. P. (1990). *Improvisational Therapy*. St. Paul, MN: Systemic Therapy Press.

Keeney, B. P. (1994). *Shaking Out the Spirits: A Psychotherapist's Entry into the Healing Mysteries of Global Shamanism*. Tarrytown, NY: Station Hill Press.

Keeney, B. P., Nolan, B., & Madsen, W. (Eds.). (1990). *The Systemic Therapist*. St. Paul, MN: Systemic Therapy Press.

Keeney, B. P., & Ross, J. (1985). *Mind in Therapy*. New York: Basic Books.

Kelly, G. A. (1955). *The Psychology of Personal Constructs* (Vols. 1 & 2). New York: Norton.

Laing, R. D. (1967). *The Politics of Experience*. New York: Pantheon.

Lax, W. D. (1992). Postmodern thinking in a clinical practice. In S. McNamee & K. J. Gergen (Eds.), *Therapy as Social Construction* (pp. 69–85). Newbury Park, CA: Sage.

Lennon, J. (1971). *Imagine*. New York: Apple Records.

Lerner, M. (1995). *The Assault on Psychotherapy*. Keynote speech, Family Networker Conference, Washington, DC. (A version appears in the *Family Therapy Networker, 19*(5), 44–52.)

Levin, C. (1993). Case studies: The enigma of EMDR. *Family Therapy Networker, 17*(4), 75–83. (With commentaries by Francine Shapiro and David Waters.)

Levin, D. M. (1987). *Mudra* as thinking: Developing our wisdom-of-being in gesture and movement. In G. Parkes (Ed.), *Heidegger and Asian Thought* (pp. 245–269). Honolulu: University of Hawaii Press.

Lewis, C. S. (1982). *The Screwtape Letters*. New York: Bantam. (Original work published 1941)

Lincoln, Y. (1990). The making of a constructivist. In E. G. Guba (Ed.), *The Paradigm Dialogue*. Newbury Park, CA: Sage.

Lipchik, E. (1994). The rush to be brief. *Family Therapy Networker, 18*(2), 34–39.

Lyddon, W. J., & Bradford, E. (1995). Philosophical commitments and therapy approach preferences among psychotherapy trainees. *Journal of Theoretical and Philosophical Psychology, 15*(1), 1–15.

Madanes, C., Keim, I., Lentine, G., & Keim, J. P. (1990). No more John Wayne: Strategies for changing the past. In C. Madanes, *Sex, Love, and Violence: Strategies for Transformation* (pp. 218–247). New York: Norton.

Madigan, R., Johnson, S., & Linton, P. (1995). The language of psychology: APA style as epistemology. *American Psychologist, 50*(6), 428–436.

Madigan, S. P. (1992). The application of Michel Foucault's philosophy in the problem externalizing discourse of Michael White. *Journal of Family Therapy, 14*, 265–279.

Madigan, S. P. (1993). Questions about questions: Situating the therapist's curiosity in front of the family. In S. Gilligan & R. Price (Eds.), *Therapeutic Conversations* (pp. 219–236). New York: Norton.

Mahoney, M. J. (1995). The psychological demands of being a constructive psychotherapist. In R. A. Neimeyer & M. J. Mahoney (Eds.), *Constructivism in Psychotherapy* (pp. 385–399). Washington, DC: American Psychological Association.

McGoldrick, M. (1995). *You Can Go Home Again.* New York: Norton.

McKibben, B. (1992). *The Age of Missing Information.* New York: Plume.

McNamee, S., & Gergen, K. J. (Eds.). (1992). *Therapy as Social Construction.* Newbury Park, CA: Sage.

Meichenbaum, D. (1977). *Cognitive-Behavior Modification: An Integrative Approach.* New York: Plenum Press.

Meichenbaum, D. (1994). *A Clinical Handbook/Practical Therapist Manual for Treating PTSD.* Waterloo, Ontario, Canada: Institute Press, University of Waterloo.

Melges, F. T. (1982). *Time and the Inner Future: A Temporal Approach to Psychiatric Disorders.* New York: Wiley.

Miller, S. D. (1992). The symptoms of solution. *Journal of Strategic and Systemic Therapies, 11,* 1–11.

Miller, S. D. (1994). Some questions (not answers) for the brief treatment of people with drug and alcohol problems. In M. F. Hoyt (Ed.), *Constructive Therapies* (pp. 92–110). New York: Guilford Press.

Minuchin, S. (1992). The restoried history of family therapy. In J. K. Zeig (Ed.), *The Evolution of Psychotherapy: The Second Conference* (pp. 3–12). New York: Brunner/Mazel.

Moore, R. L. (1994). Series foreword. In M. P. Somé, *Ritual: Power, Healing and Community* (pp. 9–10). Portland, OR: Swan/Raven.

Neimeyer, R. A. (1995). Constructivist psychotherapies: Features, foundations, and future directions. In R. A. Neimeyer & M. J. Mahoney (Eds.), *Constructivism in Psychotherapy* (pp. 11–38). Washington, DC: American Psychological Association.

Neimeyer, R. A., & Mahoney, M. J. (Eds.). (1995). *Constructivism in Psychotherapy.* Washington, DC: American Psychological Association.

Nylund, D., & Smith, C. (Eds.). (in press). *Narrative Therapy with Children and Adolescents.* New York: Guilford Press.

O'Hanlon, W. H. (1994). The third wave. *Family Therapy Networker, 18*(6), 18–29.

O'Hanlon, W. H., & Beadle, S. (1994). *A Field Guide to PossibilityLand: Possibility Therapy Methods.* Omaha, NE: Center Press.

O'Hanlon, W. H., & Hudson, P. O. (1995). *Love Is a Verb.* New York: Norton.

O'Hanlon, W. H., & Weiner-Davis, M. (1989). *In Search of Solutions: A New Direction in Psychotherapy.* New York: Norton.

Omer, H. (1993). Quasi-literary elements in psychotherapy. *Psychotherapy, 30,* 59–66.

Omer, H. (1994). *Critical Interventions in Psychotherapy.* New York: Norton.

Omer, H., & Strenger, C. (1992). The pluralist revolution: From the one true meaning to an infinity of constructed ones. *Psychotherapy, 29,* 253–261.

Papadakis, A., Cooke, C., & Benjamin, A. (Eds.). (1989). *Deconstruction: Omnibus Volume.* New York: Rizzoli.

Parry, A. (1991). A universe of stories. *Family Process, 30,* 37–54.

Parry, A., & Doan, R. E. (1994). *Story Re-Visions: Narrative Therapy in the Postmodern World.* New York: Guilford Press.

Penn, P. (1985). Feed-forward: Future questions, future maps. *Family Process, 24,* 289–310.

Pittman, F. (1992). It's not my fault. *Family Therapy Networker, 16*(1), 56–63.

Pollan, M. (1991). *Second Nature.* New York: Dell.

Polster, E. (1987). *Every Person's Life Is Worth a Novel.* New York: Norton.

Polster, E. (1992). The self in action: A gestalt outlook. In J. K. Zeig (Ed.), *The Evolution of Psychotherapy: The Second Conference* (pp. 143–151). New York: Brunner/Mazel.

Ponce, M. H. (1993). *Hoyt Street: Memories of a Chicana Childhood.* New York: Doubleday/Anchor.

Ray, W. A., & Keeney, B. P. (1993). *Resource Focused Therapy.* New York: Brunner/Mazel.

Redekop, F. (1995). The "problem" of Michael White and Michel Foucault. *Journal of Marital and Family Therapy, 21*(3), 309–318.

Ricoeur, P. (1983). *Time and Narrative.* Chicago: University of Chicago Press.

Roberts, J. (1994). *Tales and Transformations: Stories in Families and Family Therapy.* New York: Norton.

Rogers, C. (1951). *Client-Centered Therapy.* Boston: Houghton Mifflin.

Rorty, R. (1979). *Philosophy and the Mirror of Nature.* Princeton, NJ: Princeton University Press.

Rosen, H., & Kuelhwein, K. (1996). *Constructing Realities: Meaning-Making Perspectives for Psychotherapists.* San Francisco: Jossey-Bass.

Rosenbaum, R., & Bohart, A. C. (1994). *Psychotherapy: The Art of Experience.* Unpublished manuscript.

Roth, S. (1993). Speaking the unspoken: A work-group consultation to reopen dialogue. In E. Imber-Black (Ed.), *Secrets in Families and Family Therapy* (pp. 268–291). New York: Norton.

Roth, S., & Chasin, R. (1994). Entering one another's worlds of meaning and imagination: Dramatic enactment and narrative couple therapy. In M. F. Hoyt (Ed.), *Constructive Therapies* (pp. 189–216). New York: Guilford Press.

Roth, S., Chasin, L., Chasin, R., Becker, C., & Herzig, M. (1992). From debate to dialogue: A facilitating role for family therapists in the public forum. *Dulwich Centre Newsletter,* No. 2, 41–48.

Roth, S., & Epston, D. (in press). Developing externalizing conversations: An exercise. *Journal of Systemic Therapies.*

Ruesch, J., & Bateson, G. (1951). *Communication: The Social Matrix of Psychiatry.* New York: Norton.

Sarbin, T. R. (Ed.). (1986). *Narrative Psychology: The Storied Nature of Human Conduct.* New York: Praeger.

Satir, V. (1993). My declaration of self-esteem. In J. Canfield & M. V. Hansen (Compilers), *Chicken Soup for the Soul: 101 Stories to Open the Heart and Rekindle the Spirit* (pp. 75–76). Deerfield Beach, FL: Health Communications.

Schafer, R. (1992). *Retelling a Life: Narration and Dialogue in Psychoanalysis.* New York: Basic Books.

Shakespeare, W. (1974). *The Tempest.* In G. B. Evans (Ed.), *The Riverside Shake-*

speare (pp. 1606–1638). Boston: Houghton Mifflin. (Original work published 1623)

Shapiro, F. (1995). *Eye Movement Desensitization and Reprocessing: Basic Principles, Protocols, and Procedures.* New York: Guilford Press.

Singer, J. A., & Salovey, P. (1993). *The Remembered Self: Emotion and Memory in Personality.* New York: Free Press.

Sluzki, C. E. (1992). Transformations: A blueprint for narrative changes in therapy. *Family Process, 31,* 217–230.

Smith, M. B. (1994). Selfhood at risk: Postmodern perils and the perils of postmodernism. *American Psychologist, 49,* 405–411.

Speed, B. (1984). How really real is real? *Family Process, 23,* 511–520.

Speed, B. (1991). Reality exists OK? An argument against constructivism and social constructivism. *Family Therapy, 13,* 395–409.

Spence, D. P. (1982). *Narrative Truth and Historical Truth: Meaning and Interpretation in Psychoanalysis.* New York: Norton.

Strauss, S. (1991). *Coyote Stories for Children: Tales from Native America.* Hillsboro, OR: Beyond Words Publishing.

Steiner, C. M. (1974). *Scripts People Live.* New York: Bantam.

Thoreau, H. D. (1975). *Walden.* In C. Bode (Ed.), *The Portable Thoreau* (pp. 258–572). New York: Penguin. (Original work published 1854)

Tomm, K. (1988). Interventive interviewing: Part III. Intending to ask lineal, circular, strategic and reflexive questions? *Family Process, 27,* 1–16.

Tomm, K. (1989). Externalizing the problem and internalizing personal agency. *Journal of Strategic and Systemic Therapies, 8,* 54–59.

Tomm, K. (1990). A critique of the DSM. *Dulwich Centre Newsletter, 2*(3), 5–8.

Tomm, K. (1993). The courage to protest: A commentary on Michael White's work. In S. G. Gilligan & R. Price (Eds.), *Therapeutic Conversations* (pp. 62–80). New York: Norton.

Watzlawick, P. (1976). *How Real Is Real?* New York: Random House.

Watzlawick, P. (Ed.). (1984). *The Invented Reality: How Do We Know What We Believe We Know?* New York: Norton.

Watzlawick, P. (1992). The construction of clinical "realities." In J. K. Zeig (Ed.), *The Evolution of Psychotherapy: The Second Conference* (pp. 55–62). New York: Brunner/Mazel.

Watzlawick, P. (1994, December). *The Construction of Therapeutic "Realities."* Workshop held at the Sixth International Congress on Ericksonian Approaches to Hypnosis and Psychotherapy, Milton H. Erickson Foundation, Los Angeles.

Watzlawick, P., Beavin, J. H., & Jackson, D. D. (1967). *Pragmatics of Human Communication: A Study of Interactional Patterns, Pathologies, and Paradoxes.* New York: Norton.

Watzlawick, P., & Weakland, J. H. (Eds.). (1977). *The Interactional View.* New York: Norton.

Watzlawick, P., Weakland, J. H., & Fisch, R. (1974). *Change: Principles of Problem Formation and Problem Resolution.* New York: Norton.

Weakland, J. H. (1993). Conversation—but what kind? In S. G. Gilligan & R. Price (Eds.), *Therapeutic Conversations* (pp. 136–145). New York: Norton.

Weakland, J. H., Johnson, L. D., & Morrissette, P. (1995). Brief strategic psychotherapy consultation: The Mental Research Institute model. *Journal of Strategic Therapies, 14*(1), 46–60.

Weakland, J. H., & Ray, W. A. (Eds.). (1995). *Propagations: Thirty Years of Influence from the Mental Research Institute.* Binghamton, NY: Haworth Press.

West, C. (1993). *Race Matters.* New York: Vintage.

Whitaker, C. A. (1976). The hindrance of theory in clinical work. In P. J. Guerin, Jr. (Ed.), *Family Therapy: Theory and Practice* (pp. 154–164). New York: Gardner Press. (Reprinted in J. R. Neill & D. P. Kniskern [Eds.], *From Psyche to System: The Evolving Therapy of Carl Whitaker* [pp. 317–329]. New York: Guilford Press, 1982.)

White, M. (1986). Negative explanation, restraint, and double description: A template for family therapy. *Family Process, 25*(2), 169–184. (Reprinted in M. White, *Selected Papers* [pp. 85–99]. Adelaide: Dulwich Centre Publications.)

White, M. (1989a). *Selected Papers.* Adelaide: Dulwich Centre Publications.

White, M. (1989b). The externalizing of the problem and the re-authoring of lives and relationships. In M. White, *Selected Papers* (pp. 5–28). Adelaide: Dulwich Centre Publications.

White, M. (1993). Deconstruction and therapy. In S. G. Gilligan & R. Price (Eds.), *Therapeutic Conversations* (pp. 22–61). New York: Norton. (Original work published in the *Dulwich Centre Newsletter,* 1991, No. 3, 1–21. Also reprinted in D. Epston & M. White, *Experience, Contradiction, Narrative and Imagination* [pp. 109–152]. Adelaide: Dulwich Centre Publications, 1992.)

White, M. (1993). Commentary: The histories of the present. In S. G. Gilligan & R. Price (Eds.), *Therapeutic Conversations* (pp. 121–135). New York: Norton.

White, M. (1995). *Re-Authoring Lives: Interviews and Essays.* Adelaide: Dulwich Centre Publications.

White, M., & Epston, D. (1990). *Narrative Means to Therapeutic Ends.* New York: Norton.

Wylie, M. S. (1994). Panning for gold. *Family Therapy Networker, 18*(6), 40–48.

Yeung, F. K-C. (1995, July). *Reflections on the Use of Solution-Focused Therapy Among the Chinese in Hong Kong.* Paper presented at the First Pan-Pacific Brief Psychotherapy Conference, Fukuoka, Japan.

Zeig, J. K., & Gilligan, S. G. (Eds.). (1990). *Brief Therapy: Myths, Methods, and Metaphors.* New York: Brunner/Mazel.

CHAPTER 2

On Ethics and the Spiritualities of the Surface
A Conversation with Michael White

MICHAEL F. HOYT
GENE COMBS

Known for the great originality, scope, and humanism of his many contributions, Michael White is the prime enunciator and a key developer of such narrative therapy practices as "externalizing the problem," "deconstructive questioning," and the "reauthoring of lives." The Codirector of the Dulwich Centre in Adelaide, South Australia, his books include his *Selected Papers* (1989) and *Re-Authoring Lives: Interviews and Essays* (1995), as well as (with his good friend, David Epston) *Experience, Contradiction, Narrative and Imagination* (Epston & White, 1992) and the widely noted *Narrative Means to Therapeutic Ends* (White & Epston, 1990).[1]

The following conversation took place on July 16, 1994, at the Therapeutic Conversations 2 conference held in Reston, Virginia (near Washington, D.C.), where White was serving as a core faculty member. Joining us for this interview was Gene Combs, another faculty member. Combs is the Codirector of the Evanston Family Therapy Center and (along with his wife, Jill Freedman) is coauthor of *Symbol, Story and Ceremony* (Combs & Freedman, 1990) and *Narrative Therapy: The Social Construction of Preferred Realities* (Freedman & Combs, 1996), as well as other works on narrative therapy (e.g., Combs & Freedman, 1994; Freedman & Combs, 1993).

An hour before our meeting, White had presented an excellent

---

[1]In addition to these works by White himself, other valuable resources from the Dulwich Centre include the publications of Durrant and C. White (1990), Epston (1989), Furman and Ahola (1992), Jenkins (1990), and the *Dulwich Centre Newsletter* (1990–ongoing).

workshop on "Consulting Our Consultants." Sitting down to talk, we
began by focusing on the heart and soul of his work.

HOYT: I was very moved by the eloquence of your presentation this
    afternoon. I thought it was *practical love*. That's what came to my
    mind: *love in practice*.

WHITE: I can relate to descriptions like this, and believe that we need to
    be reclaiming these sorts of terms in the interpretation of what we
    are doing—*love, passion, compassion, reverence, respect, commitment,* and
    so on. Not because love and passion are enough, but because these
    terms are emblematic of certain popular discourses; because they
    are associated with discursive fields that are constituted of alterna-
    tive rules about what counts as legitimate knowledge, about who is
    authorized to speak of these knowledges, about how these knowl-
    edges might be expressed (including the very manner of speaking
    of them), about in which contexts these knowledges might be
    expressed, and so on. And these discursive fields are also constituted
    of different technologies for the expression of, or for the perform-
    ance of, these knowledges—different techniques of the self, and
    different practices of relationship. So what I am saying is that terms
    of description like *love* and *passion* are emblematic of discourses that
    can provide a point of entry to alternative modes of life, to specific
    ways of being and thinking—which will have different real effects on
    the shape of the therapeutic interaction, different real effects on the
    lives of the people who consult us, and different real effects on our
    lives as well.

    The rise of the "therapeutic disciplines" has been associated
    with extraordinary development in the discourses of science, and,
    of course, in the modern technologies of relationship. So notions of
    love and of passion haven't been considered relevant to what we
    might do in the name of therapy. Because we have become alienated
    from terms of description such as these, the popular discourses that
    they are emblematic of have not been all that constitutive of our
    work; these discourses have not had a significant effect on the shape
    of mainstream therapeutic practices in recent history.

HOYT: Watching you work, I had the thought that in India people put
    their hands together and they say, "*Namaste*"—"I salute the divine in
    you"—meaning "Whatever the story on the surface is, I see some-
    thing holy or special." If you're a Christian you'd say, "It's the Christ
    in you"—although I'm not particularly Christian. Watching you work,
    I keep seeing over and over in the tapes and the discussion with the
    audience how you hear the positive. I just want to ask you, how do
    you keep doing that? This has been a very congenial audience, but

sometimes the patients are unpleasant, they are challenging, they've done miserable things, they've hurt people, abused people, and yet you're able to meet them with this respect—to kind of separate them from the culture that's been imposed on them. Where does that come from? How can I, how can other people, do more of that? Is there sort of a key or clue that would help us look at people more that way?

WHITE: These are important questions. You have asked two questions. The first was about the spiritual piece, is that right?

HOYT: Yes. What I'm getting at is not necessarily that we have to be "spiritual" or "religious," but it's looking at people and seeing something in them that's more than the story they're presenting, being able to see the positive underneath all this misery and stuff, seeing there's something good there.

WHITE: The notion of spirituality does interest me. In the histories of the world's cultures, there have been many different notions of spirituality. I won't attempt to provide an account of these, as I've not had the opportunity to study them, and I don't believe that I have even established an adequate grasp of the dominant notions of spirituality in the recent history of my own culture—or, for that matter, in the history of my experience. But I am aware of the extent to which spirituality, in this Western culture, has been cast in *immanent forms*, in *ascendant forms*, and in *immanent–ascendant forms*.

Ascendant forms of spirituality are achieved on planes that are imagined at an altitude above everyday life. It is when people succeed in rising to these altitudes that they experience God's blessing, whomever that God might be. It is on these planes that an understanding of what would approximate a direct correspondence between God's word and one's life is attainable; it is on this plane that it becomes possible to achieve a relatively unmediated expression of God's word.

Immanent forms of spirituality are achieved not by locating oneself at some altitude above one's life, but by descending the caverns that are imagined deep below the surface of one's life. This is a spirituality that is achieved by "being truly and wholly who one really is," "by being in touch with one's true nature," by being faithful to the god of self. Much of popular psychology is premised on a version of this notion of an immanent spirituality—to worship a self through being at one with one's "nature."

And then there are *immanent–ascendant forms* of spirituality, in which spirituality is achieved by being in touch with or having an experience of a soul or the divine that is deep within oneself and that is manifest through one's relationship with a god who is ascendant.

These and other novel contemporary notions of spirituality are of a nonmaterial form. They propose spiritualities that are relatively intangible; that are split apart from the material world, that manifest themselves on planes that are imagined above or below the surface of life as it is lived. Although I find many of the contemporary immanent–ascendant notions of spirituality to be quite beautiful, and the notion of the soul far more aesthetically pleasing than the notion of the psyche, and although I remain interested in exploring the proposals for life (or, if you like, the ethics) that are associated with these notions of spirituality, I am more interested in what might be called the material versions of spirituality. Perhaps we could call these the *spiritualities of the surface.*

The spiritualities of the surface have to do with material existence. These are the spiritualities that can be read in the shape of people's identity projects, in the steps that people take in the knowing formation of the self. This is a form of spirituality that concerns one's personal ethics; that concerns the modes of being and thought that one enters one's life into; that is reflected in the care that one takes to attain success in a style of living. This is a transformative spirituality, in that it so often has to do with becoming other than the received version of who one is. This is a form of spirituality that relates not to the nonmaterial, but to the tangible. And I believe that this is the sort of spirituality to which Foucault [1980] referred in his work on the ethics of the self.

So, to return to your question, when I talk of spirituality I am not appealing to the divine or the holy. And I am not saluting human nature, whatever that might be, if it does exist at all. The notion of spirituality that I am relating to is one that makes it possible for me to see and to appreciate the visible in people's lives, not the invisible. It is a notion of spirituality that makes it possible for us to appreciate those events of people's lives that just might be, or might provide for, the basis for a knowing formation of the self according to certain ethics. The notion of spirituality that I am relating to is one that assists us to attend to the material options for breaking from many of the received ways of life—to attend to those events of people's lives that provide the basis for the constitution of identities that are other than those which are given. And in this sense it is a spirituality that has to do with relating to one's material options in a way that one becomes more conscious of one's own knowing.

I hope that this answer to your question is not too obscure, but this provides some account of what spirituality is about for me.

HOYT: No, your response is not obscure. I get the essence. It is about knowing self-formation.

WHITE: Yes. For me a notion of spirituality would have to be about this. It is about the exploration of the options for living one's life in ways that are other in regard to the received modes of being. It is to do with the problematizing of the taken-for-granted, the questioning of the self-evident. At times it is about the refusal of certain forms of individuality; about the knowing transgression of the limits of the "necessary" ways of being in the world; about the exploration of alternative ways of being, and of the distinct habits of thought and of life associated with these ways of being. In many ways it is about seizing upon indeterminacy, and about the reinvention of who we are. And it is about prioritizing the struggle with the moral and ethical questions relating to all of this.

COMBS: The thing I'm interested in is how people decide which of those possibilities to privilege, and I think that's one of the places where therapists, whether they want to or not, are given power. To become one who one has not been could go in an infinite number of directions.

WHITE: It could, I agree.

COMBS: What can you say about what your experience is, what you're guided by? Which of those directions to privilege?

WHITE: In the work itself, this is achieved by consulting people about the particularities of those alternative ways of being. This is to be in ongoing consultation with people about the real effects of specific ways of being in their relationships with others and on the shape of their lives generally. I don't think the goal is to settle on some specific "other" way of being in the world, to "fix" one's life. This work engages people with others in ongoing revisions of their images about who they might be, and about how they might live their lives. And it engages people in an ongoing critique of notions of identity that are based on our culture's many naturalized ideas about this. In fact, this work opens options for people to divest their lives of many of these notions. And in so doing, it raises options for people to explore the possibilities for disengaging from the sort of modern practices of self-evaluation that have them locating their lives on the continuums of growth and development, of health and normality, of dependence and independence, and so on. These options can also constitute a refusal to engage in those modern acts of self-government that have us living out our lives under the canopy of the bell-shaped curve.

HOYT: So we offer them, "You know, you don't have to be this way. You could continue in the path you're on, but there are alternatives. Would you like to look at those?" Is that . . .

WHITE: Yes. Well, I guess so, in a fairly crude way of putting it. I think it is about actually joining with people in the knowing exploration of, and the performance of, options for ways of being in life that might be available to them. It is to engage with people in a choice making, about these options, that is based on expressions of their lived experience and on expressions of alternative knowledges of life.

HOYT: When we use invitations or wondering or externalizing or any kind of deconstructing,[2] it seems to me we're still in some way highlighting certain options or suggesting, "You may want to consider this"—putting it crudely—and that gets into the power differential. Are we in some way subtly suggesting which alternatives they might take?

WHITE: Of course we are influential, and of course there is a power differential. And it has often been claimed that because of this there can be no way of differentiating between different therapeutic practices on the basis of subjugation; that because of this fact of influence and because of this fact of power, one therapeutic practice cannot be distinguished from another; that there is a certain equity between all therapeutic practices in terms of their real effects. But this blurring of important distinctions around forms and degrees of influence within the therapeutic context is unfortunate. In fact, I believe the blurring of this distinction to be a profoundly conservative act that permits the perpetration of domination in the name of therapy, and excuses those actions that establish therapists as unquestioning accomplices of the status quo.

It has also been said that because we are of our culture's discourses and that we cannot think and act outside of them, that

---

[2]As White (1991/1993, p. 34) has written: "According to my rather loose definition, deconstruction has to do with procedures that subvert taken-for-granted realities and practices: those so-called 'truths' that are split off from the conditions and the context of their production; those disembodied ways of speaking that hide their biases and prejudices; and those familiar practices of self and of relationship that are subjugating of persons' lives. Many of the methods of deconstruction render strange these familiar and everyday taken-for-granted realities and practices by objectifying them." He goes on (1991/1993, pp. 35–36) to explain: "Deconstruction is premised on what is generally referred to as a 'critical constructivist,' or, as I would prefer, a 'constitutionalist' perspective of the world. From this perspective, it is proposed that persons' lives are shaped by the meaning that they ascribe to their experience, by their situation in social structures, and by the language practices and cultural practices of self and of relationship that these lives are recruited into. The narrative metaphor proposes that persons live their lives as stories—that these stories are shaping of life, and that they have real, not imagined, effects—and that these stories provide the structure of life."

we are condemned to reproduce in therapy the very relations of power and experiences of self, or subjectivities, that it might be our intent to assist people to challenge. What an extraordinarily reductionist, unitary, global, and monolithic account of culture, of life, we are being encouraged to embrace by this account. What are the real effects of this sort of argument? How does it mask contestation and undermine struggle? In what ways does it contribute to the further marginalization of alternative knowledges of ways of being in the world, of alternative subjectivities?

In terms of practice, there is a very significant difference between, on the one hand, delivering interventions that are based on some external formal analysis of a problem, or suggesting to people that they should work on their "independence" or "growth" or whatever, and, on the other hand, encouraging people to attend to some events of their lives that just might be of a more sparkling nature—events that just might happen to contradict those plots of their lives that they find so unrewarding and dead-ended—and to ask them to reflect on what these events might say about other ways of living that might suit them and that might be available to them; to join with people in the exploration of the knowledges and practices of life that might be associated with these alternative plots; to contribute to their exploration of the alternative experiences of the self that might be associated with these knowledges and practices; and to encourage them to take stock of the proposals for action that might be associated with all of this. There is an important distinction to be drawn in regard to these two classes of response.

Aside from such distinctions, we can't pretend that we are not somehow contributing to the process. We can't pretend that we are not influential in the therapeutic interaction. There is no neutral position in which therapists can stand. I can embrace this fact by joining with people to address all of those things that they find traumatizing and limiting of their lives. I can respond to what people say about their experiences of subjugation, of discrimination, of marginalization, of exploitation, of abuse, of domination, of torture, of cruelty, and so on. I can join them in action to challenge the power relations and the structures of power that support all of this. And, because the impossibility of neutrality means that I cannot avoid being "for" something, I take the responsibility to distrust what I am for—that is, my ways of life and my ways of thought—and I can do this in many ways. For example, I can distrust what I am for with regard to the appropriateness of this to the lives of others. I can distrust what I am for in the sense that what I am for has the potential to reproduce the very things that I oppose in my relations with others. I can distrust what I am for to the extent that what I am for has a distinct location in the worlds of gender, class, race, culture, sexual preference, etc. And so on.

I can take responsibility in establishing the sort of structures that contribute to the performance of this distrust. As well, I can find ways of privileging questions in therapy that reflect this distrust over ways of asking questions that would propose my favored ways of living. I can make it my responsibility to deconstruct my notions of life, to situate these in structures of privilege, in regard to which I can engage in some actions to dismantle.

HOYT: Let me read you a quotation, if I may: "There is a power differential in the therapy context and it is one that cannot be erased regardless of how committed we are to egalitarian practices. Although there are many steps that we can take to render the therapeutic interaction more egalitarian, if we believe that we can arrive at some point in which we can interact with those people who seek our help in a way that is totally outside of any power relation, then we're treading on dangerous ground" [White, quoted in McLean, 1994, p. 76]. In addition to reflecting on and asking them to reflect on, how else can we stay aware of the ethics of our influence?

WHITE: I think through a significant confrontation with this fact—that there is a power imbalance. When I propose this confrontation, I am not suggesting that this fact be celebrated, and I am not suggesting that the acknowledgment of this fact is a justification for the use of power by the therapist. And in proposing this confrontation, I am not suggesting that distinctions can't be made in regard to different therapeutic interactions on the basis of the exercise of power and on the basis of subjugation. Instead, I am proposing a confrontation that opens possibilities for us to take steps to expose and to mitigate the toxic effects of this imbalance. I am proposing a confrontation that encourages us to explore the options that might be available to us to challenge the interactional practices and to dismantle the structures that support this power relation.

For example, we can set up the sort of "bottom-up" accountability structures that I have discussed elsewhere [see McLean, 1994]. We can talk with the people who consult us about the dangers and the possible limitations of that power imbalance, and we can engage them in the interpretation of our conduct with regard to this. But I have also made the point that it would be dangerous for us to believe that it is possible to establish a therapeutic context that is free of this power relation. This would be dangerous for many reasons. It would make it possible for us to avoid the responsibility of monitoring the real effects of our interactions with people who seek our help. It would make it possible for us to deny the moral and ethical responsibilities that we have to people who seek our help, and that they don't have to us. It would make it possible for us to avoid persisting in the exploration of options for the further dismantling of the structures and the relational practices that constitute this power imbalance.

HOYT: It is through accountability structures that this can be achieved?

WHITE: Well, this is part of accountability: doing whatever we can to render transparent some of the possible limitations and dangers of that power imbalance, and setting up structures that encourage people to monitor this. In this way we are able to more squarely face the moral and ethical responsibilities that we have in this work. And I would again emphasize that it would be perilous to attempt to obscure, to ourselves, the fact of this power imbalance. This would only make it possible for us to neglect the moral and ethical responsibilities that we have to the people who consult us.

HOYT: At the beginning of the conference, we were asked how would we know by the end if we "got it." I've come during the conference more and more to think of therapy as "empowerment through conversation." I just want to ask you to reflect on that. How are you defining *therapy* these days? Or what's an alternative word?

WHITE: First, I'd like to address your initial comment. This idea of being able to predict where we might be at the end of a process if all goes well is, I believe, a sad idea. It is my view that this is an idea that is informed by the dominant ethic of control of contemporary culture, although I do know that many would debate this point. I figure that conferences probably wouldn't be worth going to if we knew, in advance, where we would be at the end of them. There is a certain pleasure or joy available to us in the knowledge that we can't know where we'll be at the end; in the sense that we can't know beforehand what we will be thinking at the end; in the idea that we can't know what new possibilities for action in the world might be available to us at that time. It seems to me that to engage in prediction about where we might be at the end of a process if all goes well is to obscure, and to close down, options for being somewhere else. And why obscure the options for being somewhere else?

HOYT: It could take away surprise and discovery, couldn't it?

WHITE: If I planned to go to a conference, and if I knew beforehand what I would be thinking at the end, then I wouldn't go. (*Laughter*) It is like that with this work. If I knew where we would be at the end of the session, I don't think I would do this work. And this is also true for the sort of reflecting teamwork[3] that is structured

---

[3]See Andersen (1991) and Friedman (1995).

according to the narrative metaphor. If reflecting team members got together and prepared their reflections ahead of their reflections—if their reflection was in fact a performance of previously articulated reflections—then it is more likely that team members will be where they predicted they would be at the end of these reflections, and the more likely it will be that everyone will become quite bored and possibly even comatose—and I have witnessed this sort of outcome. On interviewing therapists about their experience of working in this fashion, I find that it is invariably constitutive of their working lives and relationships in ways that are experienced as undesirable.

However, if team members don't undertake these preparations—if they don't know what they will be thinking about and talking about by the time that they arrive at the end of their reflections, and if the teamwork is structured in a way that facilitates this sort of interaction—then it is more likely that their work together will contribute to the shaping of their own lives and relationships in preferred ways.

HOYT: In Zen, they might say you need to keep a "beginner's mind" [Suzuki, 1970]—a fresh look, not having things preconceived.

WHITE: So that's my response to the first part of your question. I think we will experience a better outcome from conferences if they contribute to some steps towards building some foundation for some other possibilities that we might not have predicted beforehand. The second part of your question had to do with how I would define therapy. Well, I define it in different ways on different days.

HOYT: What's today's date?

COMBS: The 16th.

HOYT: At this point in time, at this moment.

WHITE: At this very moment, just for today, I think it has to do with joining with people around issues that are particularly relevant and pressing to them. It has to do with bringing whatever skills we have available to assist people in their quest to challenge or to break from whatever it is that is that they find pressing. It is our part to work with people to assist them to identify the extent to which they are knowledged in this quest. And it is to join with people in the exploration of how their knowledges might be expressed in addressing the predicaments that they find themselves in.

In this work, people experience being knowledged, but this is not the starting point. Experiencing this is the outcome of a process that is at once characterized by *resurrection* and *generation*. As therapists, we play a significant role in setting up the context for this. We assist people to gain access to some of these alternative knowledges of their lives by contributing to the elevation the substories or subplots of their lives, by contributing to the resurrection of some of the knowledges of life that are associated with historical performances of these subplots. And we join with people in the generation of knowledges of life through the exploration of the ways of being and thinking that are associated with these subplots. I have shared my proposals for this process at some length in a number of publications, and will not reiterate them here. Perhaps it would be sufficient to say here that the subplots of people's lives provide a route to the exploration of alternative knowledges of life.

It is our part to assist in the identification of possibilities for action that are informed by these other knowledges of life. It is also our part to encourage people to evaluate the desirability of these other ways of being and thinking, through an investigation of the particularities of the proposals for action that are informed by them—through the exploration of the particularities of a life as it is lived through and constituted by these alternative knowledges.

I don't know if this answer to your question is a particularly good or appropriate answer. And if it's not a good answer, it's my answer for today at least. Perhaps if we do this interview again tomorrow, I just might be able to answer your question differently at that time. This is my hope.

COMBS: I guess I just want to make sure I was tracking what you were saying. So, as a therapist, you're curious about and listening for what are at the moment lesser plots, subplots, counterplots, whatever, and kind of sorting through those and exploring some of those with the person, and asking them which of those might be interesting to them or useful to them?

WHITE: Yes, I guess so. People are explicitly consulted about these subplots of their life. If the therapist's position on these subplots is privileged—if the therapist's position is primary—then imposition will be the outcome, and collaboration will be not be achieved. To avoid this imposition, and to establish collaboration, before proceeding we need to know how people judge those developments that might provide a gateway to the identification and exploration of these subplots: Do they see them as positive or negative developments, or both positive and negative, or neither positive nor negative? And we need to engage people in the naming of these subplots of their lives. Apart from this, it is also important that we have some understanding of why it is that people so judge these developments and these subplots of their lives. How do these developments fit with their preferred accounts of their purposes and values and so on?

But this is not the whole story. It is never just a matter of determining what developments might be interesting or useful to people. This is not predominantly a cognitive thing. In this work, these subplots of people's lives are actually experienced by those who consult us. In the course of the work itself, people live these subplots. Or, if you like, people's lives are embraced by these subplots. These subplots are not stories about life; they are not maps of the territory of life; they are not reflections of life as it is lived. These subplots are structures of life, and in fact become more constitutive of life.

And one further point about what is at work here. There is much that remains to be said about the language of this work, about how it evokes the images of people's lives that it does. Many of the questions that we ask about the developments of people's lives are powerfully evocative of other images of who these people might be, and other versions of their identities. These images reach back into the history of people's lived experience, privileging certain memories, and facilitate the interpretation of many previously neglected aspects of experience. So the language of the work, of the very questions that we ask, is evocative of images which trigger the reliving of experience, and this contributes very significantly to the generation of alternative story lines.

COMBS: So the expertise you bring . . .

HOYT: Well, Michael made a very good distinction, I thought, in the last presentation between *expert knowledge*, meaning "I am the expert here," versus an *expert's skills*, as I took it, meaning knowing how to ask questions in a way that will let the clients experience *their* local expertise, their local knowledge [see Wood, 1991]. I think that is very different from the dominant voice.

COMBS: So the knowledge you bring is knowledge about how to evoke in an experiential way these alternative images.

WHITE: Yes. I have often been misrepresented on this point. I have never denied the knowledgeableness of the therapist. And I have never denied the fact of therapist skillfulness. I have, however, challenged the privileging of the therapist's knowledgeableness above the knowledgeableness of people who consult therapists. And I have critiqued the "expert knowledges." I have critiqued expert knowledge claims, including those that make possible the imposition of global and unitary accounts of life and the development of formal systems of analysis. I have critiqued the power relations by which these expert knowledges are installed, including those that are essential to the normalizing judgment of the subject, that are so effective in the government of people's lives. Throughout this critique, I have supported what is generally referred to as, after Clifford Geertz [1983], the "interpretive turn."

HOYT: I had the idea that in looking for the "sparkling moments," looking for the "unique outcomes," looking for the "exceptions," in a way what we're trying to do is help the person build a past to support a better future [see White, 1993]—create some kind of structure under them, "thickening," I think you were using as a phrase, kind of fleshing it out or filling it in. Do I have that idea right?

WHITE: I'm really interested in the conditions under which people might "take a leaf out of their alternative books," rather than defining a goal and determining what steps might be necessary to reach that goal. When people get to the point of experiencing the unfolding of preferred developments in the recent history of their lives, they have some sense of where their next step might be placed. Such steps are informed by a developing appreciation of a preferred story line.

HOYT: We're making it up as we go along?

WHITE: Yes, to an extent, yes. I say "to an extent" because, although there might be certain circumstances under which we might witness what we assume to be clear breaks from the "known," it is rather difficult to think outside of what we specifically know, and, more generally, rather impossible to think outside of knowledge systems.

In regard to the knowing formation of our lives, it seems that we are, to an extent, dependent upon developing an account of how some of our recent steps fit together with classes of steps that can be read as unfolding in sequences through time according to some theme or perhaps plot. Even upon stepping into unfamiliar territories of identity, coherence appears to be a guiding criterion. And because of this, so is culture and its knowledges of ways of being and thinking in the world.

HOYT: Although sometimes as an alternative to the idea of evolution being a continuous process, I think we're getting now into the idea of evolution not being continuous but being discontinuous, punctuated evolution.[4] Stephen Jay Gould [1980], for example, talks about how things are steady-state, and something extraordinary comes along—like meteorites strike the earth, stirring up dust which kills the plant-eating dinosaurs, then that wipes out the meat eaters, and that opens the niche for mammals. There can be a sudden shift or something can be discontinuous. I relate this to page 6 of *Narrative*

_____
[4]See Rosenbaum, Hoyt, and Talmon (1990).

Means to Therapeutic Ends [White & Epston, 1990], in that table where you talk about "before and after," "betwixt and between," the whole "rites of passage" idea.[5] Sometimes we see people who feel prisoners of the path they have been on it so long, and how can they leap off it? So there are these submerged paths, I take from what you're saying, that remind them of other routes.

WHITE: Yes, there are these sudden shifts, these apparent discontinuities. And at these junctures we can feel quite lost. Perhaps it is useful to think of this experience as a liminal or betwixt-and-between phase, one that is understandably confusing and disorienting. There is always a distance between the point of separation and the point of reincorporation. But the question remains. Is it possible to break with something without stepping into other ways of being and thinking that are not in some way continuous with something else? Is it possible to step apart from familiar modes of life and of thought and to step into some cultural vacuum, one that is free of contexts of intelligibility? Historical reflection suggests that there are very few sites of radical discontinuity. But there are always margins of possibility.

HOYT: I see what you are saying. We take something up as well as separate from something.

WHITE: Yes. We step into other modes of life and of thought that go before us. But I believe that there are opportunities for us to contribute to the "drift" of these modes of life and of thought, as we live them, through processes that relate to the negotiation of the different subjectivities or experiences of the self that are associated with these, through interpretation, and through the management of indeterminacy.

Perhaps we could say that within continuity there is discontinuity. And this consideration takes us back to the discussion that preceded these comments. I have a problem with the idea of converting metaphors that come from the nonliving world, and from biology for that matter, into the realm of human life, which is the realm of practice and of meaning, and a realm of achievement.

---

[5] Building on the work of van Gennep (1960) and Turner (1969), White and Epston (1990; see also Epston & White, 1995) suggest that rather than attempting to return a patient in crisis to a "good enough" status quo, if one thinks of the crisis in terms of a "rite of passage," then a different construction of the problem is invited; different questions may be asked; and progressive movement is fostered in a different direction. By locating the crisis in relation to a *separation phase*, a liminal or betwixt-and-between phase, and a *reincorporation phase*, the person can determine (1) what the crisis might be telling him or her about separating from what was not viable for him or her, (2) what clues the crisis gives about the new statuses and roles that might become available, and (3) how and under what circumstances the new roles and statuses might be realized.

I don't believe that this is ever a realm of how things just happen to be. For example, the achievement aspects of this realm can be witnessed in the work that people put into attributing meaning to a whole range of experiences, and the extent to which many of their actions are prefigured on this.

HOYT: Rather than mechanizing or animalizing or taking us to where we're not.

WHITE: Exactly. And I can't think of one metaphor from the nonliving world that I think is appropriate to human life and human organization—to people who live in culture, who live in language, who participate in making meanings that are constitutive of their lives together. But I don't know if this is relevant to this interview or not.

HOYT: It is now. (*Laughter*)

WHITE: Can I just come back to a point that was made earlier? Gene, around the time that we were talking about the image, you asked me about the nature of this work. What was the question again?

COMBS: I was trying to imagine how it is that you conceptualize what it is that you do, what it is that you bring to the therapy situation, and I was also just trying to experience as much as I could for myself what it would be like to be you being a therapist. What am I thinking I should do next? To what am I listening?

HOYT: What is going on in Michael's head when he is working?

COMBS: Yeah.

WHITE: "To what am I listening?" is a good question. And I would say that my listening is informed by some of my preferred metaphors for this work. I particularly relate to poetics. I could read you a piece on poetics by David Malouf, because it fits so well with my conception of this work, and because he says it so much better than I could.

HOYT: Please.

WHITE: (*Searches in his bag and pulls out a typewritten page*) This is a piece from a book called *The Great World* [Malouf, 1991, pp. 283-284]. This book is substantially about men's experience of Australian men's culture. In it David Malouf talks about how poetry speaks:

How it spoke up, not always in the plainest terms, since that wasn't always possible, but in precise ones just the same, for what is deeply felt and might otherwise go unrecorded: all of those unique and repeatable events, the little sacraments of daily existence, movements of the heart and intimations of the close but inexpressible grandeur and terror of things, that is our *other* history, the one that goes on, in a quiet way, under the noise and chatter of events and is the major part of what happens each day in the life of the planet, and has been from the very beginning. To find words for *that*; to make glow with significance what is usually unseen, and unspoken to: that, when it occurs, is what binds us all, since it speaks immediately out of the centre of each one of us; giving shape to what we too have experienced and did not till then have words for, though as soon as they are spoken we know them as our own. [emphasis in original]

I so relate to this invocation of the "little sacraments of daily existence." The word *sacrament* invokes mystery. And it evokes a sense of the sacred significance of the little events of people's lives; those little events that lie in the shadows of the dominant plots of people's lives, those little events that are so often neglected, but that might come to be regarded with reverence, and at times with awe. These little sacraments are those events that have everything to do with the maintenance of a life, with the continuity of a life, often in the face of circumstances that would otherwise deny this.

These little sacraments of people's lives can be read for what they might tell us all about existence, about the particularities of how we exist. I don't believe that there is such a thing as "mere existence." Existing is something that we all do, and have obviously been doing now for many, many years. But it has, in so many ways, had such bad press in recent decades. Why is this the case? Why is it becoming so hard for us to read and to appreciate the little sacraments of daily life? Perhaps this is because these sacraments are on the other side of our culture's ethic of control. Perhaps it is because these little sacraments of daily life don't relate all that well to the accepted goals for life in this culture—like demonstrating "control over one's life." And perhaps it is because they don't fit with contemporary definitions of the sort of actions that count as responsible actions. I believe that through the metaphor of poetics it becomes possible for us to challenge the marginalizing of existence, and to all play some part in the honoring of those facts that Malouf refers to as the "little sacraments of daily existence."[6]

COMBS: When you say "the little sacraments of daily existence" and you talk about finding the words, I find myself thinking about the close of Ken Gergen's (1994) talk this morning. I don't know that it in any way relates to this. He was talking about inchoate experience, that experience that's not yet quite language and yet that is just before. Does that in any way relate to what you're talking about, sort of the

---

[6]Along related lines, Bruner (1986, p. 153) reminds us of James Joyce's phrase "epiphanies of the ordinary." Mary Catherine Bateson's (1995, p. 56) comment is also cogent: "As a society, we have become so addicted to entertainment that we have buried the capacity for awed experience of the ordinary. Perhaps the sense of the sacred is more threatened by learned patterns of boredom than it is by blasphemies."

next step of making that—sitting with somebody and then bringing that in a language, bringing that into society?

WHITE: What Malouf is saying about the little facts of daily life fits, I believe, with the notion of the "spiritualities of the surface" that we have been discussing. But I don't know whether or not what I am saying here has any relation to what Ken Gergen was saying. But it might, and I would like to understand more about what he is proposing before responding to your question.

HOYT: It's the "poetics of experience" as well as the "politics of experience."

WHITE: Yes, it is that as well.

HOYT: I heard Robert Bly, the poet, read a long, beautiful, evocative poem, and someone stood up in an audience and said, "Robert, what did it mean?" Bly said, "If I knew what it meant I would have written an essay, not a poem!" (*Laughter*) I thought what Gergen was getting at was that same special moment, the sacrament, I think some people call it the spirit of life, when it's *happening* rather than just . . . I'll have to ask him.

WHITE: It will be interesting to hear what he says.[7]

HOYT: I once asked Ronnie Laing what he thought of transference. I said, "What's your definition of it, or what do you think of it?" He said, "Oh, it's posthypnotic suggestion with amnesia." (*Laughter*) Posthypnotic suggestion with amnesia, which I relate to the whole idea of *mystification* [Laing, 1967]—that we've been sort of programmed or given this suggestion of how to take things, and we don't even remember that we were given it, so we're kind of locked in. I just wanted to ask if that, from a very different frame, is a way of talking about deconstructing? Does deconstruction get one to the consciousness where you recognize you've been, to use a modern word, programmed?

WHITE: Yes. This is a take on the practices of deconstruction that I can relate to. And I would like here to pick up Laing's contribution to the deconstruction of what we are talking about when we are talking about the phenomenon of transference. The notion of "posthypnotic suggestion with amnesia" does bring forth the history of the interactional politics that are generative of this phenomenon, and this encourages us to think of the "technologies of transference" as technologies of power. And, needless to say, since transference is a phenomenon that is invariably psychologized, to bring forth the technologies of transference does serve to deconstruct this.

[7]See Chapter 16 (pp. 364–365) for Gergen's comments.

But these technologies of transference are not just the historical conditions for the constitution of the transference phenomenon. Transference can also be read as the "trace" of very present power relations. People experience what they call "transference" most strongly in hierarchical situations when they are in the junior or subject position, and, of course, ideally (although it does occur in less formal contexts), when they are supine and in a state of vulnerability in relation to another person who is sitting erect—one who is considered an established authority on life, and who denies the subject any information that would situate this authority in his or her lived experience, intentions, or purposes. Here I describe just a few of the conditions and technologies of transference.

Perhaps it would be more appropriate to say that the experience of transference is the trace of power relations that are relatively fixed and approaching a state of domination. So, a strong and ongoing experience of transference can cue people to the fact that they are in a subject position in an inflexible power relationship that could lead to domination. This reading of transference opens possibilities for action that can include a refusal of this power relation.

I don't want to be misrepresented on this point. I'm not saying that there is no such phenomenon as transference. And I do understand that there are those who would justify bringing forth this phenomenon with the idea that this establishes a context for working though issues of personal authority, and so on. But I do think that there is a politics associated with this phenomenon, and [I] would raise questions about the deliberate and not so deliberate reproduction of these politics in the therapeutic context. And I would also want to explore the sort of questions that could contribute to a dismantling of the therapeutic structures that reproduce this phenomenon.

HOYT: How would you describe the ethic of your work?

WHITE: To answer this question, we should talk about what is generally meant by *ethics*. As Foucault [1980] observed, mostly, these days, when people are talking about ethics they are referring to rules and codes, and no doubt these have a place. But it is unfortunate that, in this modern world, considerations of the rule and the code have mostly overshadowed and even replaced considerations of personal ethics. Something precious is lost when institutional codes and rules for the government of conduct supplant notions of personal ethics. It is in the professional disciplines that we see this taken to its limits, and it is done so in the name of assuring appropriate professional conduct.

Invariably, it is argued that the privileging of matters of rule and code is preventative of the exploitation of people who consult therapists. But I don't believe that the elevation of the rule or code has achieved this anywhere in the modern world. In fact, it can be argued that such a reliance on the sort of top-down systems of accountability that are associated with systems of rule and code provide fertile ground for the very perpetuation of such injustices, of such exploitation.

At other times, when people are referring to "ethics," they are formulating questions about their existence that are informed by what Foucault refers to as a "will to truth," and, in this modern world, there has been a fantastic incitement to this will to truth. This is a notion of ethics that gives primary consideration to whatever it might be that is understood to constitute expressions of the truth of "who we are." The notions of rule and code are central to this version of ethics as well, as whatever it is that constitutes an expression of the truth of who we are is what is informed by the rules of human nature—however nature might be constructed, and however these rules might be determined.

Modern versions of this center on notions on the rule of needs: "How might we keep faith with our deepest needs?" It is chilling to consider the sorts of actions that can be justified according to modern need discourses. It is not difficult to apprehend the extent to which this will to truth marginalizes considerations of personal ethics, and obscures matters of discourse in the constitution of peoples lives. And this will to truth is still about the rule of law, only in this case it is a "natural law."

Then there is another style of ethical consideration that has a long history in Western culture, one that is referred to at those times when clashes of interest become apparent between people. This is the sort of consideration that makes it possible for people to discern between actions that are informed by selfishness on the one hand, or by altruism on the other. According to this determination, if altruism can be discerned in the actions in question, then such actions are judged to be ethical. Sarah Hoagland [1988] observes that this style of ethical consideration is one that women have principally been subject to, and that it has played a central role in women's subordination. She powerfully deconstructs this consideration in her book *Lesbian Ethics*.

And other times the criterion of ethical action is not altruism, but "responsible behavior": people can be considered to be behaving ethically when they are taking responsibility in and for their lives. So often, the version of responsibility that is referred to here is one that is informed by the ethic of control. According to this ethic, responsible action is that version of action that reflects independent and singular action on the world that succeeds in bringing about some goal in the relatively short term, and when these actions are referenced to some universal notion of the good, or some principle, like "justice" or "rights." To behave ethically is to take action that counts in the sense that it "measures up." This notion of responsible action that is informed by the ethic of control is the version that Sharon Welch [1990] deconstructs in her book, *A Feminist Ethic of Risk.*

HOYT: So, what is your account of the ethic of the work we have been discussing?

WHITE: In different places, including during this interview, I have endeavored to draw out the version of personal ethics that frames the work that I do. I have talked of the *knowing formation of the self.* I have talked of a version of *responsibility* which supports a commitment to identifying and addressing the real effects or the consequences of one's actions in the lives of others. And because this is not something that we can independently determine, either by our own interpretations of our immediate experience, or through recourse to some guiding principle, I have talked of the necessity of *accountability*. This is a specific notion of accountability—a bottom-up version, rather than a top-down version—and it is a version of accountability that is available in partnership with other people, or groups of people. It is an accountability that is in fact constitutive of our lives, one that brings many possibilities for us to become other than who we are.

I have also talked of the principle of *transparency*. This is a principle that is based on a commitment to the ongoing deconstruction of our own actions, of our taken-for-granted ways of being in this work, of our taken-for-granted ways of thinking about life. This is a principle that requires us to situate our opinions, motives and actions in contexts of our ethnicity, class, gender, race, sexual preference, purposes, commitments, and so on.

I have talked of ways of being in the world that have to do with working with others to establish what we could call the "foundations of possibility" for their lives and for ours. This is not about acting independently on the world to achieve some predicted goal in a proscribed time, but about *working collaboratively in the world* in taking steps to prepare the foundations for new possibilities in the time that it takes to do this.

And I have talked about many of the other aspects of this ethic, including the extent to which we can make it our business to develop an *attitude of reverence* for what Malouf calls "the little sacraments of daily existence," and the extent to which we can enter into a *commitment to challenge the practices and the structures of domination of our culture.*

HOYT: So, this ethic suggests a course of action that is distinct from one that is informed by a traditional goal orientation.

WHITE: Yes. It is on the other side of this. But there are important distinctions to be made here. Not all practices that invoke the notion of goal wittingly or unwittingly reproduce this culture's dominant ethic of control. I doubt that anyone would read the work of Steve de Shazer and Insoo Berg in this way.[8] And I also want to state that this is not an argument for a return to long-term therapy. To the contrary. While the ethic of control structures a context in which there are not many events that really count for all that much, this alternative ethic structures a context in which just so much that couldn't be acknowledged previously can be acknowledged. And, in so doing, it provides for an antidote to despair, for a sense of possibility in regard to one's life going forward, and for a broad range of options for further action.

HOYT: Why do you do therapy? Why do you do this work?

WHITE: This is not a new question. Way back in my social work training, which I began in 1967, we were required to address this question. This was in the heyday of structuralist thought. At that time, in response to such questions, only certain accounts of motive were considered acceptable. These were psychological accounts of motive. Accounts of motive that features notions of conscious purpose and commitment were not fashionable and were marginalized. Responses to this question that emphasized a wish to contribute to the lives of others in some way, or that were put in terms of a desire to play some part in addressing the injustices of the world, were considered expressions of naiveté. Attempts to stand by such expressions were read as examples of denial, lack of insight, bloody-mindedness, etc. On the other hand, to traffic in psychologized accounts of motive was to display insight, truth saying, a superior level of consciousness, of maturity, and so on. And invariably, the psychologizing of motive translated into the pathologizing of motive. "Which of all of one's neurotic needs was being met in stepping into this profession?" "How did this decision relate to unresolved issues in one's family of origin?" "Did this decision relate to one's attempts to work through an enmeshed relationship with one's mother?" "Or did this decision relate to one's attempt to work through a disen-

---

[8]See Berg (1994), Berg and Miller (1992), Chang and Phillips (1993), de Shazer (1985, 1988, 1991, 1993), and White (1993).

gaged relationship with one's mother?" And so on. I'm sure that you are familiar with questions of this sort, and that we could easily put a list together.

I always believe that this privileging of psychological accounts of motive to be a profoundly conservative endeavor, one that is counterinspiration, one that could only contribute significantly to therapist experiences of fatigue and burnout. For various reasons, I could never be persuaded to step into the pathologizing of my motives for my interest in joining this profession, and mostly managed to hold on to what were my favored notions of conscious purpose and commitment. I have no doubt that over the years that expressions of these notions have been a source of invigoration to me, and in recent years I have been encouraging therapists to join together in identifying, articulating, and elevating notions of conscious purpose and commitment. To this end I have developed an exercise that you can include along with the publication of this transcript. Readers might be interested in meeting with their peers and working through this together. [The exercise immediately follows this interview.]

HOYT: At the beginning of this conference, they showed a short tape that was made two weeks ago of John Weakland greeting the conference, and John invited us to consider what are the priorities in the field now. What is important and what isn't? I want to ask if you have a sense of where we're headed, what you think is important, what we need to be doing more of, what you want to privilege?

WHITE: I never want to make a prediction.

HOYT: Not a prediction of where we're going to wind up, but more a sense of . . .

WHITE: What's important for us to be looking at?

HOYT: Yeah.

WHITE: It is necessary for us to be taking more seriously what many have been saying about race, culture, gender, ethnicity, class, age, and so on. For too long we have operated with the idea that the people who seek our help have ethnicity and we don't. (*Laughter*) Not only do we need to join with people in assisting them to locate their experiences in the politics of these contexts, but we are challenged to break from the sort of practices that obscure our own location, and to find ways of engaging with others in reflecting on how this location might be affecting how we interpret our experiences of other people's lives—and, of course, how it might be affecting our conduct.

HOYT: I heard Joseph Campbell [1983], when someone asked him his definition of *mythology,* say it's "other people's religion," which we kind of dismiss as superstition.

WHITE: Unlike ours. Yeah.

HOYT: Let me read a quotation that gets to something I want to ask. In *Experience, Contradiction, Narrative and Imagination*—a wonderful title as I've come to understand it—you and David Epston [Epston & White, 1992, p. 9] comment, "One of the aspects associated with this work that is of central importance to us is the spirit of adventure. We aim to preserve this spirit and know that if we accomplish this, our work will continue to evolve in ways that are enriching to our lives and to the lives of persons who seek our help." My question is, what's next in your adventure? What's sparking your interest now? I know you began to speak earlier today about some social justice projects.

WHITE: This is a difficult question for me. There are so many things that have my attention at the moment, and they are all things that I want to step more into. Yes, some of these activities do have to do with what we have often formally referred to as "social justice projects." But this is not a discontinuity. I've always refused the sort of distinctions that put what is commonly referred to as "clinical practice" in one realm, and "community development and social action" in another.[9] This is not a distinction that I can relate to. It is a distinction that makes it possible for therapists to treat the therapeutic context as if it is exempt from the relational politics of culture, and to disavow the fact that therapeutic interaction is about action in the world of culture.

Perhaps I can answer your question about "where to from here" in a different way. I recently saw a movie called *Schindler's List,* and then read a piece about the latter years of Schindler's life. At the time he was living in a bedsitter somewhere in southern Germany, I think in Munich. He would frequent the local bars, and on those occasions when he found himself in the company of people of his own generation, he would ask the simple question: "And what did you do?"—referring, of course, to the Holocaust. Now it was my understanding that this was a genuine question, not a claim to moral superiority. I don't know how many people he found who had answers to this question. I found myself reflecting on this question, and thought it relevant to my life. It is a question that could be asked

---

[9]In discussing White's (1991/1993) masterful paper "Deconstruction in Therapy," Tomm (1993) comments on what he calls White's "courage to protest," to speak out effectively against oppression and injustice. Tomm makes a point of noting that White not only deconstructs but also helps clients to *re*construct, and says about White, "as a therapist he is an applied deconstruction activist" (1993, p. 174).

of me in relation to the many abuses of power and privilege, in relation to the many injustices, that I witness in my immediate world. But if anyone approached to ask this question of me right now, I would request a moratorium on it. I would say, "Please don't ask me this question yet, it is too soon. I'll keep working on the answer, but please come back later in my life. I hope to have an answer, one that is to my satisfaction, at that time." And I don't think that it will have to be a big answer, or a grand answer.

COMBS: I was just the other day at the Holocaust Museum in Washington, D.C. I don't know if you've been there yet, but at the end of the museum you come to a Hall of Remembrance. It's a large open space where there are no flash cameras or loud noises. And when I got there I sat and found myself making a pledge, to myself or God or whatever. It wasn't even in specific words, but it was a clear pledge or a promise.

HOYT: I know what you mean.

WHITE: It takes us back to this issue of elevating and honoring the spirit of love and passion and conscious commitment.

HOYT: Michael, in Australia, what does *fair dinkum* mean?

WHITE: It means something said that is absolutely true, deeply genuine.

HOYT: Michael, Gene: Fair dinkum!

CONSCIOUS PURPOSE AND COMMITMENT EXERCISE

Introduction: We have discussed the extent to which the privileging of psychological accounts of motive has marginalized statements of conscious purpose and commitment in this work. We have reviewed the extent to which such statements are pathologized in the culture of psychotherapy, as well as the implications of this in regard to the stories that we have about who we are as therapists. The following exercise will engage you in acts of resistance to this—acts that are associated with the elevation and reclamation of statements of conscious purpose and commitment. I suggest that you invite another person or two to join you in this exploration, for the purposes of sharing your responses to this exercise, or for the purposes of being interviewed about these responses.

1. Talk about any experiences that you have had that relate to the psychologizing and the pathologizing of your motives for choosing this work, or any reinterpretations of this choice that may have encouraged you to mistrust your statements of conscious purposes or your personal commitment to this work.

2. Review what you can assume to be some of the real effects or consequences, in your work and your life, of this psychologizing of your motives, and of this pathologizing of your accounts of your conscious purposes and commitments.

3. Identify and retrieve some of your very early statements of conscious purpose that relate to your chosen work, however unsophisticated these might have been, and reflect on what they suggest about what you are committed to in this work.

4. Share some information about the significant experiences of your life that have contributed to a further clarification of your conscious purposes and commitments in taking up this work—that have generated realizations about the particular contribution that you have a determination to make during the course of your life.

5. Discuss the experiences that you are having in the course of this exercise: those experiences that are associated with engaging in giving testimony and in bearing witness to expressions of conscious purpose; those experiences that are associated with the honoring of statements of commitment.

6. Talk about how the elevation of your notions of conscious purpose and the honoring of your statements of commitment could affect:

    a. Your experience of yourself in relation to your work.

    b. Your relationship to your own life.

    c. Your relationship to your colleagues and to the people who seek your help.

    d. The shape of your work and of your life more generally.

REFERENCES

Andersen, T. (Ed.). (1991). *The Reflecting Team: Dialogues and Dialogues about the Dialogues*. New York: Norton.

Bateson, M. C. (1994). *Peripheral Visions: Learning Along the Way*. New York: HarperCollins.

Berg, I. K. (1994). *Family Based Services: A Solution-Focused Approach*. New York: Norton.

Berg, I. K., & Miller, S. D. (1992). *Working with the Problem Drinker*. New York: Norton.

Bruner, J. (1986). *Actual Minds, Possible Worlds*. Cambridge, MA: Harvard University Press.

Campbell, J. (1983). *Myths to Live By*. New York: Penguin.

Chang, J., & Phillips, M. (1993). Michael White and Steve de Shazer: New directions in family therapy. In S. G. Gilligan & R. Price (Eds.), *Therapeutic Conversations* (pp. 95–111). New York: Norton.

Combs, G., & Freedman, J. (1990). *Symbol, Story, and Ceremony: Using Metaphor in Individual and Family Therapy*. New York: Norton.

Combs, G., & Freedman, J. (1994). Narrative intentions. In M. F. Hoyt (Ed.), *Constructive Therapies* (pp. 67–91). New York: Guilford Press.

de Shazer, S. (1985). *Keys to Solutions in Brief Therapy*. New York: Norton.

de Shazer, S. (1988). *Clues: Investigating Solutions in Brief Therapy*. New York: Norton

de Shazer, S. (1991). *Putting Difference to Work*. New York: Norton.

de Shazer, S. (1993). Commentary: de Shazer and White: Vive la difference. In S. G. Gilligan & R. Price (Eds.), *Therapeutic Conversations* (pp. 112–120). New York: Norton.

Dulwich Centre Newsletter (1990–ongoing). (Available from Dulwich Centre Publications, Hutt Street, P.O. Box 7192, Adelaide, South Australia 5000, Australia)

Durrant, M., & White, C. (Eds.). (1990). *Ideas for Therapy with Sexual Abuse*. Adelaide: Dulwich Centre Publications.

Epston, D. (1989). *Collected Papers*. Adelaide: Dulwich Centre Publications.

Epston, D., & White, M. (1992). *Experience, Contradiction, Narrative and Imagination: Selected Papers of David Epston and Michael White, 1989–1991*. Adelaide: Dulwich Centre Publications.

Epston, D., & White, M. (1995). Termination as a rite of passage: Questioning strategies for a theory of inclusion. In R. A. Neimeyer & M. J. Mahoney (Eds.), *Constructivism in Psychotherapy* (pp. 339–354). Washington, DC: American Psychological Association.

Foucault, M. (1980). *Power/Knowledge: Selected Interviews and Other Writings 1972–1977*. New York: Pantheon.

Freedman, J., & Combs, G. (1993). Invitations to new stories: Using questions to suggest alternative possibilities. In S. G. Gilligan & R. Price (Eds.), *Therapeutic Conversations* (pp. 291–303). New York: Norton.

Freedman, J., & Combs, G. (1996). *Narrative Therapy: The Social Construction of Preferred Realities*. News York: Norton.

Friedman, S. (Ed.). (1995). *The Reflecting Team in Action: Collaborative Practice in Family Therapy*. New York: Guilford Press.

Furman, B., & Ahola, T. (1992). *Pickpockets on a Nudist Camp: The Systemic Revolution in Psychotherapy*. Adelaide: Dulwich Centre Publications.

Geertz, C. (1983). *Local Knowledge*. New York: Basic Books.

Gergen, K. (1994). *Between Alienation and Deconstruction: Re-Visioning Therapeutic Communication*. Keynote address, Therapeutic Conversations 2 Conference, Institute for Advanced Clinical Training, Weston, VA.

Gould, S. J. (1980). *The Panda's Thumb: More Reflections in Natural History*. New York: Norton.

Hoagland, S. (1988). *Lesbian Ethics*. Palo Alto, CA: Institute of Lesbian Studies.

Jenkins, A. (1990). *Invitations to Responsibility: The Therapeutic Engagement of Men Who Are Violent and Abusive*. Adelaide: Dulwich Centre Publications.

Laing, R. D. (1967). *The Politics of Experience*. New York: Pantheon.

Malouf, D. (1991). *The Great World*. Sydney: Pan Macmillan.

McLean, C. (1994). A conversation about accountability with Michael White. *Dulwich Centre Newsletter*, No. 2–3, 68–79.

Rosenbaum, R., Hoyt, M. F., & Talmon, M. (1990). The challenge of single-session therapies: Creating pivotal moments. In R. A. Wells & V. J. Giannetti (Eds.), *Handbook of the Brief Psychotherapies* (pp. 165–189). New York: Plenum Press.

(Reprinted in M. F. Hoyt, *Brief Therapy and Managed Care: Selected Papers* [pp. 105–139]. San Francisco: Jossey-Bass, 1995.)

Suzuki, S. (1970). *Zen Mind, Beginner's Mind.* New York: Weatherhill.

Tomm, K. (1993). The courage to protest: A commentary on Michael White's work. In S. G. Gilligan & R. Price (Eds.), *Therapeutic Conversations* (pp. 62–80). New York: Norton.

Turner, V. (1969). *The Ritual Process.* Ithaca, NY: Cornell University Press.

van Gennep, A. (1960). *The Rites of Passage.* Chicago: University of Chicago Press.

Welch, S. (1990). *A Feminist Ethic of Risk.* Minneapolis, MN: Fortress Press.

White, M. (1989). *Selected Papers.* Adelaide: Dulwich Centre Publications.

White, M. (1993). Deconstruction and therapy. In S. G. Gilligan & R. Price (Eds.), *Therapeutic Conversations* (pp. 22–61). New York: Norton. (Original work published in the *Dulwich Centre Newsletter,* 1991, No. 3, 1–21. Also reprinted in D. Epston & M. White, *Experience, Contradiction, Narrative and Imagination* [pp. 109–152]. Adelaide: Dulwich Centre Publications, 1992.)

White, M. (1993). Commentary: The histories of the present. In S. G. Gilligan & R. Price (Eds.), *Therapeutic Conversations* (pp. 121–135). New York: Norton.

White, M. (1995). *The Re-Authoring of Lives: Interviews and Essays.* Adelaide: Dulwich Centre Publications.

White, M., & Epston, D. (1990). *Narrative Means to Therapeutic Ends.* New York: Norton.

Wood, A. (1991). Outside expert knowledge: An interview with Michael White. *Australian and New Zealand Journal of Family Therapy, 12*(4), 207–214. (Reprinted in M. White, *Re-Authoring Lives: Interviews and Essays* [pp. 60–81]. Adelaide: Dulwich Centre Publications, 1995.)

CHAPTER 3

Solution Building
and Language Games
A Conversation with Steve de Shazer

MICHAEL F. HOYT

How language is used to construct useful realities, and how this can be facilitated purposefully in therapy, are central concerns in the work of Steve de Shazer. A longtime leader in the field of brief therapy, de Shazer is Senior Research Associate at the Brief Family Therapy Center (BFTC) in Milwaukee, Wisconsin. His books have included *Patterns of Brief Family Therapy* (1982), *Keys to Solution in Brief Therapy* (1985), *Clues: Investigating Solutions in Brief Therapy* (1988), and *Putting Difference to Work* (1991). His quest for simplicity and minimalist elegance has increasingly led him to focus on the ideas of linguistic theorists (especially Ludwig Wittgenstein, Jacques Derrida, and Jacques Lacan). The title of de Shazer's (1994) most recent book borrows a phrase from Sigmund Freud to attest to his views regarding the power of language: *Words Were Originally Magic*.

The following conversation took place on April 10, 1994, in de Shazer's BFTC office in Milwaukee.

HOYT: The first thing I want to ask, Steve, is how has what you mean by *brief therapy* changed over the years? What are some of the things that you've given up or you've added, and why?

DE SHAZER: Well, I guess that when it first started, there was really no definition whatsoever, except "brief." I don't think "brief" was ever defined in any way at all. Then, doing what I was calling "brief therapy," I ran into John Weakland and his gang at MRI [the Mental Research Institute in Palo Alto, California] with their 10-session limit. I knew 10 was an arbitrary number. I also knew it didn't fit with my experience. So we started a research project: we tossed a coin and decided whether to have a 12-session or 6-session limit. And we found out that in the 12-session limit, they waited until session 10 to do anything.

HOYT: Parkinson's law.[1]

DE SHAZER: With a 6-session limit, they only waited until session 5. And the outcomes were no different. So we added a third condition—which was we wouldn't say anything about a time limit. It turned out that the average number of sessions with no time limit was less than with either 6 or 12, and the outcomes were slightly better.[2] So I abandoned having a numbered session limit in 1973 or 1974 or something like that. That was the first change. For some years it's been that brief therapy means, among other things, "as few sessions as possible and not one more than necessary." Who knows how many that may actually be, over how many years? The average number of sessions dropped to about four about 10 years ago. It's been relatively stable at around four.[3] Of course, it switched from problem solving to solution building in the early '80s. That switch is in the books.[4] "You can look it up," as Casey Stengel used to say.

HOYT: In reading the early books and following the progression, it seems there's been a shift away from strategy and power.

DE SHAZER: Certainly away from strategy. You don't need strategies, or you don't need "strategic maneuvers" à la Haley or Haley's interpretation of Erickson, or even the earlier MRI stuff. I found out that when we switched from problem solving to solution development, you just don't need to do that sort of thing. You don't need these fancy interventions. You don't need all this elaborate stuff. It's no more effective than the simple things we are doing, maybe even less effective. Certainly they are far more work than what we're doing now. We were pretty good at it in the '70s; the early books and papers illustrate that we became pretty damn good at that style of intervention. We still have to resist doing it now and then, because we know it's no better than finding something the client already is doing that they can do more of.

---

[1]Appelbaum (1975; see also Hoyt, 1990) has noted what he calls "Parkinson's Law in Psychotherapy," the idea that therapeutic work expands or contracts to fit the time allotted for it.

[2]This project was never written up or published. Similar results have been reported by Fisher (1980, 1984).

[3]Actually, for the past two years the average has dropped to three!

[4]In addition to those authored by de Shazer himself, other books especially aligned with the solution-focused model include those by Dolan (1991), Walter and Peller (1992), Berg and Miller (1992), and Berg (1994).

HOYT: It's the temptation you write about as "Erickson-the-clever."[5]

DE SHAZER: Yeah, absolutely. We set out to emulate that. I don't mind being thought clever, it's just hard as hell to teach it.

HOYT: Where does hypnotic induction fit in now in your work?

DE SHAZER: As far as anything formal, it doesn't fit at all.

HOYT: Why have you moved away from it?

DE SHAZER: Solution-focused brief therapy is easier on the therapist; it's less work for the therapist; it actually takes fewer sessions; and it has as least as good results. The problem with hypnosis, no matter how "naturalistic," etc., etc., it might be, how unobtrusive it might be, the client thinks it's "hypnosis." My conversations with clients later on indicate that they blame the hypnosis (and/or the therapist) for the "success" or "failure," no matter how little hypnosis you actually do. It's the magic of hypnosis.

HOYT: So it's disempowering.

DE SHAZER: Yeah.

HOYT: "I didn't do it; I don't have any control."

DE SHAZER: Right. That's another reason I moved away from it, aside from the fact that this works better.

HOYT: You said it's easier on the therapist as well as getting better results. I see it as also resulting in less burnout. We're not fighting the client; we're not having to work through a hard "resistance."

DE SHAZER: Yeah, we don't have to be clever. It takes a lot of work for most people to be clever.

HOYT: What about reframing techniques that we've all used? Is that something else that you've given up or don't see as useful?

DE SHAZER: I certainly won't go through and do any kind of reframing like we used to do, where we would invent a new frame à la MRI or our early work. I think that the compliments and the way we do the interview—our "procedural interventions," as Dick Fisch calls them— will lead the clients to spontaneously reframe things for themselves.

---

[5]In *Words Were Originally Magic* (1994), de Shazer describes different ways of relating to clients. He contrasts Erickson's "expert" stance with other, less hierarchical and more egalitarian positions, including "de Shazer-the-stupid." He goes on to add: "Actually, I should have seen all of this long ago, since the two major influences on my interviewing style have been John Weakland's persona 'Weakland-the-dense' and Insoo Kim Berg's persona 'Insoo-the-incredulous' " (p. 34). Later (p. 266), he adds: "Having spent most of the '70s and part of the '80s designing 'novel tasks in the Erickson style,' I still find it difficult at times to restrain myself from proposing such interventions to clients. However, these fancy tasks are very difficult to design; furthermore, teaching therapists to design such clever tasks is not an easy job. In the great majority of cases these clever tasks seem to be no more, perhaps even less, effective than simpler ones based principally on what the clients have already said they know how to do."

The only reframe that counts is if the client buys it. So the best ones are the ones they come up with.

HOYT: I might express it as you're punctuating and they're changing the meaning.

DE SHAZER: Yeah, okay.

HOYT: Underscoring certain experiences for them or getting them focused on certain experiences.

DE SHAZER: Yeah.

HOYT: What about the use of paradox?

DE SHAZER: That went away a long time ago. By that I assume you were asking about paradoxical interventions?

HOYT: Right. Can you recall an episode that told you, "Enough of this"?

DE SHAZER: Well, I remember we used to do paradoxical interventions or attempt to do them [de Shazer & Nunnally, 1991]. But most of what I see people doing that they call "paradoxical interventions" are not. Most of them are reverse psychology; they are not paradoxical interventions.

HOYT: What's the distinction?

DE SHAZER: Well, a paradoxical intervention has to be exactly counter to what it is you're going after. The reverse double-bind kind of thing. There has to be no escape. Most of the "paradoxical interventions" don't have that feature.

HOYT: Where reverse psychology is just, "Keep doing it."

DE SHAZER: Yeah. So most of what people call "paradoxical interventions" are not paradoxical interventions. We used to do some, and we came to the conclusion that paradoxical interventions were unnecessary for several reasons, the main one being that we aren't trying to stop anything. Paradoxical interventions are designed to stop something, and we aren't trying to stop anything. What we are doing is trying to start something or increase the frequency of something. So there's no need for paradoxical interventions. If you do it right, they work if you want to stop something. Doing it right actually involves following the rules, and I think Watzlawick, Beavin, and Jackson [1967] put down the rules quite nicely in *The Pragmatics of Human Communication*. That was the most evolved version of it, I think. I don't think there's been any refinements of it after that.

HOYT: When you're trying to start something rather than stop something, will we still encounter what is sometimes called "resistance"? The client doesn't want to start?

DE SHAZER: Well, if I were to use the word *resistance*—I wouldn't, but if I were—it would translate in my vocabulary as *therapist's error*. That would mean to me that the therapist wasn't listening, and therefore he told the client to do something the client didn't want to do. That means he wasn't listening during the interview. Most of our stuff is based on the fact of something they told us about, that they did such and such and it worked in some situation, so it's just a matter of transferring that from situation A to situation B. So there's nothing new. Most of our interventions are nothing new for them.

HOYT: It's, as the title of that Zen book has it, *Selling Water by the River* [Kennett, 1972].

DE SHAZER: Yes. Or selling water *to* the river.

HOYT: It's selling them themselves, in a sense. Something that's felt good before, so why resist it?

DE SHAZER: So we don't have that kind of difficulty ("resistance") very often, but if we do we know why. It means we weren't listening. We may have gotten ourselves into an Erickson mode.

HOYT: Where we were trying to maneuver them into something they weren't ready for or wanting.

DE SHAZER: Right.

HOYT: Can you give an example that brought home to you "the death of resistance" [de Shazer, 1984], where it could have been done one way but you did it another way and then you had to deal with resistance—you created resistance?

DE SHAZER: I haven't thought about "resistance" in so many years, it's hard. I don't think I can come up with anything.

HOYT: It's not a very solution-focused question.

DE SHAZER: I don't have any idea how to answer that question. I can't remember.

HOYT: I think another advantage, then, to a solution-focused approach, is that it doesn't stimulate noncompliance because there's nothing they have to noncomply with. It makes it more user-friendly for both the therapist and for the client. It's less likely to drive clients away.

DE SHAZER: Less likely. What I see sometimes is the amateurs, so to speak—the beginners, who somehow think more is better and, therefore, they give this endless stream of compliments and bore the client silly with them and, therefore, the client stops taking them seriously. That's one thing I see happen with beginners, in particular: There's just too damn many compliments, and that will drive the client away.

HOYT: I think there's an ethical position that it's very respectful. I know we talked with John Weakland in that other interview about the importance of taking the client seriously [Hoyt, 1994]. The person feels heard, validated, appreciated for who they are. How do we separate the idea of "influence" from "brainwashing," to call it that? We're influencing but not imposing our values, manipulating them?

DE SHAZER: There's that line, all right. Clients hire us to influence them; that's why they come. The more you are using their stuff, the less danger you are in of moving into brainwashing. The more you are putting in your stuff, the closer you're getting to brainwashing. That's pretty clear to me. Those are the two ends of it, perhaps. I'm not sure if it is a continuum, but there certainly is a line in between. And, frankly, I see many, many of the psychotherapy models as being closer to brainwashing than to anything else.

HOYT: I think the respectful ethic is that it's truly informed consent. We're identifying what their goals are and helping them meet their goals, rather than imposing our agenda.

DE SHAZER: Right. You know, we have a saying around here—there used to be a sign made by somebody on the team (probably Gale Miller): "If the therapist's goals and the client's goals are different, the therapist is wrong."

HOYT: I don't know if you've seen it yet, but in the latest issue of the *Family Therapy Networker*, Eve Lipchik [1994] has an article called "The Rush to Be Brief." She makes the point that sometimes therapists trying to be brief go forward before they have validated and before they've heard or acknowledged the client.[6] They are not being respectful in that sense. It's much like giving too many compliments, leaping ahead.

DE SHAZER: John Weakland's first law of brief therapy still applies. He promulgated it for many years and I have continued to. It's a two-word law: "Go Slow."

HOYT: What's another of John's laws?

DE SHAZER: The first one is very clear: "Go slow." The second one is "If you don't know what to do, the best thing to do is nothing." You'll notice if you watch either his interviews or mine that the therapist

[6]There are many ways to achieve alliance and connectedness. In *Words Were Originally Magic*, a man starts to "present" himself as a clinical "case," and de Shazer (1994, p. 241) nicely interrupts him by saying, "No, no, not about that. . . . Tell me something about you, who you are . . . what you enjoy doing." For further discussion of the importance of acknowledgment and validation in strategic and solution-focused therapy, see Hoyt (1994) as well as articles by Aponte (1992), Duncan (1992), Held (1992), Kiser, Piercy, and Lipchik (1993), Nylund and Corsiglia (1994), Real (1990), and Solovey and Duncan (1992).

is doing relatively nothing much of the time, including just sitting there and not saying anything. Weakland and I have talked about this many times—what I call "actively doing nothing." Weakland was trained, at least in part, as an anthropologist, then married a Chinese family. I don't know if he knew he was marrying the whole family, but that's what happens when you marry an Asian woman. You marry the whole family. Then you get a position in the family. I did the same thing, married a Korean woman. So you marry this whole family and you get a position in the family that is uniquely yours, particularly because you're not Asian. But nonetheless, you have a position in the family that is absolutely unique. Nobody can tell you what the rules are, because you're supposed to know these things. You're supposed to know them. Your position in that family starts from the moment you're born, and you're still there in that same position relative to the rest of the hierarchy. But coming in there as an adult, you're assumed to know all these rules. Therefore, the likelihood is very high that whatever you decide to do in any given situation is going to turn out wrong—this likelihood is very, very high, and you're going to pay for it for years. So, as I learned from John Weakland, the best thing to do in that situation is nothing. If you do it often enough and long enough, eventually you acquire the label of "wise"!

HOYT: (*Laughter*) In talking about treating people respectfully, I just recently finished reading Insoo's *Family-Based Services* [Berg, 1994]. If there's the book *Pragmatics of Human Communication* [Watzlawick et al., 1967], I think this book could be subtitled *Pragmatics of Therapeutic Communication*. I thought it was an extraordinarily fine book. I was struck over and over how in these very multiproblem, painful family situations, Insoo was able repeatedly to form alliances with the people and work *with* them, where many of us just would have attempted to protect the children from the parents, thinking, "These are bad people; there's something that they've done wrong." We would be in a judgmental frame. How do you work with folks? What helps you form alliances in difficult situations?

DE SHAZER: Well, I guess that there's two parts to that. Since you framed it around Insoo, I'll start there. She was raised in a different culture, and I've been studying that culture for 20 years or whatever it is now. There are big differences between Asian and American families. Both of them in general produce reasonable, functional adults. The difference between the two can be sketched this way. In the United States, if a kid does something wrong, he is likely to be grounded. That is, he is imprisoned within the family. Therefore, being with the family is negative—it's a punishment. In Asia, this same kid for the same offense is likely to be expelled from the family in some way. So being with the family is a positive. And we wonder why our families are disintegrating. Why kids can't wait to get away. The Koreans wonder how they will ever get rid of their kids. It does seem to be exactly the opposite. They both work in the long run; they produce reasonable adults. That was the first clue that led us (as a group, 20 years ago) away from something like Minuchin's [1974] structural family therapy that postulates some kind of ideal family. There ain't no such critter, so we moved away from that very quickly; it made no sense to us. I was doing brief therapy before I heard about family therapy. When I heard about family therapy, one of the ones I looked at was Minuchin's because I knew from its reputation that it actually worked, but I couldn't hold to its value system.

HOYT: I understand what you're saying about the difference between the Asian and the American family, but how does that connect to alliance?

DE SHAZER: It allows us to accept whatever people are doing as having the potential of working. Let's go back into sociology, and there one talks about personality as being situationally determined or constructed, as opposed to psychology, where it's intrapsychically determined. Sociology more likely talks about it being situationally determined. Therefore, "If I was in this client's shoes, saw things the way this client does, I would be doing the same thing he's doing." That's the central constructivist principle. We can accept it and, therefore, we can develop an alliance with it.

HOYT: It's recognizing the difference in "state" versus "trait."

DE SHAZER: Yeah, sort of.

HOYT: They are in a state where this is appropriate behavior.

DE SHAZER: They're doing what they think is the best thing to do, given their situation. We would probably do the same if we were in their shoes.

HOYT: It's recognizing people as problem solvers rather than as evil— that they are trying to cope as best they can with what they've been taught and their resources and the options they are creating that they see available.

DE SHAZER: So, therefore, we can develop an alliance with anybody who wants to develop an alliance with us. And do it very quickly, because this is something we take for granted. We just act as if we have an alliance right from the moment one.

HOYT: What indicates, then, a difficult case?

DE SHAZER: That's not in our vocabulary.

HOYT: If there hasn't been some change by a certain number of sessions, are there strategies?

DE SHAZER: Usually the people who ask that question have something in mind—something that they think is a difficult case, like a flasher or something. What makes it a difficult case in that instance is that you're thinking it's a difficult case. We did this project a couple of years ago because people often asked this question. We sat down and tried to operationalize the concept "difficult case" in order to have an answer for this question. Since our average is around four sessions, we decided that a difficult case must be one in which they are not reporting a significant change at the third session. That seemed a reasonable point. So we decided that that would be a "difficult case" for the sake of this project. We decided that we would then scrupulously work with the team with the next 50 intakes, we'd videotape, make predictions, etc., etc. In the first session, what is it that gave us the idea this would or would not be a difficult case? At the end of this, we had our 50 cases, 50 intakes in a row, and we looked at them all. There wasn't a single case that didn't report significant change by the third session. Well, what the fuck, now what? We decided that we'd look at all the second sessions and see if there was something there. We found, I think there were four cases, all of them had turned around in session 3. What we found out was that these were the four cases where we did something different from the standard protocol during or at the end of the second session. Therefore, we went right back to rule 3: "If what you're doing isn't working, do something else."[7] One thing that happened is with one case the therapist reassembled the client group after the break in a different room than he'd done the therapy in. The intervention message was exactly the same kind of thing we usually do, no different. Case number 2, I saw just the mother and left the kids out of the room. Case number 3, the person who was doing the interview stood up delivering the intervention message rather than sitting down. And case number 4, someone else from the team went in and delivered the message.

HOYT: "If it's not working, do something different."

---

[7]The basic rules of solution-focused therapy: (1) If it ain't broke, don't fix it. (2) Once you know what works, do more of it. (3) If it doesn't work, don't do it again; do something different. Following from these rules, some heuristic questions: *First session*—What do(es) the client(s) want? What can the client(s) do (toward what is wanted)? What needs to happen? *Later (second and subsequent) sessions*—What is better? What did the client do (toward better)? What happened (to make it better)? What compliments and tasks can be given (staying within the client's expertise)? Is it "better" enough—when should therapy stop?

DE SHAZER: No matter how trivial—standing up, somebody else going in, sitting in a different chair. So if you're stuck, the first thing you want to do is ask, "What part of this do I have control over?" You have control over where you meet, when you meet, where you sit, where they sit. You have some control over whether you're standing or sitting, a different office. Just anything that you have control over, you can do something, and therefore you stand a chance of having an impact.

HOYT: Change the context, break the set, punctuate it differently. More of the same does not make a change.

DE SHAZER: It's very simple, sometimes.

HOYT: If we're required to do an evaluation, it's good then to move to another room or change seats, to give the sense of "Now we're going to do something different" rather than "It's going to be more pathology talk."

DE SHAZER: Right. Absolutely. That's what people always ask, "How do we do solution-focused when we gotta do all these God-damned forms for managed care or the hospital or whatever?" Well, the simplest thing is, you can change rooms like that. If you're a medical doctor in the hospital, wear your white coat for the diagnostic part; take it off when you start doing therapy. Or switch. If you have a partner you trust, have them do the first part and you do the second, and for their cases you reverse.

HOYT: That's a switch from being a mental illness professional to a mental health professional.

DE SHAZER: It's easy, by just taking off the white coat.

HOYT: When would you bring in more people? If we're stuck, should we bring in other family members?

DE SHAZER: Almost never.

HOYT: Would you bring in less family?

DE SHAZER: I would be more tempted to bring in less.

HOYT: You said you saw her [the mother in case 2] without the kids.

DE SHAZER: Much more likely to go that direction.

HOYT: Simplify rather than bringing in more complexity?

DE SHAZER: As I see it, the idea of bringing more people in is based on the idea that you're stuck because you don't have enough information. That's the premise behind it. My idea, following Wittgenstein, is "The problem is you have too *much* information already, but you just don't know how to organize it." Or, furthermore, from Wittgenstein again, "You're in this situation and you've got what you got and that's all there is. There ain't no more."[8] All you got is a problem of organization. So get people out and talk to just one person at a time, and maybe you can simplify it enough to do something. I haven't invited—I can't remember when last I said, "Bring your husband," or something like that. I can't remember that happening.

HOYT: What about the situation of the so-called "multiproblem family" when they are presenting a number of issues at once, competing informations? How do you organize that? Ask them what their first goal is?

DE SHAZER: Oh, God, no. Then you just have another argument. First of all, I think it is perfectly normal and reasonable for any family to have everybody disagreeing about what the rules are; I think that's perfectly reasonable. So I don't consider that a problem. We think about them as "multigoal families." So I guess basically what we do is something like his in that kind of situation. First of all, if you ask the miracle question[9] early enough in the session, you oftentimes avoid that difficulty—having all these multiple goals. Sometimes.

HOYT: Who do you ask the miracle question of?

DE SHAZER: Everybody.

HOYT: And if everyone gives a different answer?

DE SHAZER: That's reasonable.

HOYT: Then you have competing goals.

DE SHAZER: That's normal and reasonable. Then you say, "Okay, 10 stands for this package—everything you've been talking about, those kinds of things. Whatever it will take for you guys to each individually and collectively to recognize that a miracle has happened, that's 10. Where are we today?" We get different estimates where each of them are. Then we sort of work on getting everybody's number on the scale and ignore, if you will, the fact that their version of 10 is probably different, because it's always going to be different with more than one person. And even with one person, he's going to have more than one goal, and they may conflict with each other anyway. So, what we do then—and again, remembering Wittgenstein, we say something like, "Well, you have a wish and you make that wish. Then at some point you're satisfied. There's no guarantee that your wish has been met, and there's no guarantee that if your

[8]"Our mistake is to look for an explanation where we ought to look at what happens" (Wittgenstein, 1968, #654).

[9]"The Miracle Question: 'Suppose that one night, while you were asleep, there was a miracle and this problem was solved. How would you know? What would be different?' " (de Shazer, 1988, p. 5).

wish had been met you'd be satisfied." As they move up the scale, we keep saying, "Is this good enough? Can we stop now?" Our studies indicate that most people—most families stop with 7 being good enough, and that 6 months later they will have frequently moved up to 8, but that is almost the outer limit. Very few people make 10. Those that do make 10 usually end up going into the teens as well—"overachievers."

HOYT: Again, the therapist has to be careful that she or he doesn't impose their perfectionism with the idea, "They're only at 8. We've got to keep working."

DE SHAZER: Oh, yeah. I remember one case fairly recently where I asked the scaling question [Berg & de Shazer, 1993], and she said she was at 2. I just sat there and didn't respond; I didn't do anything. I can imagine the people behind the mirror saying, "Oh, Christ, she's only at 2." I was just sitting there. But I was just waiting for her to expand some on what "2" might mean, without having to ask her. Then after a short pause, she said, "You know, that's pretty damn good for me." I shook her hand. She thought it would be a God-damned miracle for her to ever reach 3 or 4. So, her 2 was halfway to her goal—she knew she would never get past 4. If she maintained that 4, she would be satisfied.

HOYT: I think we get into a therapeutic Xeno's fallacy, having to get halfway there, and then half of that, then half of that, etc., so that you can never get there.

DE SHAZER: Yes. You can never get there.

HOYT: "I'm good enough, I made it, this works for me. I'm satisfied."

DE SHAZER: That's usually around 7.

HOYT: Some patients come in and say they have a personality problem: "There's something wrong with me." And some therapists talk about Axis II [American Psychiatric Association, 1994] or a "personality disorder" diagnosis. How do you react to that?

DE SHAZER: In what sense?

HOYT: I've been at workshops presenting, and somebody says, "Well, what about brief therapy with Axis II? How does brief therapy address the underlying personality problem?"

DE SHAZER: It doesn't. I'll frequently say something like, "I have no idea what you're talking about. Give me a case example so I can understand what you're talking about."

HOYT: Deconstruct the diagnosis into what it really is.

DE SHAZER: I have no idea what "Axis II" might mean, and I don't want to know.

HOYT: I remember one time hearing [Jay] Haley say to someone at a conference, "I wouldn't let that be the problem."

DE SHAZER: Yeah. Absolutely.

HOYT: Find a problem that can be solved rather than a hypothetical construct.

DE SHAZER: Years and years ago, I saw a lot of research about the unreliability of diagnostic categories.

HOYT: Especially when they're highly hypothetical and based on somebody's theory.

DE SHAZER: So the answer is, "Tell me about a case and I'll tell you how I might work with that case."

HOYT: Let me read you a quotation from *Words Were Originally Magic* [de Shazer, 1994, p. 267]: "The miracle question was not designed to create or prompt miracles. All the miracle question is designed to do is to allow clients to describe what it is they want out of therapy without having to concern themselves with the problem and the traditional assumption that the solution is somehow connected with understanding and eliminating the problem." How do you see the role of causation and determination?

DE SHAZER: Absolute idiocy. I think the concept of causation, given the kinds of things that we deal with, is absolute nonsense.

HOYT: What if the client wants or feels they need an explanation: "I need to figure out where this came from, why I do this"?

DE SHAZER: Well, actually, that's more of a hypothetical than a real client. That's the kind of thing a therapist would suspect clients are going to say. I think that's happened to me twice in my career. And both times I said, "Will it be all right if we solve the problem and then come back to that, if you are still interested?" And they both agreed. That doesn't really happen, and I'm talking, oh, how many cases? Ten thousand cases plus. I think it's happened twice that I can recall.

HOYT: Some patients I've encountered have been convinced by popular media or something that "I have to get to the root of it," or "Until I really understand where it came from, I'm not really going to solve it; it's just putting a Band-Aid on it." It's almost like an agricultural metaphor: "I want to dig it up by the root and pull it out completely."

DE SHAZER: Well, as I said, that doesn't seem to happen to me. I can't explain why it doesn't happen. But I suspect that part of the reason it doesn't happen is that I never ask them what the problem is. I say, "What brings you here?" and then I go into the miracle question and start dealing with where we're going. Sometimes I realize at the end of the therapy I never did find out what the problem was.

HOYT: I sense that when most clients come in, they want to be happy; they want relief from pain. And if we can focus on that, they may have had the theory "I need to dig it out," but once the pain goes away it's irrelevant to kind of dig around in archeology.

DE SHAZER: Right, and I think that people become very interested in where they're going in the future. If you can do that, you avoid all this stuff about causation, etc. But there's no way we can get at what might have caused something. There's no way we can get at that. Even the ideas of linear or circular causation—neither of them apply within this domain.

HOYT: How did Freud and Wittgenstein go in different directions? What was the question for which they got such different answers?

DE SHAZER: They were both trying to figure out what the hell was going on at a particularly difficult time during history—turn-of-the-century Vienna, where you had this regal empire that was going around spending a lot of money on masked balls and all the great things that the Viennese monarchy did, with a country that was disintegrating and a country with no common language.[10] The Austrian–Hungarian empire had many, many languages, so there was a question about what in the world is language. That's why the Austrians are the ones who developed philosophies of language. You had to look behind and beneath whatever the monarchy was doing to find out what the hell was going on. So I think it's just two alternatives to the same difficulty. One being less obvious than the other, I suppose.

HOYT: The two alternatives?

DE SHAZER: One being Freud's idea that "Whatever is going on is a mask for what's really going on." And Wittgenstein's idea that "It's just a matter of we can't decipher it," which is different.[11]

HOYT: "Shadows on the wall that mean something else," as opposed to "All you have is what you have," not looking for a meaning beyond it.

DE SHAZER: "It's all there, it's just that you can't put the pieces together"— that's Wittgenstein. You have this puzzle on the table that's upside down; you have the gray side. You may suspect at times that you don't have all the pieces. Freud would assume immediately that you don't

[10]Primary sources for Wittgenstein's thought include *The Blue and Brown Books* (1958), *Philosophical Investigations* (1968), and *Culture and Value* (1980). To learn more about his life and times, interested readers may want to consult Bartley (1985), Duffy (1988), Janik and Towlmin (1974), and Monk (1990), among others.

[11]"There must not be anything hypothetical in our considerations. We must do away with all explanation, and description alone must take its place" (Wittgenstein, 1968, #109).

have all the pieces, that there must be a reason why it's on its face, gray side up rather than picture side up.

HOYT: In a practical sense there may be enough there to solve it, rather than saying, "What else? What's missing?"

DE SHAZER: There are people who can solve jigsaw puzzles gray side up.

HOYT: Why not look at the doughnut rather than the hole? Even Lacan's [w]hole.[12]

DE SHAZER: Yes.

HOYT: Let me read another quotation I want to ask your thoughts about. In the article "Doing Therapy: A Post-Structural Revision" that you and Insoo wrote together, you say, "The user only discovers the meaning of his words in the act of using them in a language game. A word is not *sent* but only *received*" [de Shazer & Berg, 1992, p. 79; emphasis in original]. What do you mean by "language game," and then how do you mean we only discover the meanings of our words after using them?

DE SHAZER: We have a language game right now that is between you and me and whatever, defined as an interview that will form a chapter in a book. That's a language game; it defines everything we're doing in this hour. So if I were to hit you over the head with this unabridged dictionary here, you can only interpret that within the context of this being an interview for this book of yours.

HOYT: It would be a "foul" in the language game! (*Laughter*)

DE SHAZER: Yeah. Therefore, an observer might say I've suddenly gone berserk, violating the rules of the language game. You can only find out what the rules are by participating. So, whatever words I choose to describe what I'm talking about, I choose these words internally somehow. Then they come out of my mouth and you react to them one way or another, and that's how I discover whether they meant what I thought they were going to mean or they meant something else.

HOYT: So you never know what question you truly ask until you see what answer you get.

DE SHAZER: Right.

HOYT: You may think you asked a certain question, but it's how it's received, how it's taken.

---

[12]An allusion to de Shazer's discussion of language, structure, and meaning in *Words Were Originally Magic*. See especially Chapter 3, "Lacan's [W]hole," and Chapter 4, "Getting to the Surface of the Problem."

DE SHAZER: Right.

HOYT: So we're creating the meaning rather than it sort of being revealed or objectively . . .

DE SHAZER: Right. Meanings evolve during the course of the activity. So you take a pair or some interlocking pairs of our conversation here and move it into a different context, it may make absolutely no sense whatsoever. Because there's no language game to define what's going on. I can refer you to that mask over there (*gestures toward a carving on the wall*), and if you look at that mask at the right angle, you'll see how much it looks like Lyndon Johnson.

HOYT: Yes, I can see LBJ. It looks like a Korean LBJ.

DE SHAZER: Yes, it's a Korean mask. We have a link then to the language game of hanging around in our living room last night, looking at masks on the wall.[13] If you include this thing about the mask in the transcript and we don't include this next part, that looks like, "What?" But *you* knew exactly what it was.

HOYT: Why suddenly we were talking about masks.

DE SHAZER: Yes.

HOYT: If the reader can't see the mask, it sounds like you've halluci- nated.

DE SHAZER: You didn't have any trouble with it, because you were part of that language game of the masks last night.[14]

HOYT: Orville Wright once said, "If we all worked on the assumption of what is accepted as true is really true, there would be very little hope of advance."

DE SHAZER: If we think it's true, then we won't ask any questions.

HOYT: So we need to recognize there's a language game rather than there's an absolute reality.

DE SHAZER: Oh, yeah. Then there's reality, and if I hit you on the knee with this, this is going to hurt you.

---

[13]Context: After a delicious home-cooked meal the night before, we had discussed some masks I had been admiring.

[14]de Shazer and Berg (1992, p. 75) explicate: "One way to begin conceptualizing, describing, and using a post-structural view of what is involved in doing therapy is to borrow a concept developed by Ludwig Wittgenstein and to look at doing therapy as an example of an activity involving a set of related, but distinct 'language games' (Wittgen- stein, 1958, 1968). For Wittgenstein (1968, #23), 'the term "language game" is meant to bring into prominence the fact that the speaking of language is part of an activity.' A language game is an activity seen as a language complete in itself, a complete system of human communication: You've got what you've got and that's all there is. There is no need to look behind or beneath since everything you need is readily available and open to view. Nothing is hidden."

HOYT: Like the Zen teacher who whacks you and says, "Is that real?"[15]

DE SHAZER: You better believe it's real. That's an entirely different domain. People who confuse the two are what we call "crazy," psychotic perhaps.

HOYT: How then can we be respectful of the client's belief, language game, the way they construct reality, and at the same time suggest things may not be as they seem to be, kind of casting doubt on or opening them to other possibilities? We're deconstructing.

DE SHAZER: Basically by emphasizing parts they aren't emphasizing. But it's something they said, so you can go with that enough to respect the whole package. That's the easiest way to say it.

HOYT: One of the problems I've had lately trying to read psychoanalytic writers is they usually seem very much to believe that they're *right*, that there's a reality there and they are uncovering it. I'm expecting to read a psychoanalytic article soon called "Postmodernism as a Defense against Reality."

DE SHAZER: (*Laughter*) I'm sure there already is such an article.

HOYT: If there isn't, I'm sure there will be. Rather than accepting the idea that it's a game, that it's being created. It can be a serious game that is being played, but it's being made rather than it's being revealed.

DE SHAZER: Any day now you'll see that article.

HOYT: I also see a danger in constructivist or postmodern views, which is some people consider that we can define anything away: "The Holocaust didn't happen, child abuse didn't happen. It's just something that you think happened, or maybe for you it did, but it didn't really." How do we protect against dismissing such important events?

DE SHAZER: There's actually a book, I'm trying to find it (*searches and pulls it off the shelf*). Here.

HOYT: It's called *Uncritical Theory: Post-Modernism, Intellectuals, and the Gulf War,* by Christopher Norris [1992]. What does it tell us about the dangers of pretending . . .

DE SHAZER: First, he's drawing a distinction between postmodernism

---

[15]The all-in-your-mind view has never really recovered from the kick it received from Dr. Samuel Johnson more than two centuries ago: "After we came out of the church, we stood talking for some time together of Bishop Berkeley's ingenious sophistry to prove the non-existence of matter, and that everything in the universe is merely ideal. I observed, that though we are satisfied his doctrine is not true, it is impossible to refute it. I never shall forget the alacrity with which Johnson answered, striking his foot with mighty force against a large stone, till he rebounded from it, 'I refute it *thus!*' " (Boswell, 1791/1980, p. 333; emphasis in original).

and poststructuralism, which is similar to the distinction I draw. I perhaps got it from him. The difference being that the postmodern is an inversion of modern, and, therefore, it is really a good question. How, as he says, how can we tell the difference between these rockets shooting over Baghdad or a video game of rockets shooting over Baghdad? He goes a lot into that. I'm not sure he comes up with a good conclusion.

HOYT: Because now there's the danger of "virtual reality," that they can make it seem so close: "Is it Memorex or is it real?"

DE SHAZER: I think it's exactly the same problem. If I hit you on the knee with this, it's going to hurt you. It's exactly the same problem. There are documents of the Holocaust, there are lots of documents, etc., etc., a preponderance of evidence. You can do an archeological study that these things actually did occur. What it may mean, of course, is open to negotiation; but the events happened, we do have the hard physical evidence. It's a really different domain.

HOYT: I recently toured the U.S. Memorial Holocaust Museum in Washington, and it was very archival. I think some of the need for the archival quality was the documentation to counter the assertions that this didn't occur—a heavy emphasis on the physical evidence. The meaning, as you say, is still subject to debate.

DE SHAZER: Yeah, and it always has been. The meaning of anything has always been subject to debate. That's why we have always had both a "true church" and "heretics," whatever that might be. There's never been a time when there was only one religious sect; there's always been a division into other truth or truths.

HOYT: History is now being rewritten around the Alamo in San Antonio, Texas.

DE SHAZER: Well, and I think it probably should be. History will always be rewritten in terms of who is writing it. History doesn't change; what you write about it changes.

HOYT: The event that occurred doesn't change, but the meaning we give.

DE SHAZER: Right.

HOYT: History is not the events; it's our recollection, report, and analysis.

DE SHAZER: History is very difficult unless there are archives, so to speak. You can't depend on asking somebody.

HOYT: So in a narrative constructive approach, we're assisting clients to write a history that works for them.

DE SHAZER: Yeah, but that is a long way, I think. You don't need to do that. All you need to do is get it started, and then get the hell out of the way. There's no reason to hang around to correct their grammar. (*Laughter*) And you can start that by pointing out the historical truth that on Tuesday he didn't pop any heroin into his arm. That's just as true as the fact that he did on Wednesday, Thursday, and Friday, but he didn't on Tuesday; that's historical truth for the guy. Let's build on that one.

The "anything goes" school—we're back to Wittgenstein, with the whole elaborate private-language argument that he engages in with his interlocutor. The premise is that there is no way you can depend on a private language. They're not valid. You can't depend on its stability. You may have this idea that the Holocaust didn't happen, but you're going to have a hell of a time when you start bringing that out . . .

HOYT: As an external reality.

DE SHAZER: When you start talking to somebody else about it, the more you maintain the Holocaust is really a "lie," the more crazy that becomes. You can't develop it. A psychotic episode is what you're having, and actually both people probably feel like they're having it. So reality, as I see it, is created by two or more people. One person can't do it by himself; if he does, he is in danger of becoming psychotic. That's the private-language argument.

HOYT: Why will some people get stuck in what I might call a "persistent negative narrative"? One person may say, "Something has happened; that's me; that's my identity. I was molested; I am ruined." Another person says, "I was molested. It was a bad thing, but it's not me; it's not my whole identity," and they go on. Some people will get locked in.

DE SHAZER: Yeah. I guess I would start with this idea. Probably the majority don't get locked in. We're talking about out there in the world. We have evidence now that's accumulating, for instance, that half of the people who quit drinking, quit using heroin, crack cocaine—half of the ones who quit do it spontaneously, with no treatment whatsoever.

HOYT: Is this Fingarette [1988]?

DE SHAZER: There are a number of studies [see Berg & Miller, 1992; Sobell, Sobell, Toneatto, & Leo, 1993].

HOYT: So half the so-called "addicts" stop . . .

DE SHAZER: No, no, the other way. Half of those who quit.

HOYT: Okay, half of those who quit, quit without "treatment."

DE SHAZER: No treatment whatsoever, right. So, I suspect that we don't know how they do it. So, that's what they, the researchers, are trying to get at. How do they actually do it? Can we design treatment along that line? Is there some way to design therapy? I don't know. Our whole model is based on this. That the people come in, and if you ask them right, they will tell you about when the problem doesn't happen and, therefore, you can increase the frequency of its not happening. It's very simple. Now, don't get confused—simple does not mean easy. It's a very simple idea. Most people whose 9-year-old boy wets the bed don't treat it as a problem to go to therapy about, and it goes away at some point.

HOYT: It's one of the dangers of locking people in with diagnosis. It doesn't just describe the present and the past, but it shapes the future.

DE SHAZER: Oh, yeah, Thomas Szasz has been talking about that for a hundred years or however long. The diagnosis is more *pre*scriptive than it is *de*scriptive. It prescribes both what the patient's going to do and how the people around him are going to react.

HOYT: So once you have diagnosed them as "alcoholic," if they come in and say, "I stopped drinking," rather than seeing it as a solution, it gets seen as a denial.

DE SHAZER: Oh, yeah, I heard this from a client years ago, who had gone into an inpatient alcohol treatment program back in the "good old days"—the 28 days business. He was telling me about this. In order to really get the benefit from going to this program, he stopped drinking three weeks before he went in. (*Laughter*) And so he told them about that . . .

HOYT: The cure precedes the treatment.

DE SHAZER: He told them about that in the first meeting that they had in the hospital, and the response from the therapist was, "You are lying. You will tell us the truth one of these days." The guy said to himself, first, "I'm not lying." Then he said, "Fuck you!" He got up and left. He came to see me. Three years later he still wasn't drinking.

HOYT: That's the opposite of shaking the person's hand, building an alliance, and complimenting them on their strengths and successes.

DE SHAZER: Most people do it on their own. Most people that we see just don't realize they've done it on their own. They don't think they've done a good enough job yet. Most people—according to this research, at least half—do it on their own, and feel that they've been successful doing it, so they don't need to get coaching somewhere. I would suspect that 50% is an underestimate. That's my hunch. I'd go up to two-thirds. That's a hunch based on the number of clients over the years who have told me about things that they have stopped doing without treatment. So I would guess that there's more out there than we know about. I don't know how you go about finding these people—advertising in the paper, I suppose.

HOYT: Let me shift and ask another question. How do you think of applying solution-focused work in supervision, training, and teaching? How does the trainer work differently when being solution-focused?

DE SHAZER: Well, you have to assume the same things about these kinds of clients as you do about clinical clients: that whatever they are doing makes sense to them. They are obviously doing something that works. Therefore, the first thing you've got to do is find out what that is, so you can build on it. If I'm doing consultation interviews, the first thing I will do is ask the client on a scale from 0 to 10 (or –10 to 0, if we're in Germany), "You started off therapy here, and here is where you want to get. Where are you now?" I do that not only to give the client the idea that he is making progress, but to give the therapist the idea that he's doing something right. You've got to be able to get that much very quickly in a consultation interview. So that the therapist you're consulting for, here's where he's doing something right. Out of the client's mouth is best, because there is the assumption that the client's going to tell you the truth, of course. So that's the first thing. You have to look at it exactly the same way. You have to find out what they're doing that's working—what are they doing right. Then you have to somehow determine how you're going to know when to stop. When is supervision done, consultation done, training done? Generally, I suppose that has to be arbitrary; somehow they determine that.

HOYT: It's establishing goals and augmenting strengths.

DE SHAZER: Yeah, it's basically the same procedure, except you haven't got a complaint, no problem to solve. So you don't have to start with that. You can just start with the miracle question without asking anything else, so to speak. There's no problem involved. So it's *not* therapy. You can't measure success in the same ways.[16]

HOYT: What's next? Do you see solution-focused therapy being developed in a different direction? The last time I asked you that question about a project [Hoyt, 1994], you said you were working on a book; you weren't sure until you were done what it would be. It turned out to be *Words Were Originally Magic*. Are you working on another one?

---

[16]See Selekman and Todd (1995).

DE SHAZER: Oh, no! I have no idea where it might go. I have no idea. I see a lot of nonsense out there. And there's a lot of "solution-focused" nonsense as well as other kinds.

HOYT: How would we recognize it?

DE SHAZER: Anybody who believes that the miracle question creates miracles is somewhere in the vicinity of talking complete nonsense. But there are therapists out there—and I didn't realize this, not being a very religious-type person—I didn't realize that there were people out there who believe in miracles. They actually either think the miracle question can or should create miracles. And there are others who ask, "What if a miracle doesn't happen?" That's also complete, utter nonsense. Miracles don't happen.

HOYT: The miracle question may be a useful tool, but it's a problem if one believes in miracles.

DE SHAZER: There is other, more subtle nonsense. The piece of nonsense I ran into most recently that is the most startling, most appalling, came from a well-known and highly-thought-of presenter who opened his presentation with the following sentence: "There is no such thing as a bad idea." I spent the rest of the day cataloging all the bad ideas I could think of, like Nazism, fascism, political correctness, and so on. I have no idea what else he had to say.

HOYT: An idea can be very dangerous, especially if you only have one.

DE SHAZER: Yeah. Or none in this case. (*Laughter*) If there are no bad ideas, then there are no ideas, I'm afraid. He doesn't have any idea.

HOYT: How shall we close?

DE SHAZER: Wittgenstein [1980, p. 77e] has some tremendous advice for all authors: "Anything your reader can do for himself, leave to him."

AFTER WORDS WITH INSOO KIM BERG

As we were getting ready to leave the office, Insoo Kim Berg joined us. de Shazer's colleague, partner, and wife, she is a major developer of solution-focused therapy and Director of the Brief Family Therapy Center. Intrigued by the clarity of her perspective (see Berg & Miller, 1992; Berg, 1994; Kean & Chang, 1994; Miller & Berg, 1995), in the course of our continuing discussion I turned the tape-recorder back on and asked:

HOYT: In a brochure description of your training staff, it says, "A native of Korea, Insoo balances her Eastern heritage with her Western scientific training in her clinical practice and teaching." How do you see that?

BERG: To me there's a clear distinction between the Eastern and Western approach to life itself. We're talking about the whole attitude toward life, the view of life. They're very different, I think. What's different about it is the whole notion of being scientific means that you go after the underlying causes. I think the whole scientific stance has been very useful because it builds on understanding the causal relationship.

HOYT: It's very Western that life is to be analyzed . . .

BERG: Analyzed and solved. I think that medicine is a good example of where that has been very terribly helpful. It has led to many, many wonderful discoveries and treatment approaches and so on. But I think that somehow when it comes to human relationships, problems of living, we tend to have the same mechanistic approach to life, the issue of life. I think that medicine sees the body as a machine-like entity. So we can take it apart, we study it and fix it, and then put it back together. I think that kind of influence, a positive scientific quality, spilled over into the psychotherapy field.

HOYT: Michael White writes a lot about this in *Narrative Means to Therapeutic Ends* [White & Epston, 1990]. He has a table of analogies [p. 6] where he spells it out very clearly. He doesn't relate it to East–West, but he talks about the positivist scientific approach of analyze it, dissect it, cure it, cut it out, fix it. This could be opposed to one of more appreciating sort of the—I don't know if you want to call it the mystery of it, but the totality of what it is.

BERG: This is life, and I think the Eastern mindset is that we rarely ask, "Why does this happen?" We say, "This happens, that's how life is."

DE SHAZER: We know from acupuncture: You stick a needle up here, it may have an effect down there.

BERG: For the first time in my life, I started going to an acupuncturist. If I went to a medical doctor he would do all the X-rays and blood tests, and blah, blah, blah, and then he will tell me the diagnosis of what my problem is. I was very dissatisfied with this acupuncturist; he sort of looked at me and he listened to my complaints, and he started to pull out his needles and he started sticking them into me. He never tells me what's wrong with me. He just sort of proceeded, "Oh, okay, seems like this could be useful for you." I'm lying there and I'm thinking with my Western mind, "Am I wasting my money? Am I throwing my money away?" But you know, that's how he proceeds. So I think that that's the kind of very different way.

HOYT: In doing therapy, do you think that carries over? With what the patient's brought in: "This is what it is."

BERG: This is what is.

HOYT: And I can kind of take it for what it is, rather than having to pull it apart and analyze it.

DE SHAZER: There's no "the way it's supposed to be."

HOYT: There's no way it's supposed to be; this is the way it is.

BERG: This is the way it is.

HOYT: You don't have to be judgmental, you have to be . . .

BERG: There's no right way to be. That's just the way it is.

DE SHAZER: Or back to the previous stuff about nonsense. All the nonsense is built upon "This is the way it's supposed to be."

HOYT: The medical model, that you should be 98.6°, you should be this shape, this way, there's a right way, and you're outside of that.[17]

DE SHAZER: It's just the way it is. Just the way it is. There's no "supposed to be" about it.

HOYT: I think when some people get nervous, they want to replace imagination with precision.

BERG: That's right. Or the illusion of precision.

HOYT: Control.

BERG: There's no precision in life, right?

HOYT: In a Greek model, we might say they're Apollonian rather than Dionysian. They want to fit everything into neat structured categories.

DE SHAZER: I had a client who said that impossibility coupled with certainty equals confirmed nonsense (*laughter*). It's a translation out of German, but nonetheless it's still the same thing.

HOYT: So the Eastern attitude is more of taking it for what it is. Some people call it being a Taoist.

BERG: That's how it's been given, and you work with it and do the best you can, and see what unfolds. Because I don't know what is going to unfold.

[17]See Hoyt (1979, 1985).

DE SHAZER: We know from lots of experimentation, we can't make those predictions, so we don't know what's going to unfold. We tried to predict but it didn't work.

BERG: Does that answer your question?

HOYT: Now I know what my question was. We don't know the answer to the question until we hear the answer. Now I know what I asked today.

REFERENCES

American Psychiatric Association. (1994). *Diagnostic and Statistical Manual of Mental Disorders* (4th ed.). Washington, DC: Author.

Aponte, H. J. (1992) Training the person of the therapist in structural family therapy. *Journal of Marital and Family Therapy, 18,* 269–281.

Appelbaum, S. A. (1975). Parkinson's law in psychotherapy. *International Journal of Psychoanalytic Psychotherapy, 4,* 426–436.

Bartley, W. W., III. (1985). *Wittgenstein.* Chicago: Open Court.

Berg, I. K. (1994). *Family Based Services: A Solution-Focused Approach.* New York: Norton.

Berg, I. K., & de Shazer, S. (1993). Making numbers talk: Language in therapy. In S. Friedman (Ed.), *The New Language of Change: Constructive Collaboration in Psychotherapy* (pp. 5–24). New York: Guilford Press.

Berg, I. K., & Miller, S. D. (1992). *Working with the Problem Drinker: A Solution-Focused Approach.* New York: Norton.

Boswell, J. (1980). *The Life of Samuel Johnson, LL.D.* (unabridged). Oxford: Oxford University Press/World's Classics. (Original work published 1791)

de Shazer, S. (1982). *Patterns of Brief Family Therapy.* New York: Guilford Press.

de Shazer, S. (1984). The death of resistance. *Family Process, 23,* 79–93.

de Shazer, S. (1985). *Keys to Solution in Brief Therapy.* New York: Norton.

de Shazer, S. (1988). *Clues: Investigating Solutions in Brief Therapy.* New York: Norton.

de Shazer, S. (1991). *Putting Difference to Work.* New York: Norton.

de Shazer, S. (1994). *Words Were Originally Magic.* New York: Norton.

de Shazer, S., & Berg, I. K. (1992). Doing therapy: A post-structural revision. *Journal of Marital and Family Therapy, 18,* 71–81.

de Shazer, S., & Nunnally, E. (1991). The mysterious affair of paradoxes and loops. In G. Weeks (Ed.), *Promoting Change through Paradoxical Techniques* (pp. 252–270). New York: Brunner/Mazel.

Dolan, Y. M. (1991). *Resolving Sexual Abuse.* New York: Norton.

Duffy, B. (1988). *World as I Found It.* New York: Ticknor & Fields.

Duncan, B. L. (1992). Strategic therapy, eclecticism, and the therapeutic relationship. *Journal of Marital and Family Therapy, 18,* 17–24.

Fingarette, H. (1988). *Heavy Drinking: The Myth of Alcoholism as a Disease.* Los Angeles: University of California Press.

Fisher, S. G. (1980). The use of time limits in brief psychotherapy: A comparison of six-session, twelve-session, and unlimited treatment with families. *Family Process, 19,* 377–392.

Fisher, S. G. (1984). Time-limited brief therapy with families: A one-year follow-up study. *Family Process, 23,* 101–106.

Held, B. S. (1992). The problem of strategy within the systemic therapies. *Journal of Marital and Family Therapy, 18,* 25–34.

Hoyt, M. F. (1979). "Patient" or "client": What's in a name? *Psychotherapy, 16,* 46–47. (Reprinted in M. F. Hoyt, *Brief Therapy and Managed Care: Readings for Contemporary Practice* [pp. 205–207]. San Francisco: Jossey-Bass, 1995.)

Hoyt, M. F. (1985). "Shrink" or "expander": An issue on forming a therapeutic alliance. *Psychotherapy, 22,* 813–814. (Reprinted in M.F. Hoyt, *Brief Therapy and Managed Care: Readings for Contemporary Practice* [pp. 209–211]. San Francisco: Jossey-Bass, 1995.)

Hoyt, M. F. (1990). On time in brief therapy. In R. A. Wells & V. J. Giannetti (Eds.), *Handbook of the Brief Psychotherapies* (pp. 115–143). New York: Plenum Press. (Reprinted in M.F. Hoyt, *Brief Therapy and Managed Care: Readings for Contemporary Practice* [pp. 69–104]. San Francisco: Jossey-Bass, 1995.)

Hoyt, M. F. (1994). On the importance of keeping it simple and taking the patient seriously: A conversation with Steve de Shazer and John Weakland. In M.F. Hoyt (Ed.), *Constructive Therapies* (pp. 11–40). New York: Guilford Press.

Janik, A., & Towlmin, S. (1974). *Wittgenstein's Vienna.* New York: Simon & Schuster.

Kean, M., & Chang, J. (1994). Outlook is everything: An interview with Insoo Kim Berg. *Journal of Collaborative Therapies, 2*(2), 1–6.

Kennett, J. (1972). *Selling Water by the River: A Manual of Zen Training.* New York: Pantheon.

Kiser, D. J., Piercy, F. P., & Lipchik, E. (1993). The integration of emotion in solution-focused therapy. *Journal of Marital and Family Therapy, 19,* 233–242.

Lipchik, E. (1994). The rush to be brief. *Family Therapy Networker, 18*(2), 34–39.

Miller, S. D., & Berg, I. K. (1995). *The "Miracle" Method: A Radically New Approach to Problem Drinking.* New York: Norton.

Minuchin, S. (1974). *Families and Family Therapy.* Cambridge, MA: Harvard University Press.

Monk, R. (1990). *Ludwig Wittgenstein: The Duty of Genius.* New York: Viking/Penguin.

Norris, C. (1992). *Uncritical Theory: Post-Modernism, Intellectuals, and the Gulf War.* Amherst: University of Massachusetts Press.

Nylund, D., & Corsiglia, V. (1994). Becoming solution-focused forced in brief therapy: Something important we already knew. *Journal of Systemic Therapies, 13,* 1–8.

Real, T. (1990). The therapeutic use of self in constructionist/systemic therapy. *Family Process, 23,* 255–272.

Selekman, M. D., & Todd, T. C. (1995). Co-creating a context for change in the supervisory system: The solution-focused supervision model. *Journal of Systemic Therapies, 14*(3), 21–33.

Sobell, L. C., Sobell, M. B., Toneatto, T., & Leo, G. I. (1993). What triggers the resolution of alcohol problems without treatment? *Alcoholism: Clinical and Experimental Research, 17*(2), 217–224.

Solovey, A. D., & Duncan, B. L. (1992). Ethics and strategic therapy: A proposed ethical direction. *Journal of Marital and Family Therapy, 18,* 53–61.

Walter, J. L., & Peller, J. E. (1992). *Becoming Solution-Focused in Brief Therapy.* New York: Norton.

Watzlawick, P., Beavin, J., & Jackson, D. D. (1967). *Pragmatics of Human Communication.* New York: Norton.

White, M., & Epston, D. (1990). *Narrative Means to Therapeutic Ends.* New York: Norton.

Wittgenstein, L. (1958). *The Blue and Brown Books.* New York: Harper.

Wittgenstein, L. (1968). *Philosophical Investigations* (3rd ed., G. E. M. Anscombe, Trans.). New York: Macmillan.

Wittgenstein, L. (1980). *Culture and Value* (P. Winch, Trans.). Chicago: University of Chicago Press.

CHAPTER 4

Welcome to PossibilityLand
A Conversation with Bill O'Hanlon

MICHAEL F. HOYT

Perhaps best known as the senior author of the classic *In Search of Solutions: A New Direction in Psychotherapy* (O'Hanlon & Weiner-Davis, 1989), Bill O'Hanlon is affiliated with Possibilities in Omaha, Nebraska. A peripatetic and much-acclaimed workshop presenter, O'Hanlon is also an accomplished songwriter and guitarist, avid computer techie, and Milton Erickson's former gardener. O'Hanlon's great energy, enthusiasm, and evolving therapeutic interest and expertise are reflected in the range of his many publications, including *Taproots: Underlying Principles of Milton Erickson's Therapy and Hypnosis* (O'Hanlon, 1987); *Shifting Contexts: The Generation of Effective Psychotherapy* (O'Hanlon & Wilk, 1987); *An Uncommon Casebook: The Complete Clinical Work of Milton H. Erickson, M.D.* (O'Hanlon & Hexum, 1990); *Rewriting Love Stories: Brief Marital Therapy* (Hudson & O'Hanlon, 1991); *Solution-Oriented Hypnosis: An Ericksonian Approach* (O'Hanlon & Martin, 1992); *Love Is a Verb* (O'Hanlon & Hudson, 1995); and *A Brief Guide to Brief Therapy* (Cade & O'Hanlon, 1993). He has also produced a computer program, *Brief Therapy Coach* (O'Hanlon & Schultheis, 1993) and a videotape, *Escape from DepressoLand: Brief Therapy of Depression* (O'Hanlon, 1993). His recent book, *A Field Guide to PossibilityLand: Possibility Therapy Methods* (O'Hanlon & Beadle, 1994), reports some of the latest refinements in his continuing search for what works.

The following conversation took place in Orlando, Florida, on February 26, 1994, where we were serving as faculty members at the New England Educational Institute Winter Symposium:

HOYT: What's the distinction between *brief therapy, solution-oriented therapy,* and *possibility therapy*?

O'HANLON: There's a whole bunch of types of brief therapy. *Brief therapy* is pretty clearly therapy that's focused, and the therapist helps provide the focus. It's usually focused on problem resolution, and it's goal-oriented. There are lots of theories—psychodynamic, solution-oriented, problem-focused, lots of family therapy approaches, systemic approaches, interactional approaches—that one can use to do brief therapy within that framework. That's what most of the brief therapies have in common. They are problem-driven; they are focused on resolving the presented problem that the person brought in; they are goal-oriented; and the therapist is responsible for creating and maintaining those focuses.

Solution-oriented therapy is more than a brand of brief therapy or just therapy that tends to be brief. It's different. Solution-oriented therapy has mainly a focus on the present towards the future, and not so much a focus on the past. It's focused on what people do well and their resources. It comes out of an Ericksonian bias that people have resources and competency, [and] that there are ways to deliberately focus them on those resources and access those resources and evoke them during treatment.[1] The therapist can actively do that, and the therapist again actively creates and maintains a focus on the present towards the future and on resources and solutions— both past solutions, present resources and solutions, and future possibilities for solutions.

Possibility therapy, for me, is where all this comes together with brief and solution-oriented therapy—what I now typically call "possibility therapy" in my approach with the aftereffects of sexual abuse. I think what bothered me a bit about the articulation of brief therapy and solution-oriented therapy is that brief therapies seem to give short shrift to feelings, to people's felt experience and sense of themselves, their own experience. What I think Carl Rogers [1951, 1961] and followers of Rogers did long ago was talk about and really articulate and emphasize how important it is for people to have a sense of being *heard*, *acknowledged*, and *validated*. I think that's done in brief therapy a lot—the kind of solution-focused, problem-oriented, problem-focused, interactional stuff that's the tradition I come from—but it's not articulated.

HOYT: Literally validated, the truth of their experience—that what's happened to them has happened to them?

O'HANLON: Oh, no, no. I'm talking about much more their felt sense of where they are now, their sense of who they are now and how

---

[1]Erickson's words: "Patients have problems because their conscious programming has too severely limited their capacities. The solution is to help them break through the limitation of their conscious attitudes to free their unconscious potential for problem solving" (Erickson, Rossi, & Rossi, 1976, p. 18).

they are now, and their ideas about the past. Being *acknowledged*, that's different from *validated*. I'm going to use the words a little differently, and we'll talk about the difference because that's part of the model or approach. But I would say that the possibility therapy approach that came clearer to me is making sure that you balance that acknowledgment and validation with the directiveness or non-directiveness that goes on with the opening of possibilities. So you're not moving on so quickly that the person gets a sense of "Wait a minute, don't you want to hear about what I feel or what I think or where I am now or where I've been?"—so that you don't minimize or invalidate that, or give the person short shrift in terms of that. You really give them a sense that they've been heard; that their experiences have been acknowledged; that who they are has been valued and validated. And then, as soon as you're clear that they've got that, then you invite them and you can do it sort of simultaneously, invite them into a future with possibilities.

HOYT: How does that juxtapose with the idea of brief therapy being quick or moving forward?

O'HANLON: I think you have to be better at acknowledging people in brief therapy, because if you don't you're going to get that bounce-back effect—where they respond, "Wait a minute, you didn't really hear me, and I'm not going to cooperate with you."[2] I think brief therapists have always had to be really good at quickly meeting people where they are and acknowledging and validating. They are much more active in doing that than most longer-term therapists, who have the sense that they have to develop the relationship over time. Brief therapy is much more like, as Nick Cummings [1990] wrote about the GP [general practice] model, that basically you're not going to go to your general physician or family practice physician and say, "Let's you and I sit down for six or seven sessions, develop a little relationship, and then we'll get on to what I'm here for." You

---

[2]This "rush to be brief," as Lipchik (1994) calls it, can be especially stimulated when an artificial, Procrustean limit is preimposed. O'Hanlon (1991, p. 108) has made his view clear in this regard: "Another thing that has become clear to me over the past ten years is that time-limited therapy is different from brief therapy . . . I am a brief therapy evangelist, to be sure, but above and beyond that, I am an advocate of respecting clients. Therefore, I stand opposed to time-limited therapy. I certainly influence my clients in the direction of completing therapy briefly, but I also attend to their responses and let those influence me. What some clients have taught me over the years is that they won't complete their therapy briefly. Not that they are resistant or dependent, but that therapy takes differing amounts and lengths of time for different people. Erickson used to see people for sessions lasting three or four hours or for 15 minutes. Modelling that, I have completed therapy with some in one session and I have completed therapy with others in 3 years of regular sessions. My experience is that the vast majority of people will complete their therapy in a relatively short time, 3 or 4 sessions, and a few, perhaps 5%, will take longer."

come in, you're hurting, and while you're working on what you're hurting about—either getting reassurance or getting some help to change it—the trust develops, the relationship develops. But if your physician doesn't hear you, then you're going to be frustrated. And that's part of the source of frustration with physicians sometimes. You have a sense they haven't really listened to you, they haven't heard you, they haven't taken you seriously. If that happens, you'll be less satisfied. But you don't spend a lot of time working on the relationship—you say, "Forget it. I'm going to go find somebody who will listen to me and who will acknowledge and validate me."

HOYT: That also gets at the concept of "resistance." The idea that "They are not seeing it the way we think they should; therefore, they are being resistant," as opposed to us recognizing the validity of their experience.

O'HANLON: This is a point that's been made by many therapists, I think, and especially more directive brief therapists. What we've called "resistance" has been a mix of a lot of things. Sometimes people bring certain issues that no matter how you approach them it's going to be difficult, you know, those so-called "borderline" or "characterological" issues, they are going to be challenging for people. There are ways to minimize that challenge. But I think some of the things that showed up as "resistance" were related to therapists' just not listening to people, not acknowledging them, not validating them, not taking them seriously.[3] And I think that people naturally respond to that with resistance. When therapists are trying to drive them in a direction they don't want to go, they show up as "resistant." When we think it really exists over there, it may be a function of the interaction.

HOYT: It's not really resistance, it's that they are being noncompliant: meaning they are not complying with our vision of their reality.

O'HANLON: That's right, or what we think they should do or feel. They are being pushed in a direction they don't want to go, so they push back. So I think that piece about making sure that you acknowledge and validate and value people that Rogers articulated influenced me a lot in the beginning of my career. Then I went into much more directive kinds of therapy. I learned family therapy, then I learned from Bandler and Grinder [1975, 1982], who later called their approach NLP [neurolinguistic programming], and then I learned Gestalt therapy along the way, then Ericksonian therapy, and brief, and solution-oriented therapies as the years went on. All of those

---

[3]The theme of taking the patient *seriously* was also a key in the de Shazer and Weakland interview (Hoyt, 1994a) reported in the first volume of *Constructive Therapies*.

really emphasize the directiveness of the therapists, and they didn't so much emphasize the nondirective aspects.

HOYT: They are all based on a foundation of careful listening.

O'HANLON: Careful listening, but they didn't articulate the *respectful* aspect so much. So I think, especially with the aftereffects of abuse, that you have to be very careful about that, because people can be very sensitive to being minimized or invalidated or not heard about that. We've certainly had a lot written and said about how society minimizes or denies or invalidates those kinds of experiences or people who have been abused, or blames some people who have been abused. So I think it's especially important for that to be articulated in the brief or solution-oriented therapy approaches. So I wanted to find some theory or some way of describing what I did that was more of a reflection of what I did. So possibility therapy is like the mutant child of Carl Rogers and Milton Erickson, in that it really places an emphasis on validating and valuing people and acknowledging their experience, the felt experience, and who they sense they are; *and* it also keeps the possibilities open for change.

HOYT: With sexual abuse survivors, beyond reflecting and clarifying, what are some of the things you do?

O'HANLON: I think if that's all one does, it's going to take a long, long time. It's going to be a pretty tortuous process, typically. So I think there are some things that one can bring from more directive and focused approaches and brief therapy approaches that can facilitate moving on and not being stuck.

HOYT: Such as?

O'HANLON: I think I need to just articulate a little bit of my understanding of the aftereffects of sexual abuse trauma especially, but trauma generally, and how it's similar to traditional models of PTSD [posttraumatic stress disorder] and sexual abuse treatment, and how it's different from those—very different. I went to graduate school in marriage and family therapy, and I got my degree in that, and I went into a child development and family studies department where I got my degree at Arizona State. They made me learn all this stuff about child development—Kohlberg and Piaget and Vygotsky and all these people—and I quickly forgot it as soon as I got out of graduate school, and it never helped me with raising my kids or anything. But I remembered a few things over the years, and one of the things that I remember is that Piaget showed through experiments that all kids are born Buddhists. What do I mean by that? All kids seem to be born with this sense of nondifferentiation with the world. They glom everything together: "I am the world; you are the world; we're all together; and I don't make a distinction between me and parents, generally, and the chair that you're sitting in." After a while, in this culture, we turn kids from Buddhists into personalities.[4] That is, we give them the sense that you sit over there in that chair, I sit over here in this chair, and we're both different from the chair.

So we start to distinguish the world, and so we develop a sense of boundaries. My boundaries end at my bag of bones typically, you end at your bag of bones, as Bateson [1972] said; that was one of his favorite phrases, "bag of bones." Some cultures give you the sense that you are the environment. Their boundaries are different. But in our culture, typically we have a sense that our boundaries end at our bodies and that's it—that I may have some connection with you, but basically you're separate from me. So, they have really good external boundaries. I have a sense that I end here and that you begin there. And I have maybe different parts of myself, but they are very diffuse internal boundaries. I have a shy part, but it's not really a personality, it's not really a separate part of me, it's just me—an expression of me that's a little different from my ham part that gets up on stage and teaches workshops. And I have a musical part and I have certain memories, but I have a sense those are *my* memories. What I think holds that inner stuff together and the boundary together is that we make a distinction between ourselves and the world, and we create a narrative: "Here's my story, here's me." And we do that when we go over the scrapbooks with our family members and they say, "That was you when you were four years old." I don't remember being there, but sure, okay, I'll accept that. We develop a sense of continuity of our lives and where we came from, what happened then, what happened then, what happened then, and how it led us to this. We develop a sort of coherent story with some noncoherent parts or parts that don't quite fit in, but a generally coherent story about ourselves, and a sense of where the story is going. So that's how this fits in with the narrative idea.

HOYT: And that's the sense of "self."

O'HANLON: That's right, a *narrative* sense of self, I think. We're going to talk about another sense of sense as well. That's the narrative self or personality identity that one constructs.

HOYT: Some parts may not fit in well, but there's a general sense of "This is Bill."

---

[4]Elsewhere in this volume, see especially Chapter 10 (Gilligan's model of the "relational self"), Chapter 11 (Rosenbaum and Dyckman's discussion of the "empty self" in psychotherapy) and Chapter 16 (Gergen's comments regarding narrative and the "postmodern self").

O'HANLON: Yes, this is me, and there are parts that I don't like too well, that don't fit in well, but generally they're me.

HOYT: Walt Whitman once said, "I am large, therefore, I have contradictions."[5]

O'HANLON: Yeah, and that will become very relevant to some of what I want to talk about next. So, when people are intruded upon physically or experientially earlier on, before they develop a coherent narrative of self— there is that "mystification" process that R. D. Laing [1967] talked about, where you tell the person what they are feeling or thinking; or "mind reading," as Virginia Satir [1967] called it.[6] I remember a story that I heard about Jay Haley—it may be apocryphal. One time he wanted to go out, and his wife wanted to have their 10- or 11-year-old daughter put on a sweater because she thought it was cold outside. The 10- or 11-year-old didn't want to put on the sweater. So mother and daughter were arguing. Haley leaned against the door jamb. He knew, "Don't triangulate." He knew enough not to get in between, and he let them argue it out. But finally he wanted to go, so he turned to the daughter and said, "Put on your sweater. Your mother's cold." So that's the opposite of that intrusion. He basically said, "Just do the behavior; you don't have to feel the feelings." Instead there are the parents who say to the kid who is kind of cranky, "Say, you know, you're really tired. You're so cranky, you're really tired." When it's time for the kids to go to bed in my house, I say, "You go to bed. *I'm* tired."

HOYT: He didn't violate her with the misattribution, "You are cold."

O'HANLON: Right, or tell the person, "You're sleepy, or you're upset or angry," or whatever. That kind of stuff. That kind of mystification or attribution of experience goes on a fair amount along with sexual abuse, I think, and physical abuse: "You really like this. This feels good," when the person is not liking it or doesn't feel good, most of the time. And so, when that physical intrusion or experiential intrusion happens early on, the person often doesn't develop a really good sense of identity, or some pieces get left out of the identity

---

[5]Whitman's actual words (from "Song of Myself" in *Leaves of Grass*, 1892/1993):

Do I contradict myself?
Very well then I contradict myself,
(I am large, I contain multitudes.)
    [Stanza 51]

In the same poem, he also says:

I am the poet of the Body and I am the poet of the Soul,
The pleasures of heaven are with me and the pains of hell are with me,
The first I graft and increase upon myself, the latter I translate into a new tongue.
    [Stanza 21]

[6]Or "mind fucking," as Perls (1969) was wont to say.

story that are actually in a person's experience. I'm going to talk about the *experiential self*, or as Rogers called it, the "organismic self," and also the *narrative self*, the identity self, the self-image, the self-identity, the one that one constructs "who I am." When one gets intruded upon early on, I think some parts get left out of that identity story; they are never included in the narrative for one reason or another. We dissociate—that's well established. We dissociate, but not only do we dissociate, we disown. We say, "It's not me." As Gestalt used to say, "Don't say *it*, say *I*." They were trying to get you to reown some things that you call the "it." Georg Groddeck [1923/1976] years ago wrote a book called *The Book of the It*, that was about the "it-ness" of some aspects of our experienced self. It was about other things, too, but I think the nice thing in that the *id* translates from German to English as the *it*. It really meant "the alien within," if you will. So, I think we develop that alien within our experience. So it's *dissociate*, *disown*, and—the third thing is critical—*devalue*. I don't experience it, I dissociate from it; and it's not me, I disown it; and it's bad, or I'm bad if I experience it.

HOYT: It reinforces the dissociation.

O'HANLON: So far, this is pretty much straightforward trauma theory. We dissociate, disown, but somehow devalue ourselves or the experience, and don't include it within the boundaries of our defined self or narrative self. We identify with certain aspects of our experience and disidentify with other aspects, and devalue those other aspects and dissociate those other aspects. When that happens, I think there are one or two aftereffects or sometimes both. One is that the symptoms that show up some time later are either *inhibited* kinds of symptoms or the opposite polarity, *intrusive* symptoms.[7] Inhibited symptoms are when you've got control of the rheostat and you turn it all the way down; the person is sexually numb, doesn't have any memories. It's like the "negative symptoms" of schizophrenia, as they are sometimes called, when there's lack of affect. Something's missing from the person's experience; it just goes missing altogether—when they would have thought they would have responded sexually or emotionally, they are just flat; they don't feel anything, sense anything; they don't remember anything, there are gaps in their memories. That's an inhibited kind of symptom. Or it's intrusive—flashbacks, not inhibited memory

---

[7]Horowitz (1986) has characterized "stress response syndromes" as alternations between phases of "denial" and "intrusion." For a comprehensive review of the PTSD literature, see Meichenbaum (1994; see also Chapter 5, this volume).

at all, intrusive memories, or compulsive behavior. Compulsive masturbation, or what Patrick Carnes [1983, 1989] calls "sexual addiction." It becomes a compulsive sexuality instead of non-sexuality or no sexual feelings.

HOYT: Why would someone become compulsive if it's devalued, disowned, put away?

O'HANLON: Precisely because it's devalued, disowned, put away. "It" goes out of relationship with your self, with your experiential self. Rogers actually had a theory that relates to this. He used to draw these two circles (or at least the way I was taught, there would be two circles). One would be the self-image, and one would be the organismic self, the experiential self, the one that actually has physiological sensory experience. And he thought that when they are far apart, the person is incongruent, and it results in neurotic behavior—for example, the guy who comes into your office and pounds on your desk, yelling, "I'm not angry." Instead of valuing one or another, Rogers would say, "I hear you saying you're not angry, and I see you pounding on the desk, and I hear you raising your voice." Not judging or valuing, but just validating both parts. Not saying one is right or one is wrong, like "You're really angry," or "Okay, your guy doesn't get angry." He wouldn't take either of those sides. He'd validate both sides, and he felt that under the warmth of that acknowledgment, the two sides, the two circles move more together and are able to merge. The closer they're together, the more congruent the person is. He had the idea that they are never going to be totally together, totally congruent, but you can get them closer together and, therefore, symptomatic experience and behavior diminishes.

It's as if the person is living in a house with a bunch of other people, and they decide there's a roommate there that they don't get along with. "Let's get rid of the bad roommate." So they throw the roommate out, change the locks. The roommate comes and pounds on the door for a while, and they say, "Don't let him in, just ignore him, he'll go away." After a while, it seems like he's gone away, because he stops pounding on the door. He slumps against the door and is tired; he can't keep it up any more; and the roommates figure, "Good, we've gotten rid of him." So he seems to go away until a day later, a year later, 5 years later, 20 years later, all of a sudden he decides, "I live there, my stuff's in there, I'm getting back in," and he crashes through the front window. That's flashbacks, or that's sexual compulsiveness. Something cues off that wakes the sleeping roommate outside the door and says, "I'm getting back in there, I belong there. I'm in your experiential life and, damn it, you're going to deal with me." So, something, you may be reading something that reminds you of the sexual abuse that you've had, or you may have been watching something on television. You go into therapy; a therapist may say, "Do you think you were abused, given your symptoms?" or whatever. And, boom, this flood of memories come back. Who knows? Something cues it off. Or, it's been happening for years, and the missing roommate has been crashing in through the window or has just gone missing for a while.

HOYT: Or there may be some innate drive to integrate, to make whole.

O'HANLON: It could be that finally when you get to a good enough place and you're ready to deal with it, who knows? I'm not precisely sure why, but that's typically the point that people come to see us—when they are being bothered by something. Either something's missing, inhibited, or something's intruding or making them feel compulsions. The idea is that it's out of relationship with your experiential organismic itself. And because it's out of relationship, it's like that movie *Dr. Strangelove*.

HOYT: With the hand that keeps coming up?

O'HANLON: Yeah. It's the hand, I think, that's clearly dissociated, devalued, and disowned, because it's a gloved, metallic kind of hand. And it's the hand, I think, that can push the button to start a nuclear war. This brilliant Cold War scientist, who is supposed to be modeled on Herman Kahn, is giving these lectures about how we can win a nuclear war, and all the time the hand is creeping up trying to choke the character (played by Peter Sellers), and the character is always pulling the hand back down. There's that sense that that hand is out of relationship with the rest of him, who is this cold intellectual. But that hand is like the disowned, devalued, dissociated part of people. Typically I find it's either sexual sensations or experience, sexual excitement, memories, anger, sadness—body feelings all together or some part of the body. Those are the typical things that I find that people have dissociated and disowned and devalued in the aftereffects of abuse. So one of those things or several of them have gone out of relationship with the person. So if it's part of your body, or your body, maybe you'll start slicing yourself up with a razor. That's how it shows up in a compulsive, intrusive way. Or you don't feel your body at all. No body. You keep running into things because you don't know where your body is, that kind of thing. So far this description sounds like fairly standard posttraumatic stress theory, especially post-sexual-abuse kind of stuff. The difference is in how do I think it can be treated? The standard idea is "You never really experienced it in the past because you dissociated from it. So in order to really heal from it, you have to go back and reexperience what you really didn't experience the first time. So you have to relive and remember the trauma." This is an "unexperienced experience" model. Typically age regression is used, with the therapist's encouragement to really reclaim and integrate those aspects of yourself that you dissociated, devalued, and disowned.

HOYT: In a way, this is Freud's [1914/1958] idea of "remembering, repeating, and working through"—that what we don't experientially complete will continue to press, that the Gestalt will be there until it's completed. What we resist persists.

O'HANLON: Right. That's the idea of the traditional treatment. What I'm suggesting is that there is an alternative, and actually the way that this occurred to me is that I've worked on this solution-oriented/brief therapy/possibility therapy wave for years. I've been hearing clients talk about sexual abuse since the mid-'70s, maybe 1974, when I started doing therapy. Also, I was sexually abused when I was younger. More recently, people have been bringing sexual abuse issues as the primary presenting problem. Before I knew much about what sexual abuse treatment experts were doing, I dealt with it in the ways that I typically did therapy, and then after about five years I got to thinking, "You know, I ought to go and find out what other people are doing, read a little more stuff." Most of it what I read was very psychodynamic and not to my liking, and I started going to more workshops and I thought, "You know, I am not doing this right. My clients seem to be getting better, and I'm not having them age-regress and I'm not having them relive the experiences, but they seem to be doing fine and they tell me it's helpful in resolving their problems." I started to be bothered that there seemed to be a monolithic approach out there, like there is typically to drug and alcohol problems: it's the Twelve-Step model or nothing else. I started to think, "Wait a minute. There's an alternative here that should be spoken about." Not everybody has to age-regress. Some of my clients do, but it's the minority of my clients that age-regress and relive it with my support and help, and that takes a long time. It's a tortuous process. Usually people decompensate and get a lot worse during that process; often they get more suicidal, more self-injurious, feel worse about themselves. If they are in relationships, their relationships are strained by either lack of sexual contact, because at that point they are so into the memories that it's very hard for them to have a sexual experience that's present; they flashback too much, so the partners are upset. Or, they are just acting out a lot more or are a lot more disturbed, so it takes a special partner to really support them through that process.

HOYT: What distinguishes the people who needed to age-regress and reexperience it fully from those people who were able to get well without it?

O'HANLON: I have no clue—that's the first answer. I say that the therapy that I do is sort of like the sport of curling. I'm sweeping in front of people, opening possibilities, while I'm acknowledging and validating them, and I'm inviting them from the present into the future. Sometimes as I do that, they zip back to the past and start to relive and reexperience their abuse or remember it in very vivid ways. If that's what they do, I better go back there and sweep in front of them and support them in doing that. So, I would say my pragmatic answer is the people that do that seem to need to do that, and most people don't, and the people that don't, don't.

HOYT: The people who don't, have you seen some long-term follow-up?

O'HANLON: Yes.

HOYT: That's convinced you that they don't really need to?

O'HANLON: That's right. That it isn't just a "Band-Aid," as people sometimes say about brief therapy—that it really doesn't last. I've been able to do that with enough people so I'm convinced.

HOYT: Some therapists hold the view that people need to fully reexperience and abreact; otherwise, they will be sealing over and be very likely to relapse, and these will be the people who later will be back, not having really resolved the problem. Yet many people report the other experience: that they are able to do the work, finish, and don't seem to have a relapse.

O'HANLON: Sure, and I'm sure that it's possible that some people do the work and then it gets undone or whatever; it's not finished, or it shows up again because it wasn't done; or the piece that they did was done and they come back for something else. I'm sure on the other side one can say that with some of those longer-term abreactive approaches, we can see some of them in which the people don't survive or they don't get better; they just keep reliving it and seem to be stuck in the experience. So I think you've got to balance that. I would be wary of anybody who said everybody has to do it without age-regressing or catharting, because that seems to me much more a function of the therapist's beliefs than the client's needs.

HOYT: Even if they don't age-regress or cathart, I think there is still a place for emotion and affect as part of the validation. If we slide past that without letting the person express their pain and validate it, it may not be the age regression that is missed, but that they haven't been heard.

O'HANLON: Yeah, I think that's an important point. And the other thing is, sometimes acknowledging the details of the abuse without having to go back and live it and reexperience it emotionally, I think is another issue. Sometimes it is very important for people to speak about their abuse to another person or write about it or speak publicly about it. That seems to be an important part for some of my clients of what they do to come to terms with it—and we'll get back into this—and bring it into their sense of identity, their narrative about themselves. That seems to be part of that renarration process. That's different from reliving it or catharting. And I think you made a good distinction there. When they express emotion, it would be disrespectful to say, "I don't do emotions. I'm a brief therapist." Really validate them as people and value them as people and make room for those emotions. But don't say, "Oh, good, now we're getting someplace. Go with it and get back into it."

HOYT: As though the emotions are the goal more than anything else.

O'HANLON: That's right. The idea that the expression of emotion is automatically curative is a dubious proposition. Anybody who has done a lot of marital therapy knows you can hear a lot of expressions of emotions and it's not necessarily curative.[8]

HOYT: You mentioned that it may be the need of the therapist or the therapist's countertransference, their theory belief. You also mentioned in passing that you had had a sexual abuse experience in your own personal life. I don't want to probe into that more personally than you want, but what I want to raise is a point about what some people call "countertransference"—that therapists working with abuse victims have to be open to the experiences that are going to be stirred in themselves. Otherwise, we oftentimes have trouble validating people's experience because we're busy invalidating our own experience.

O'HANLON: Guarding against our experiences.

HOYT: So, in a way, one has to have done the work with oneself to be clear enough to hear so that we can let the other person be who they are; otherwise, we're going to restimulate our stuff in a way we don't want.

O'HANLON: Sure, or in the other way—if we've actually come to terms and resolved it in some particular way, assuming that our clients are going to do it in the same way. It's like the AA [Alcoholics Anony-

---

[8]For more discussion of O'Hanlon's views regarding marital therapy issues, see Gale and Newfield (1992), Hudson and O'Hanlon (1991), and O'Hanlon and Hudson (1994, 1995).

mous] model saying, "I went through AA, so you're going through AA because that's the way that worked for me." Maybe there are other ways that people can stop drinking. It's important to be able to provide those alternatives, rather than saying this is the only way to do it. If I went through a regressive cathartic therapy and it was greatly helpful for me, or long-term therapy was and I loved it and thought it was great, it may not be that that's what my clients need. And it doesn't have to invalidate that long-term, wonderful therapy you went through. That's the caution of what I've called "theory countertransference."[9]

HOYT: Because if you're talking about the idea of a narrative theory of repression, then there's also the possibility of countertransference repression—that I'm going to collude with you to keep this from your story because it's too close to my story, or will interfere with me believing in my story.

O'HANLON: I think we're talking about two different ideas. One is sort of unfinished stuff of the therapist that might get in the way. The other one is an attachment to a theory or a method that might get in the way.

HOYT: One is much more a personal problem, and the other is more theoretical.

O'HANLON: That's right—getting attached to a certain theory. Or, "I learned it in graduate school or this was helpful for me personally," so it's a little more of a personal issue there. But I think those are two different concerns and possible traps that I'm trying to warn against. What I'd like to say is one of the bottom lines, one of the basic ideas that I want to get across here is *variability*. In agriculture, they have this idea that if you only have one strain of a crop, like the Irish potato or whatever, there's a potential for agricultural disaster because you don't have enough biodiversity. I think in therapy methods it's the same way: If there's not enough diversity in therapy approaches available, you're going to be invalidating and minimizing some people. When all the therapy theories were written by straight heterosexual white middle-class or upper-class men, it didn't bode well for other experiences being validated. I think the same thing about the sexual abuse aftereffects. Where there's only one way to do it—the unexperienced experience model, age regression, cathar-sis, working through—then it's going to work wonderfully for the people for whom that really fits, and it's not going to have room for the other people; so I want to speak for an alternative that's worked

[9]Advocating openness to various possibilities, O'Hanlon (1991; Hubble & O'Hanlon, 1992) has warned against "theoretical countertransference" and "delusions of certainty."

for me and my clients. The alternative is valuing, going like brief therapy does for change through the door of the present problem or complaint. That is, instead of going globally after it, by "working through" the aftereffects of sexual abuse or going after the memories, get specific.

Because I do hypnosis, sometimes people come to me: "Can you hypnotize and help me remember?" No. Number one, I'm not a good directive hypnotist. I'm more of a permissive hypnotist, so I don't say, "Go back through the pages of time—you're five years old now and you will remember." It gives me the creeps, that stuff, anyway. It's too intrusive and too directive for my tastes. And the other thing is that I don't think typically it's helpful to remember that way. Some people do and some people will remember through hypnosis, and that's fine. But typically in both situations, whether they come for hypnosis or whether they don't, go through the door of the presenting complaint. I focus on the question: what are they complaining about? That is, when someone comes in and says, "I think I was sexually abused," or "I know I was sexually abused," or "I was sexually abused and I want to work on this," I say, "Okay, what's bothering you now? That is, what's your concern? What's your complaint? What do you want to resolve?" That makes it more brief, more focused, and you have some sense of when you get there. So typically they're going to complain about one thing or another. They are going to say, "Well, it bothers me because when I start to have sex with my partner, I go numb. I get scared right before I have sex, and I can push myself through that, but then I get numb."

HOYT: So, "What are the particular impairments or residuals?"

O'HANLON: "What's bothering you now? And how will you know when that's resolved?" That's the goal-oriented part: "How will you know when we've actually resolved it?" "Well, when I have sex with my partner and I'm there during the experience and I actually experience sexual sensations, and I don't go away any more, I don't get numb, I don't age-regress and feel like a little kid being raped." Okay, that's a pretty good hint. We are starting to clarify what the goal is and how you'll know when you're done. Again, it's going back to that GP-model physician. You come in with a concern, and either you want reassurance that you don't have a brain tumor or cancer or something, and sometimes we can give reassurance: "Yes, a lot of people have been sexually abused, you're not strange, you're not out of the ordinary." And many people have these kinds of worries about themselves or experiences with themselves. Sometimes they think they were to blame; sometimes they think they should have been able to stop it even though they were a child; sometimes they had sexual sensations during the abuse, and then they feel guilty because they think they enjoyed it. We can normalize a lot of that stuff, like the book *The Courage to Heal* [Bass & Davis, 1994] can. You read that and you think, "I'm not so weird; other people experience this, too," so sometimes that's our function, to normalize and reassure. Like your physician would say, "It's going to pass in a couple of days; it's just a simple flu. It doesn't mean you have meningitis. I've checked for the warning signs and you probably don't have it. But if it persists, call me back." Sometimes we go for reassurance and sometimes we go for change. What are people complaining about and what do they want? Those are the things that typically drive brief therapy and goal-focused therapy. So that's the door in, because I find that when you go in through that door, that's where the dissociative, devalued, disowned parts are. How do I work in a present to future-oriented way rather than a past way? By valuing the person and valuing the part. So the part comes back into the person's experience by helping them acknowledge it and by me acknowledging it.

HOYT: Can you give a brief example of valuing the person and the part?

O'HANLON: Yeah. I had a person who came to see me who was dissociated to the point of multiplicity, multiple personality. During one of the conversations that we had in therapy, a part showed up, a personality that had never showed up—before. It was very hostile; as is often the case in multiple personality, there's a hostile, angry part. And that part was "Astoroth," the devil. Astoroth, when Astoroth emerged, basically started growling and threatening me and her, threatened to do terrible things to my genitals (I won't detail it here), and threatened to do terrible things to her, and threatened that therapy will get nowhere: "I will do everything I can to stop it. I'm going to defeat you. I'm more powerful than you. I'm more powerful than her." I said, "Okay, thank you for sharing." I was a little surprised because he emerged very quickly and he was gone as quickly as he came, and she was back, and she was disturbed by this—she was "Wow, what happened?" She said, "I think that that's the part that the people who tortured me put in me, the devil. So do you think you could do an exorcism?" Just for a second, I was thinking, "You know, I've never done an exorcism, and I have a priest friend who would probably do this; that would be kind of neat." Just for a second I thought that. Then I thought, "No, wait a minute. I think Astoroth *is* her. I don't want to get rid of Astoroth—that's her." My idea is that it is part of her experience, and I don't want to devalue or throw it out; it's the missing roommate thing. So I talked to her a little bit about it. I said, "Let's go a little farther. I think that's you." She said to me, "Me? No, thanks."

So over the next couple of sessions, Astoroth came out and visited with me—at first threatening me, and then I would say, "Well, what's going on? Why do you want to do this?" And I would talk to Astoroth like I would if a client came in and said, "I want to go out and kill everybody." Basically, Astoroth became my client, if you will. As Astoroth and I started talking—I'm kind of lively in therapy and can be humorous—and Astoroth, despite his hostility, liked my jokes, he would find himself laughing despite himself. So I'd say, "I got you, didn't I? You laughed at that one." He and I would start to joke together. For a devil, he had a pretty good sense of humor! (*Laughter*) So we started to become friendly, and he started telling me, "I have to kill her to protect her." I said, "Okay, we have to protect her, but if you kill her you'll die too, and that seems kind of weird," and we talked about all that, and the strange logic of that. And then we found that that was some decision he'd made or she'd made a long time ago, and that we could retalk about that decision in light of current reality, and he got a lot more cooperative. He thought I was his ally after a while, not his enemy, so we started working together. She still didn't want have anything to do with him; she didn't want to touch him with a 10-foot pole. But he became less threatening to her, and after a while she was willing to approach him, and they started to develop a conversation—an internal and external dialogue—and they started to get along a little better. He became her real protector inside instead of torturer and threatener, and then he turned into a scared little girl which she protected, and then the scared little girl turned into her over time. So under the conversation in which Astoroth isn't blamed, isn't devalued, and isn't kicked out, if you will, *that* Astoroth starts to become part of her ongoing narrative of who she is and turned into her. So that's a sense of it. She didn't regress to do that.

HOYT: You provided enough of a container and made friends with parts of herself so she could, one might say, "metabolize."

O'HANLON: That's a nice analogy. And I guess the difference between the traditional model is—the way to metabolize in the traditional model is you have to go back. In possibility therapy, you value the aspect, like anger was valued. You do not value some expressions of anger. You do value some expressions of anger, that's different. You know, she wanted to hurt me; that wasn't any good, I didn't want that. The containment, as you say, is the behavioral containment, saying, "It's not okay to hurt yourself, it's not okay to hurt me; it's not okay to hurt the body; it's not okay to hurt other people; *and* you can feel like hurting other people." But an active encouragement of that in saying, "That's okay, it's fine"—permission and validation for the experience, not the action. Under that valuing in the present, details about the abuse did emerge. Astoroth told me some things that had been done to him—and, of course, to her—and that acknowledgment was part of that validation. Acknowledgment about what happened, and acknowledgment of his or her feelings and rage; anger gone out of relationship with self turned up as rage.

So if you have no room for anger—anger is devalued, invalidated, dissociated, disowned—it shows up every once in a while as rage in what is most of the time the sweetest, nicest person. I had a client who was nicknamed Sunshine when she was growing up. She was being massively abused, but she was always nicknamed Sunshine and she smiled. And even as an adult when she got mad at someone, she was one of those people who would smile at you while she was mad, so you didn't really get the full impact of her anger. She would tell you that she was angry, but you didn't really get a sense of it. It would even be hard for her to tell you that she was angry. And then every once in a while, she would be in a rage with her kids or her husband over a seemingly little thing. So when something goes out of your narrative or out of relationship with your experiential self, and you don't include it in your self-identity, then I think that it starts to develop a life of its own.

HOYT: What we might call "in the shadow."

O'HANLON: And it's not only shadow stuff, too, because sometimes you get people who do multiple personality that have wonderful musical abilities or artistic abilities. They are not just shadow stuff.

HOYT: Not all evil or bad.

O'HANLON: That's right. It's all out of relationship with self because it seems to have a mind of its own. Artists often have that experience. That brings up the question of how do you explain repression or forgotten memories in this narrative model? I think that there is a hint of this in Judith Herman's [1992] really nice book, *Trauma and Recovery*, that people have this whole narrative of who they are and where their life has been and where they are going; and that there are these pieces that are "unmetabolized," if you will, that aren't included in the narrative; and so if they never get in the narrative, they're not remembered very well. Why are more and more people experiencing and remembering sexual abuse and coming to terms with it more recently? Because our narratives aren't only individual narratives; they're influenced by cultural and social narratives. Many feminists and many theorists of trauma have pried open a space and said, "Oh, let's include in her story posttraumatic stuff, rape, and domestic violence, violence against women, sexual abuse against children," and that's become a lot more accepted and acknowledged. So we have the movie stars that come out and say they were sexually abused, they talk about it a lot more; the movie-of-the-week has a lot more of this stuff. There's many more books about it, a lot of books about multiple personalities. So we're going to see a lot more multiple personalities in the next 20 years, because the kind of problems that we see in therapy do not occur in isolation; they occur in cultural context as well. And when there's no room for a multiple personality in the cultural narrative, it shows up never or very rarely, as it has from the 1800s to the 1960s. It showed up so rarely it was not in the general therapeutic narrative.

HOYT: What's the cultural milieu that's allowing us to recognize "multiple personalities" and allowing them to "come out," so to speak?

O'HANLON: Or be *constructed* much more. As I said at the very beginning—and I want to emphasize this—I think personality is constructed, and I think multiple personalities are constructed, so they are the same degree of "real" as far as I'm concerned. I experience myself as a personality, even though I think that's clearly a construct, and I think most people would agree that it's a theoretical construct; they can't do an autopsy and find a personality inside me. I think it's really a function of some people being very persuasive at selling the narrative called "multiple personality." As more and more people get convinced of it, they become teachers and writers, and they convince other people, and that's how diagnoses get popular. I think that "borderline personality" having the stock that it does, being so popular, is a lot a function of some very articulate theorists. Kernberg [e.g., 1975] and Masterson [e.g., 1976] and other people who have done a lot of work became fascinated with them, became convinced that this was true—not that it was a good idea, but that it was true. It may or may not be a good idea, but very few other theorists have this idea that it is constructed; they think they discovered a new truth, and then they put it out there, and they become so persuasive and have conferences on it, and then they convince other people and it becomes "true" in our culture. Where were all the "codependents" 25 years ago? We didn't have them. It doesn't mean that that doesn't really explain a lot; it does explain a lot, and it's helped a lot of people. Is it "true"? Who knows? All we can say is we can't get rid of it now.

HOYT: Do you think there's an external reality? I know that sounds like back in college, Descartes and Locke and Hume, or maybe Carlos Castaneda [1968] saying, "But, Don Juan, did I *really* fly?"

O'HANLON: I know what you're talking about. Yes, I think there's a sensory-based reality. It's the interpretation of that reality that is variable. And, also, I don't think we can just make any construction.

You can't just make any construction and sell it, because there are two constraints on it. One is that physical reality, sensory-based reality.

HOYT: Gravity and the sharp edges will keep you honest.

O'HANLON: Right. You'll knock into them no matter how you make up reality. If you're on LSD and you don't see them, you'll still get knocked over and you'll cut your leg, although you may not be aware of it. If you walk out into the middle of the freeway and the cars are going fast, no matter what your state of subjective reality, physical reality will run you over. That kind of physical reality is one of the constraints to what kind of narratives can be made up.

HOYT: "My karma just ran over your dogma!"

O'HANLON: (*Laughter*) That's right. So the second constraint is, I think, there are cultural traditions and explanations—what Heidegger [1962] calls the "throwness." You're not born as a blank slate. You're born into a culture that already shapes you by language and by practice, by interactions. So I don't know how Heidegger meant it, but I think of "throwness" like the clay being thrown on the wheel, the potter's wheel. And it's already shaped; there's a certain throwness to it. You're thrown in the middle of it, and you're not just bringing any possibility to it; the pot already has a shape before you get there. So there's only such much leeway there, because of the physical reality and because of the cultural social practices and traditions.

HOYT: Not *tabula rasa*.

O'HANLON: No, not that kind of radical constructionism. Because if that were the case, I'm really good at creating therapeutic realities, and all my clients would be cured in one session. They're not. They bring their own traditions and their own narratives, and then we have to be co-narrative.

HOYT: That really speaks to the question of why can't people just change their mind or look at it differently or reframe it or say, "Oh, that was me then but this is me now"? Why do we sometimes get stuck in a persistent negative narrative?

O'HANLON: I have no idea, and I'm not very interested in that question. I think that's a psychologist's question, to tell you the truth. I think that a therapist's question is "How do we change that?"

HOYT: I agree. Why build between us a narrative that will not get us to a better answer?

O'HANLON: Right. Asking change-oriented questions is much more interesting to me than asking explanation-oriented questions—although some explanation-oriented questions get you to change.

HOYT: How do people free themselves when they've been stuck? How does it happen that they get unstuck? By owning the parts that have been devalued, disowned, and . . .

O'HANLON: . . . Valuing it, owning, associating to and taking actions to change the current situation to their goal. The other thing is changing their stories or their narrative so that there's possibilities for actions and possibility for a future that will be more of what they want. So changing the doing and changing the viewing. And the prerequisite for that is, I think, valuing and validating experience before that, or along with that.

HOYT: What else?

O'HANLON: I think one more element. I say this is a present and future-oriented approach; how is it future-oriented? There are exceptional survivors—people that seem to belie the rule that this stuff messes you up for life and holds you back and keeps you stuck. There are some people who clearly have been massively abused or devalued, and that somehow do pretty well in the present and the future. How come that is? Some become presidents of the United States, and some really deteriorate and go into the psych hospital. What's the difference? Why, given similar kinds of backgrounds, and how do we encourage more people to live those better futures?

I think one of the places I learned that was from Viktor Frankl at the second Evolution of Psychotherapy Conference [Zeig, 1992]. He came and gave a keynote address and told the story about how he was in the Nazi death camp, several Nazi death camps, being marched through the field in the middle of Poland; and he fell down in a fit of coughing and couldn't get up. He's being beaten by a guard who said, "Get up and keep marching to this work detail or you're going to die." He just thinks, "Okay, that's it. I thought I was going to survive, but I'm not going to. I just don't have the physical wherewithal to get up and keep moving." All of a sudden, he's no longer in a field in Poland, he's standing at a lectern in postwar Vienna, giving a lecture which he had been working on all the time he'd been in the death camp, on the psychology of death camps [see Frankl, 1963]. He's giving this brilliant lecture to this imagined audience of about 200 people who are listening in rapt attention as he explains how people can dehumanize people so much to put them in death camps and treat them so terribly, and also how some people psychologically and spiritually and emotionally survive. He came up with the "will to meaning," and having found some purpose and meaning, those people seem to survive better than those people who didn't have any purpose and meaning and gave up hope. So he's talking in his imagined lecture about the day he almost died in the death camp, outside the death camp in Poland. The day he was walking through the snowy field with not enough clothes on, and he was ill in the middle of winter in Poland, and he said, "And I thought I was going to die there, and then I found myself getting up surprisingly and walking; I don't know how I did it, but I did it." Meanwhile, his body is still in Poland and it stands up, and he walks to the work detail, does the work, and comes home. All the time, he's just doing the work automatically by his body, not really experientially there any more, still giving his lecture when he gets back to the death camp; he collapses in the bed, and he survives another day. At the end of his imagined lecture in postwar Vienna, he got a standing ovation. In 1990, many, many years later in Anaheim, California, he got a standing ovation from 7,000 people.

HOYT: I was in that audience.

O'HANLON: Frankl did something different from what most of us do who are traumatized. He didn't stay stuck in the past and keep repeating it again and again in flashbacks, with the disowned and dissociated and devalued parts kind of coming and haunting him. He projected into a future where things worked out; it had meaning and had purpose. A future in which this terrible experience had contributed to him getting to that future, and he imagined back from the future to the present; he oriented himself to a future with possibilities, and let that future pull him out of the terrible present. Many sexual abuse survivors, victims, come in saying "Nothing is right. I'm terrible. I'll never survive this. There's no reason to be alive." And I always think and somehow ask, "What are you doing in my office? Some part of you, some aspect of you, has a vision of a future where things work out, or you wouldn't be here. Why would you bother getting out of bed?"

HOYT: They were hanging on until the time when it would pass and they would be survivors.

O'HANLON: And they sometimes have, if you can help them articulate it, a very clear Viktor Frankl-like vision of a future where things work out.

HOYT: In a way, a crystal-ball-type thing [Erickson, 1954].

O'HANLON: Yes, very much like the crystal ball.

HOYT: Looking to a time when the problem is no longer a problem.

O'HANLON: Erickson would have people project into a future and tell him how they worked out the problem, and then he would bring them out of a trance with amnesia for that fantasized future, and then he would often tell them to do the things that they told him that they would do in that imagined future. Most of us have the notion that the present determines the present and the future, but what if the future determined the present? Think about it, if you knew you would win the Lotto tonight, would you be here interviewing me? Perhaps, but maybe not.

HOYT: So if you have a different image of your future, you will conduct your life differently in the present.

O'HANLON: That's right. It becomes a self-fulfilling prophecy sometimes. It definitely becomes presently oriented.

HOYT: So it's not really the future; it's our image. There's only the present, but when we think of the future, that's expectation, and our expectation will lead us to do certain things.[10]

O'HANLON: Right. So what I want to do as a therapist is open up a future with possibilities, instead of having the future be a repeat of the past. I think people come in "frozen in time." That is, they froze their sense of themselves or some aspect of themselves at that moment in time when they were abused. They froze and they keep doing the same experience over and over again through flashbacks, muscle behavior, interactions. They keep doing the same damn thing over and over again, as John Weakland calls it, instead of one damn thing after another, which is what life usually is. It's not a flow, it's a repetition. It's frozen in time. Under the thawing of the therapist valuing and going through the door of the presenting complaint and focusing on a future with possibilities, it becomes less frozen in time and thaws out and starts to flow.

HOYT: So it's the warmth of validation, and then they can begin to see a future and move into it.

O'HANLON: Right. I think they already have a sense of that future, and under the warmth of the validation of their experience of who they are, of the disowned and devalued and dissociated parts, and under the questioning of the therapist and the focus of the therapist on that future, they become a lot more articulate about that future. And it becomes more available to them, and they become a lot more committed to it.

---

[10]St. Augustine observed in his *Confessions*: "What is by now evident and clear is that neither future nor past exists, and it is inexact language to speak of three times—past, present, and future. Perhaps it would be exact to say: there are three times, a present of things past, a present of things present, a present of things to come. In the soul there are these three aspects of time, and I do not see them anywhere else. The present considering the past is the memory, the present considering the future is expectation" (quoted in Boscolo & Bertrando, 1993, p. 34).

HOYT: Some therapy theories have the idea that people have a script or an unconscious plan, a vision of the future, and a drive toward health or wholeness, but something can block it. Fear of pain, something I can't experience, so I can't get to the future because it's too painful to walk across what I have to go through first. But if I can have the promise of getting there, I'll do almost anything to get there. But I don't want to just take the pain to be in pain; I'd rather be numb.

O'HANLON: Right. It's like having some pain in labor that you know is going to produce a child is much different from just having abdominal pain that's extreme and thinking, "What's happening here? It's terrible. Am I going to die?" or whatever. It's a different sense and it's still the same kind of sensations, but a different sense of anticipation.

HOYT: As a general idea, people when they are depressed foreshorten the future; they don't have a future. They don't see it.[11]

O'HANLON: I think many people who come into therapy with the aftereffects of abuse are depressed.

HOYT: In Zen they say, "Burn clean and leave no ashes." Metabolize the experience completely, like the saying, "Time flies when you're having fun"—living in the now, the endless now.

O'HANLON: That's nice. And I think for people who are stuck with the aftereffects of abuse, it's the endless repetition of the past. It's showing up in the present and a foreshortened sense of the future.

HOYT: It's not "burning clean," it's "frozen in time."

O'HANLON: It's frozen in time. That's right.

HOYT: What do we learn from people who are not permanently victimized by sexual abuse?

O'HANLON: I think this whole vocabulary of "victim" and "survivor" and all that stuff is difficult. Some people say they should acknowledge the pain and the victimization of it, make sure the people who were abused don't get blamed. Some people call them "survivors," to emphasize the fact that they survived. I would say let people call themselves what they will and give them the options and possibilities. I would rather call them "people who have been sexually abused," rather than "survivors" or "victims," because I think you're right: Some people come out of it not seeming to be in that victim stance or victim experience. So I think what I learned from some of the people that have survived it a little better or thrived, even though

---

[11]For discussions of therapy and the temporal structuring of experience, see Bertrando and Boscolo (1993), Hoyt (1990), Melges (1982), and Ricoeur (1983).

they have been abused and victimized—what I've learned from those people as adults (I mostly treat adults, who have gone through sexual abuse experiences when they were younger) is that the ones that seem to have done better seem to have four things happen for them, or some combination or some parts of these four. If they have all four, they seem to survive it a lot better. One is that somehow, somewhere, they acknowledged the abuse to themselves and/or to somebody else. They didn't not know about it.

HOYT: So it's owned.

O'HANLON: It's acknowledged. It's a little different from owned. Acknowledged: it happened.

HOYT: If it's interpersonal, then it's even more acknowledged.

O'HANLON: That's right. It's out there in the public dialogue world; even if they only tell one person, it's out of their bag of bones into external reality. So if they *acknowledge* it to themselves and/or to somebody else, they seem to suffer less. The quicker they do that, the sooner they do that, they seem to suffer less of the lasting effects. Second thing is, once they acknowledged it or if it's been acknowledged, do they get *validated* or do they get invalidated or blamed? Because sometimes people will go to a parent or somebody, and they won't be believed, so they will be invalidated: "You're making that up. It never happened. That couldn't have happened." Or they'll be blamed: "You should have stopped him. You're walking around here in those skimpy clothes. You made it happen," or "If you weren't a bad girl, this wouldn't have happened to you." Did they get blamed or invalidated for the experience during the experience, and/or if they ever acknowledged it, did they get blamed or invalidated?

Third thing is, once they acknowledged the abuse, once they went public with it, did they get *protected*? Did it stop? Sometimes it's acknowledged and they are validated, but not protected: "Yes, honey, I know. The same thing happened to me when I was younger, and it's not your fault, but I can't meet your stepdad's needs and you're going to have to meet his needs," or "I can't stop him; he's beating me, too. Sorry," or "We need the money. We need to keep him around. I'll try to keep him from you, but I can't guarantee it," and they don't. Or they are put in foster care and abused there. Or the other person [the abuser] is brought back into the home, and the abused person doesn't feel safe or there's no protection. So, was and is the person protected?

Fourth one is, did someone ever give them the *message that they were worthwhile and lovable*, and did they get that experientially—not just have somebody mouth the words, but did they really get that from somebody somewhere along the line before the abuse? I think it's an inoculation; after the abuse, it's somewhat reparative and healing. I was teaching with Patrick Carnes, who is a sexual addiction therapist, and he was talking about the abuse that he went through as a kid, and his escape was in books. He found a librarian at school who took a great interest in him, and through her eyes, he starting seeing himself as a valuable, worthwhile person. She'd save out special books for him. When he showed up at the library she'd say, "Patrick, I held this one for you because I know you like this kind of book; it just came in." He developed a relationship with her, and through that relationship, he started to see himself as a worthwhile person. What did he do? He grew up and got a PhD and wrote books [Carnes, 1983, 1989].

HOYT: He developed the primary self-narrative that he's a worthwhile person, validated, respected, who had bad things happen to him—not that he's a bad person. He organized his identity.

O'HANLON: That's right. Or at least he had an alternate story available. If you talked to him, I suspect he would say his primary narrative was he was bad and evil and had all the shadow stuff to deal with. His alternate model, though—which was an alternate voice, if you will, an alternate vision—said "I think you're okay." And that's the spiritual aspect of him. That's the librarian message to him. So, because that alternate was available, the one that said, "You're bad; you're devalued; you're terrible; you'll never do anything with your life," wasn't the only narrative. So there were alternative narratives available, and he would switch back and forth. In recent years, I think he would say that the librarian/spiritual/lovable narrative became his primary identification. And the other stuff was "Yes, and this happened to me and it's a part of my identity now, but it's not all of who I am and it doesn't define who I am and it doesn't define my worth." So did anybody ever give them the sense of worth?[12]

HOYT: What is the role of diagnosis and assessment in possibility therapy? What do you look for?

O'HANLON: Well, first of all, I want to say I think there are labels and diagnoses that open up possibilities, and there are ones that close

---

[12]See O'Hanlon (1992) for a case study of helping a woman who had been sexually abused reclaim her own identity: "We worked together to cocreate a new view and experience for S. She had been living a life that was in many ways determined by her history, by what someone who had abused her had done to her in the distant past. She was living *his* story. We collaboratively opened the possibility for her to start to live *her* story, to take back her life and to create new chapters in the future" (p. 147, emphasis in original). An analysis of how to use an externalization approach to separate the problem from the personal identity of the patient is presented in O'Hanlon (1994). For other discussions of constructive approaches to treating the aftereffects of sexual abuse, see Dolan (1991, 1994) and Durrant and White (1990).

down. There are labels that respect people and validate people, and there are labels that invalidate people, I think. Some years ago, I did therapy in the prehistoric days that I call "BBB." This was "before borderlines and bulimics." There were no bulimics when I first started therapy. And "borderline" was an existent category, but it was rarely used; it was an obscure analytic concept that basically meant the border between psychosis and neurosis. Very rare. I saw a person who did bulimia, but was diagnosed as having anorexia based on DSM-II; there was no diagnosis for bulimia for that time. It was seen as a subset or part of anorexia—a phase or one of the symptoms of anorexia, that people would sometimes binge or purge—and it was called bulimia. But it wasn't a special diagnosis. I saw a woman who did bulimia, and I helped her stop bingeing and vomiting; she did stop bingeing and vomiting.

Some time later, I read an article . . . [Boskind-Lodahl & Sirlin, 1977; see also Boskind-White & White, 1983], and they were talking about how 11% of the females they saw in college did bulimia. "Eleven percent?" I thought. "That's a lot". I lived right next to a college, I was in a community mental health center. I was fascinated with this. I read everything I could about it. I put an ad in the college newspaper saying, "Do you binge and vomit or take laxatives or diuretics? If you do, there's a treatment or support group starting at Tri-City Mental Health Center. Call Bill O'Hanlon." I got one of my colleagues to do it with me; we did the group together. Over the next three days I got perhaps 50 phone calls, lots of phone calls. What was striking about those phone calls was that the people, all young women, said one or two or all three of these variations on the theme. One is "I never knew there was a name for what I did." They often cried on the phone, just out of relief of someone to talk to about this and get help from: "I never knew there was a name for it. I never knew that anybody did it. I always thought I was weird and strange and nobody else did this. And I never knew there was any help for it. Thank you." And, you know, sometimes that was what they needed to do, just tell me and acknowledge and that was it.

About 20 people ultimately came into the group out of that group of 50. And when they got to the group, about five people had stopped bingeing and vomiting—it took a month to get the group together. I'd read the literature and this wasn't to be expected. Bulimia is considered an intractable problem. I asked them, "What's that about?" Some of them said, "Just to know that there was a name for it and there was help for me helped me stop." Now, that's a label that empowers. Some of them said, "I was too embarrassed to tell anybody that I did this, so I determined that I would stop it before I came in here so I wouldn't have to tell you all I was still doing this.

I was so embarrassed about it." And some people said, "It just helped me get a handle on it, and I knew I was coming here, and it helped me just get over the edge." So, that's a label that empowered, like going to an AA meeting and saying, "I'm Bill and I'm alcoholic." That can free me, save my life. Now, if I say to you, "You're Michael and you're alcoholic. Go get some help for your drinking"—if you don't believe it and you resist it, then it becomes a label that doesn't empower. It becomes a political matter between the two of us, a way for me to blame you or push you in a direction you don't want to do. It doesn't have that same empowering effect as if you went to an AA meeting and really chose it and said, "I'm Michael and I'm an alcoholic."

HOYT: The politics of experience [Laing, 1967].

O'HANLON: Yeah, the politics of experience and the politics of diagnosis. There are some labels that don't seem to empower. Some are mixed, like if you go to a codependency group and realize that, "Gee, after all these years I realize I'm codependent, and that's really great. I don't feel so weird." So that's one of the values of a label—it can validate or normalize your experience: "Other people feel this, other people experience this and I'm not so different or strange or bad or weird because of it." I think that sometimes, though, what goes on with this is "Once an alcoholic, always an alcoholic; once a bulimic, always a bulimic," and you never recover. You'll never really be able to drop this identity label: "You'll always be bulimic whether you do bulimia or not. You'll always be alcoholic whether you drink alcohol or not. And you'll always be codependent whether you're doing codependent behaviors or not." And I think that way sometimes closes down possibilities.

HOYT: I have just written an article called "Is Being 'In Recovery' Self-Limiting?" [Hoyt, 1994b]. I see many people in recovery and it's helpful, but I almost never see anybody say, "I am recovered." If you have to admit that you are weak and will always have this problem, then it becomes this self-limiting kind of thing.[13]

O'HANLON: Yes, and there are some people who in their private moments will tell you, "I haven't had the urge for a drink for years, and I'm never going to drink again." They are truly not alcoholic any more, but the narrative in that subculture says that if you ever say

---

[13]As Kaminer (1992, p. 26) has commented: "It is an odd program in self-esteem that rewards people for calling themselves helpless, childish, addicted, and diseased and punishes them for claiming to be healthy. Admit that you're sick and you're welcomed into the recovering persons fold; dispute it and you're 'in denial.' Thus the search for identity is perversely resolved: all your bad behaviors and unwanted feelings become conditions of your being."

that, that's a sign of trouble, so they are not going to say it out loud. That's a way that kind of story or that kind of diagnosis invalidates that person's experience. I think also when I said "BBB"—"before borderlines and bulimics"—sometimes one suspects that the label "borderline" is overly applied, sometimes because of therapist errors that create troubling situations or in which it is then applied to people who are just considered a pain in the butt. They call us a lot, or get too needy or dependent on us, or threaten suicide a fair amount in response to whatever we do, or maybe they were going to do that anyway. But that label doesn't typically empower and help people move on. It may help the therapist figure out what's going on and find some maneuvers, and if it does, that's a little better. But if you have the label for one of your clients as "borderline" and your colleagues commiserate and say, "Don't get too many in treatment and don't expect much," then it's not such a great label.

HOYT: Do you know where the word *diagnosis* comes from? *Diagnosis* is *via gnossis*; it means "way or path of knowledge," or in modern parlance, information [Hoyt, 1989]. A good diagnosis should be information that points a path or way to being helpful; it's not simply pejorative or pathologizing.

O'HANLON: Or just good explanation. Bateson [1972] used to make fun of that in the "dormative principle" that came from the Molière play in which this sort of shoot-the-breeze kind of BS'ing medical resident is asked by the learned doctors what is it in morphine that makes people go to sleep, and he says, "It's the dormative principle." That's just Latin for "It makes him go to sleep." The learned doctors all nod their heads, saying, "Yes, that's it." So if it's an explanation that doesn't give you anything to do, I think that's not so good. The other thing is sometimes the label that validates one person invalidates or blames another.

HOYT: "ACA"—"adult child of alcoholic"—can be very useful: "I've had an experience other people have had; I picked up certain tendencies or made decisions." But sometimes people come in and say, "I can never be relaxed or enjoy spontaneity . . . "

O'HANLON: " . . . because my parents did it to me."

HOYT: It's disempowering, rather than it giving me a handle that I can work this better.

O'HANLON: Yeah, that's right. Or it blames somebody else and externalizes your power. So I think there are some problems with diagnoses. Do they validate and capture people's experience in such a way that they say "Yes" with that nod of recognition, and it keeps the possibilities open and doesn't blame or invalidate the person getting the label or the other people around them? That's the role of diagnosis in therapy. The role of assessment is to figure out what they're complaining about and what they want. That's the quick version of the role of assessment. I think assessment is different from diagnosis. Assessment is assessing what is going on, not necessarily what the diagnosis is.

HOYT: Not putting a word or a label on it.

O'HANLON: That is diagnosis, and that's necessary to get insurance reimbursement, so that's a very helpful thing. Sometimes it's necessary to help us organize our thinking about the case, and also to communicate in code words to our colleagues so we don't have to explain in detail all the time.

HOYT: What about "false memory syndrome"?

O'HANLON: There's a lot of debate even about that term, whether there's such a syndrome or not. I think that that's a little bit of a nitpicking thing. People in the sexual abuse field, of course, are concerned that if we get into this false memory syndrome idea that we might undo a lot of the cultural work that's been done to open up the narrative to recognizing knowledge that kids have been abused, and how much progress we've made in getting the society to recognize that. So they are concerned that people will get continually invalidated or more invalidated, or denial or minimization will take place. I think that's a good concern. I've seen many, many people who said they've been abused, and generally I don't lead people in that direction, I don't think. Because I'm briefly oriented and very problem-focused, I don't typically introduce the topic of abuse, and still I've heard from people that they've been abused; years ago, even before it was a popular thing, I heard it. I think people have been abused and a fair amount of people have been sexually abused—many more than we imagined, I think, in the years past.

I also think that not everyone who says they were abused was abused. Partly, I am really disturbed by this notion of "believe the children." Having four children of my own, I can tell you very clearly that if you get rid of the violent rhetoric on either side and you raise a child, you'll know that a child does not always tell the strict reality truth about things. A child can fabricate things; a child mixes stories together. Adults mix stories together; I mix stories together. What the heck, we do make some mistakes, or reshuffle our narratives and our memories, so I think that you can't always "believe the children." You'd better err on the side of caution in believing the children; I think that's a good idea. Adults remembering childhood events, I think, are a little shakier, and I think that we need to distinguish between a couple of things. One is, most of us who are doing clinical work are not forensic investigators. It's never going to be our role; we're not going to have the resources to do it; we don't have the expertise to do it. We're not trained in forensic psychology or psychiatry. If we are, we probably can't do clinical work with the same person, because you have to have a different stance to do forensic investigations. When you do clinical work you're advocating for them, you usually try for them. In forensic work you have to be a little more objective, a little less sided, I think, and you're also using different methods for investigation. So I think people who investigate factual truth are different from people who are investigating narrative truth. That is, "This shows up in your experience, and I'm not going to say it didn't happen, that you made it all up. And I'm also not going to say I'm a psychological forensic investigator, and the way you present your symptoms shows me clearly you have been sexually abused."

HOYT: What do you do when the client says, "My experience is, my memory is, my recall is, this happened to me. Do you believe me?" Do you say, "I believe you experienced it that way"?

O'HANLON: "Seems like it happened to me, and I don't know for sure; I wasn't there and I'll never know for sure." I'm not going to get into "Yes, I believe that," or "No, I don't."

HOYT: And if they say, "You have to believe me"?

O'HANLON: I say, "Look, it seems to me like it happened from the way you say it. It doesn't seem like you made it up to me, and I don't know." I have a client who I mentioned before, the Astoroth person, who went through an extended and, in part, regressive therapy. She "remembered" being abused by a cult; family members were involved in this cult activity. Treatment is over, has been over for some time, the multiplicity is resolved. The therapy went well. Recently there came a situation in which the person was confronted with the possibility of going public, the invitation to go public, with the story. And she said, "You know, I don't know whether this strictly happened or not." It wasn't the same as during treatment, when she said, "I must be making this up. I must be making this up," which she said quite a bit, and I said, "I don't know. It sounds like you're experiencing something and I don't know where it's coming from, but it's pretty heavy-duty stuff." She just said, "I think it happened; I'm pretty sure it happened. I'm not positive." Now, some people would say treatment is incomplete. The treatment issues that she came in for are resolved, the multiplicity is resolved, and she's still not sure it's true reality.

HOYT: But she's functioning well. She got her therapy.

O'HANLON: She's a very sophisticated person and is saying this with a very informed judgment. She knows a lot about the field of abuse herself and doesn't say it lightly.

HOYT: There are also forensic issues, if I understand, that once someone has used hypnosis it may qualify or disqualify the possibility of her testimony.

O'HANLON: My brother is a district court judge in West Virginia, and he had a case in which a man was accused of rape by two women. This was one of the first cases of DNA testing, where they were trying to use it to establish identity because they had DNA samples from him and from the sperm from both women. These two women became convinced that this guy was the rapist. In part it appears they became convinced because they were hypnotized, and in the hypnosis they remembered the details of it in much more detail, and they became convinced that the guy who was now arrested and accused of it was the guy. And when it was reported in court that the DNA ruled out the possibility that it could be the guy, my brother had to rule whether that could be allowed in because it was controversial new evidence, and the women were still convinced it was the guy, even in the face of this. Then it was discovered that they had been hypnotized. They didn't throw out all the testimony, but they disqualified all the testimony that was reported after the hypnosis. Now, in some jurisdictions, they throw out all the testimony. So, yes, one has to be careful.

Martin Orne [1979] and other people have done experiments that they say show that when one is hypnotized, that what one remembers isn't necessarily strict reality memory, but narratively influenced by the therapist's expectations, by the client's current conditions. And more than that, the client becomes more convinced because it happens experientially, and things that happen experientially seem to be much more potent for people, so they become more convinced even though it's not necessarily true memories. What the advocates of trauma work often say is that "We think experimental evidence is different than what we see in our clinical offices—that we think that traumatic memories may get encapsulated in a special way, so they are not influenced." As I was saying, "frozen in time." Perhaps that's true. Not influenced so much by current narrative, by current conditions. So they are sort of intact memories. But, of course, as soon as one started to remember them, they'd be influenced by current contexts.[14] How come the average number of personalities discovered in multiple personality was several, two to three, until the '70s and '80s, where now it's 36? Those were people who initially were investigating multiple personality who believed in multiplicity, but they didn't discover or know so many multiple personalities. Were there really more personalities? Were there not? I don't know. I just know that it's inextricably bound up with current ideas and current narratives, and you can't separate those things. It's the same as sexual abuse memories. They are inextricably bound up with current narratives as soon as you start to speak about them and bring them into an interactional setting.

In regard to the so-called "false memory syndrome," yes, I think some overzealous therapists can lead clients in the direction of believing that they were sexually abused when they weren't. Do I think it happens a lot? I don't know how much it happens. I think most people you talk to about sexual abuse were sexually abused. And I think what will come out of this polarized debate, which I'm sorry is so polarized, will be some better things for most of us who are in the middle ground. We will be more cautious about introducing those ideas and inadvertently or advertently influencing people, and we'll be more cautious about invalidating people. The people who take a polarized position are saying, "Oh, all this stuff is a bunch of hogwash and it never happened, and you've just been reading too many books or you've read *The Courage to Heal* [Bass & Davis, 1994], so therefore all your memories are invalid." Or, on the other extreme, "Believe the children; this false memory stuff is a conspiracy perpetrated by women-haters and perpetrators." I think that there will be a nice middle ground that will be reached by most of us, and the extremists will fight it out for years. Because they are true believers.

HOYT: What's next, Bill? What's your current interest?

O'HANLON: I think this sexual abuse stuff is very interesting, because it seems to me that, like hypnosis, the field of posttraumatic stress—and especially the aftereffects of sexual abuse—really is a proving ground or an experimental ground or learning ground that can shed light on the rest of therapy. This is a particularly difficult situation, the aftereffects of sexual abuse. I think I have learned so much from doing this work that then goes back and applies to general therapy work. I also think it's a very good way to get across to people who typically wouldn't approach anything called "brief therapy" or "solution-oriented therapy." I think it's a really good way to smuggle in some of these ideas about respectful and effective treatment that I've

---

[14]For further discussion of the "true and false memories" controversy, see Courtois (1988, 1992), Loftus (1980; Loftus & Ketcham, 1991), Terr (1990, 1994), and Yapko (1994).

been trying to smuggle into psychotherapy for a long time, through the rubric of treating the aftereffects of sexual abuse. Because I think you can show how respectful and effective these approaches can be, and therapists are desperate for anything that can help the clients that are really hurting so much and are often in physical danger through self-abuse and mutilation and suicidal tendencies and impulses. That's really exciting.

HOYT: What's the message from your work?

O'HANLON: Businesses are big on mission statements. Because I read a lot of business books, I decided to sit down and write my mission statement a while ago. I was shocked that it didn't have anything to do with Ericksonian approaches or brief therapy or solution-oriented or even possibility therapy.[15] I really want to transform the field of psychotherapy, change it. I want to oppose and stand against ideas and practices that are disrespectful or harmful and discourage people. I want us to be even better. There are people still hurting out there in the world that we haven't found ways to help. Various theorists and practitioners are coming up with promising ideas that if they really work, some of them are going to revolutionize our work—make it more brief, make it more effective, and really contribute to people, and so I'm really excited about that. I think it's important to stay flexible and stay interested, not just develop your narrow view of things. I have interest in any ideas that I think are respectful and encouraging, and also effective. I'm sure that the approaches that I use aren't as effective as they could be. I want to learn some more over the years, and I have learned more over the years. My contribution to the field of treating the aftereffects of sexual abuse is one of my ways of trying to make the field more diverse and effective, allowing different ideas and combining those ideas with people in ways that work, hopefully.

[15]In another interview (Bubebzer & West, 1993, pp. 370–371), O'Hanlon commented: "Mainly, what I read for pleasure or interest are business books. Therapy books are usually so pathologically oriented and although I occasionally find a good one, most of them are fairly boring to me. Business books are really good because I learn about creating results, quality, and customer relationships. They talk about getting close to the customer and finding out what the customer's perception is, what the customer's ideas are about, where they want to be, and what constitutes good results."

REFERENCES

Bandler, R., & Grinder, J. (1975). *The Structure of Magic*. Palo Alto, CA: Science & Behavior Books.

Bandler, R., & Grinder, J. (1982). *Reframing*. Moab, UT: Real People Press.

Bass, E., & Davis, L. (1994). *The Courage to Heal* (3rd ed.). New York: HarperCollins.

Bateson, G. (1972). *Steps to an Ecology of Mind*. New York: Ballantine.

Boscolo, L., & Bertrando, P. (1993). *The Times of Time*. New York: Norton.

Boskind-Lodahl, M., & Sirlin, J. (1977, February). The gorging–purging syndrome. *Psychology Today*, pp. 50–56.

Boskind-White, M., & White, W. C. (1983). *Bulimarexia: The Binge–Purge Cycle*. New York: Norton.

Bubenzer, D. L., & West, J. D. (1993). Interview with William Hudson O'Hanlon: On seeking possibilities and solutions in therapy. *The Family Journal: Counseling and Therapy for Couples and Families, 1*(4), 365–379.

Cade, B., & O'Hanlon, W. H. (1993). *A Brief Guide to Brief Therapy*. New York: Norton.

Carnes, P. (1983). *Out of the Shadows: Understanding Sexual Addiction*. Minneapolis: CompCare.

Carnes, P. (1989). *Contrary to Love: Helping the Sexual Addict*. Minneapolis: CompCare.

Castaneda, C. (1968). *The Teachings of Don Juan: A Yaqui Way of Knowledge*. New York: Ballantine.

Courtois, C. (1988). *Healing the Incest Wound: Adult Survivors in Therapy*. New York: Norton.

Courtois, C. (1992). The memory retrieval process in incest survivor therapy. *Journal of Child Sexual Abuse, 1,* 15–32.

Cummings, N. A. (1990). Brief intermittent therapy throughout the life cycle. In J. K. Zeig & S. G. Gilligan (Eds.), *Brief Therapy: Myths, Methods, and Metaphors* (pp 169–184). New York: Brunner/Mazel.

Dolan, Y. M. (1991). *Resolving Sexual Abuse: Solution-Focused Therapy and Ericksonian Hypnosis for Adult Survivors*. New York: Norton.

Dolan, Y. M. (1994). Solution-focused therapy with a case of severe abuse. In M. F. Hoyt (Ed.), *Constructive Therapies* (pp. 276–294). New York: Guilford Press.

Durrant, M., & White, C. (Eds.). (1990). *Ideas for Therapy with Sexual Abuse*. Adelaide: Dulwich Centre Publications.

Erickson, M. H. (1954). Pseudo-orientation in time as a hypnotic procedure. *Journal of Clinical and Experimental Hypnosis, 6,* 183–207.

Erickson, M. H., Rossi, E., & Rossi, S. (1976). *Hypnotic Realities*. New York: Irvington.

Frankl, V. E. (1963). *Man's Search for Meaning: An Introduction to Logotherapy*. New York: Washington Square Press.

Freud, S. (1958). Remembering, repeating and working-through. In J. Strachey (Ed. and Trans), *The Standard Edition of the Complete Psychological Works of Sigmund Freud* (Vol. 12, pp. 145–156). London: Hogarth Press. (Original work published 1914)

Gale, J., & Newfield, N. (1992). A conversation analysis of a solution-focused marital therapy session. *Journal of Marital and Family Therapy, 18,* 153–165.

Groddeck, G. (1976). *The Book of the It*. New York: International Universities Press. (Original work published 1923).

Heidegger, M. (1962). *Being and Time*. New York: Harper and Row.

Herman, J. L. (1992). *Trauma and Recovery*. New York: Basic Books.

Horowitz, M. J. (1986). *Stress Response Syndromes* (rev. ed.). Northvale, NJ: Jason Aronson.

Hoyt, M. F. (1989). Psychodiagnosis of personality disorders. *Transactional Analysis Journal, 19*, 101–113. (Reprinted in M. F. Hoyt, *Brief Therapy and Managed Care: Readings for Contemporary Practice* [pp. 257–279]. San Francisco: Jossey-Bass, 1995.)

Hoyt, M. F. (1990). On time in brief therapy. In R. A. Wells & V. J. Giannetti (Eds.), *Handbook of the Brief Psychotherapies* (pp. 115–143). New York: Plenum Press. (Reprinted in M. F. Hoyt, *Brief Therapy and Managed Care: Readings for Contemporary Practice* [pp. 69–104]. San Francisco: Jossey-Bass, 1995.)

Hoyt, M. F. (1994a). On the importance of keeping it simple and taking the patient seriously: A conversation with Steve de Shazer and John Weakland. In M. F. Hoyt (Ed.), *Constructive Therapies* (pp. 11–40). New York: Guilford Press.

Hoyt, M. F. (1994b). Is being "in recovery" self-limiting? *Transactional Analysis Journal, 24*, 222–223. (Reprinted in M. F. Hoyt, *Brief Therapy and Managed Care: Readings for Contemporary Practice* [pp. 213–215]. San Francisco: Jossey-Bass, 1995.)

Hubble, M., & O'Hanlon, W. H. (1992). Theory countertransference. *Dulwich Centre Newsletter*, 1: 25–30.

Hudson, P. O., & O'Hanlon, W. H. (1992). *Rewriting Love Stories: Brief Marital Therapy*. New York: Norton.

Kaminer, W. (1992). *I'm Dysfunctional, You're Dysfunctional: The Recovery Movement and Other Self-Help Fashions*. New York: Vintage.

Kernberg, O. (1975). *Borderline Conditions and Pathological Narcissism*. New York: Jason Aronson.

Laing, R. D. (1967). *The Politics of Experience*. New York: Pantheon.

Lipchik, E. (1994). The rush to be brief. *Family Therapy Networker, 18*(2), 34–39.

Loftus, E. (1980). *Memory*. Reading, MA: Addison-Wesley.

Loftus, E., & Ketcham, K. (1991). *Witness for the Defense*. New York: St. Martin's Press.

Masterson, J. F. (1976). *Psychotherapy of the Borderline Adult: A Developmental Approach*. New York: Brunner/Mazel.

Meichenbaum, D. (1994). *A Clinical Handbook/Practical Therapist Manual for Treating PTSD*. Waterloo, Ontario, Canada: Institute Press, University of Waterloo.

Melges, F. T. (1982). *Time and the Inner Future: A Temporal Approach to Psychiatric Disorders*. New York: Wiley.

O'Hanlon, W. H. (1987). *Taproots: Underlying Principles of Milton Erickson's Therapy and Hypnosis*. New York: Norton.

O'Hanlon, W. H. (1991). Not strategic, not systemic: Still clueless after all these years. *Journal of Strategic and Systemic Therapies, 10*, 105–109.

O'Hanlon, W. H. (1992). History becomes her story: Collaborative solution-oriented therapy of the after-effects of sexual abuse. In S. McNamee & K. J. Gergen (Eds.), *Therapy as Social Construction* (pp. 136–148). Newbury Park, CA: Sage.

O'Hanlon, W. H. (1993). *Escape from DepressoLand: Brief Therapy of Depression* [Professional training videotape]. Omaha, NE: Possibilities.

O'Hanlon, W. H. (1994). The third wave. *Family Therapy Networker, 18*(6),18–26, 28–29.

O'Hanlon, W. H., & Beadle, S. (1994). *A Field Guide to PossibilityLand: Possibility Therapy Methods.* Omaha, NE: Center Press.

O'Hanlon, W. H., & Hexum, A. L. (1990). *An Uncommon Casebook: The Complete Clinical Work of Milton H. Erickson, M.D.* New York: Norton.

O'Hanlon, W. H., & Hudson, P. O. (1994). Coauthoring a love story: Solution-oriented marital therapy. In M. F. Hoyt (Ed.), *Constructive Therapies* (pp. 160–188). New York: Guilford Press.

O'Hanlon, W. H., & Hudson, P. O. (1995). *Love Is a Verb.* New York: Norton.

O'Hanlon, W. H., & Martin, M. (1992). *Solution-Oriented Hypnosis: An Ericksonian Approach.* New York: Norton.

O'Hanlon, W. H., & Schultheis, G. (1993). *Brief Therapy Coach* [Computer program, Macintosh or IBM-compatible]. Omaha, NE: Possibilities.

O'Hanlon, W. H., & Weiner-Davis, M. (1989). *In Search of Solutions: A New Direction in Psychotherapy.* New York: Norton.

O'Hanlon, W. H., & Wilk, J. (1987). *Shifting Contexts: The Generation of Effective Psychotherapy.* New York: Guilford Press.

Orne, M. (1979). The use and misuse of hypnosis in court. *International Journal of Clinical Hypnosis, 27,* 311–341.

Perls, F. S. (1969). *Gestalt Therapy Verbatim.* Lafayette, CA: Real People Press.

Ricoeur, P. (1983). *Time and Narrative.* Chicago: University of Chicago Press.

Rogers, C. (1951). *Client-Centered Therapy.* Boston: Houghton Mifflin.

Rogers, C. (1961). *On Becoming a Person.* Boston: Houghton Mifflin.

Satir, V. (1967). *Conjoint Family Therapy* (rev. ed.). Palo Alto, CA: Science & Behavior Books.

Terr, L. (1990). *Too Scared to Cry: Psychic Trauma in Childhood.* New York: Harper & Row.

Terr, L. (1994). *Unchained Memories: True Stories of Traumatic Memories, Lost and Found.* New York: Basic Books.

Whitman, W. (1993). *Leaves of Grass* (rev. ed.). New York: Random House/Modern Library. (Original work published 1892)

Yapko, M.D. (1994). *Suggestions of Abuse: True and False Memories of Childhood Sexual Trauma.* New York: Simon & Schuster.

Zeig, J. K. (Ed.). (1992). *The Evolution of Psychotherapy: The Second Conference.* New York: Brunner/Mazel.

CHAPTER 5

Cognitive-Behavioral Treatment of Posttraumatic Stress Disorder from a Narrative Constructivist Perspective
A Conversation with Donald Meichenbaum

MICHAEL F. HOYT

One of the founders of the "cognitive revolution" in psychotherapy and a major proponent of the constructivist perspective, Donald Meichenbaum is Professor of Psychology at the University of Waterloo in Ontario, Canada. A prolific writer, researcher, and international lecturer, he is the author of the classic *Cognitive-Behavior Modification: An Integrative Approach* (1977). His other books include *Stress Reduction and Prevention* (Meichenbaum & Jaremko, 1983), *Pain and Behavioral Medicine: A Cognitive-Behavioral Perspective* (Turk, Meichenbaum, & Genest, 1983), *The Unconscious Reconsidered* (Bowers & Meichenbaum, 1984), *Stress Inoculation Training: A Clinical Guidebook* (1985), and *Facilitating Treatment Adherence: A Practitioner's Guidebook* (Meichenbaum & Turk, 1987).

The following conversation took place in San Francisco on May 4, 1994, where Meichenbaum was to present a two-day workshop on "Treating Patients with Posttraumatic Stress Disorder" for the Institute for Behavioral Healthcare. We had just been looking at the typescript of his forthcoming magnum opus, *A Clinical Handbook/Practical Therapist Manual for Treating PTSD* (1994),[1] an extraordinary compendium of information for clinicians and researchers working with persons suffering the effects of traumatic stress.

---

[1]This 600-page manual is now available directly from Donald Meichenbaum (University of Waterloo, Department of Psychology, Waterloo, Ontario N2L 3G1, Canada).

HOYT: The first question I want to ask you, Don, is how did you come to think of treating PTSD [posttraumatic stress disorder] as a narrative constructive endeavor?

MEICHENBAUM: For a number of years, I have been involved in treating adults, adolescents, and children with behavioral and affective disorders who were depressed, anxious, angry, and impulsive. Based on my research and clinical experience with these populations, I was invited to present a number of training workshops. Then a very interesting set of invitations came my way when I was given the opportunity to consult and conduct research on a variety of different distressed populations. I was asked to consult on a treatment program within the U.S. military on spouse abuse. I also consulted with mental health workers who conducted debriefing of natural disasters, occupational accidents, and combat. I also consulted at residential treatment programs for children and adolescents, some 40% of whom met the DSM criteria for PTSD. In addition, I was supervising various mental health workers (psychiatrists, psychologists, social workers, family physicians) who were treating clients who had a history of victimization experiences—child sexual abuse, rape, domestic violence. As I became more and more involved with these populations and spent many hours listening to the therapy tapes, looking at the debriefing experiences, I became quite fascinated with the nature of the "stories" that people offered to describe their traumatizing experiences and how they coped—that is, the narratives and the accounts that they constructed.

HOYT: What about the stories?

MEICHENBAUM: I became fascinated with how people describe their experience and how their accounts changed over time. While victimization experiences can affect individuals at various levels (e.g., physiologically, behaviorally, socially), given my cognitive-behavioral background and my interest in cognition and emotion, I became particularly interested in the nature of the "stories" that people tell themselves and others, and the manner in which they offer accounts of their experience. When something bad happens to you, when some natural or man-made disaster occurs, when some form of victimization experience occurs to you or to your family, ordinary language and everyday vocabulary seem inadequate to describe your experience and reactions. In their own ways, these "victimized" individuals became "poets" of sorts, using metaphors to describe their experiences. They conveyed their experiences by using phrases such as "This is like . . . ," "I feel like a . . . ," and so forth. The victimized individual may describe herself as a "prisoner of the past," as a "doormat," a "whore," as a "time bomb ready to explode," and the like. Just imagine the impact on yourself and on others if you go about describing your experiences in such metaphoric terms.

As a result of these initial clinical impressions, I undertook the task of analyzing the nature of the metaphors and the narrative accounts that clients offered over the course of their therapeutic sessions. I also analyzed the literature on PTSD in order to discern what were the narrative features of individuals who did *not* suffer PTSD following exposure to traumatic events [Meichenbaum, 1994; Meichenbaum & Fitzpatrick, 1993]. Based upon both the clinical analysis and the literature review, I came to appreciate the heuristic value of a constructive narrative perspective, not only for PTSD, but for other clinical disorders as well. Obviously, I am not the first to propose such a constructive narrative perspective. Let me note that there are people like Harvey [Harvey, Weber, & Orbuch, 1990], Gergen [1991; McNamee & Gergen, 1992], Schafer [1992], White and Epston [1990], and O'Hanlon [O'Hanlon & Weiner-Davis, 1989] who have also advocated for a constructive narrative perspective.

HOYT: Let me read you a quotation from an article you wrote with Geoffrey Fong [Meichenbaum & Fong, 1993, p. 489]. You said, "The constructivist perspective is founded on the idea that humans actively construct their personal realities and create their own representational models of the world. There is a long tradition of philosophical and psychological authors who have argued that the paradigms, assumptive worlds, and schemas that individuals actively create, determine, and in some instances constrain how they perceive reality."[2] When someone becomes a victim, has a horrible trauma, how does that affect them? What changes, especially in terms of their world view?

MEICHENBAUM: The answer to what changes after you've been victimized depends on which piece of the puzzle you look at—sort of like the old metaphor of the elephant, whether you examine the tusk, the tail, or whatever. Clearly, there is increasing evidence that something changes physiologically [see van der Kolk, 1994]. This is especially true of chronic, prolonged exposure, or what are called *Type II stressors* (e.g., abuse, domestic violence, Holocaust victim). Such

---

[2]Meichenbaum and Fong (1993, p. 489) go on: "Common to each of these proponents is the tenet that the human mind is a product of constructive symbolic activities and that reality is a product of the personal meanings that individuals create. Individuals do not merely respond to events in and of themselves, but they respond to their interpretation of events and to their perceived implications of these events. . . . Constructivists assume that all mental images are creations of people, and thus, speak of 'invented reality.' How individuals construct such meanings and realities, how they create their world view is the subject of narrative psychology."

exposure leads to what are called "disorders of extreme stress" that affect one's sense of trust in family and beliefs about self and the world. To use Janoff-Bulman's [1985, 1990] model, traumatic events can "shatter" your basic assumptions about the world; traumatic events can violate and invalidate your core beliefs. Another thing that trauma does is overly sensitize you to trauma-related cues, and this hypervigilance feeds into, and is in turn affected by, the ruminations, flashbacks, and avoidance behaviors that characterize PTSD. Trauma biases the ways in which you selectively attend to events. There is a great deal of data that I review in the PTSD clinical handbook [Meichenbaum, 1994] that examines the impact of trauma from an information-processing and a constructive narrative perspective.

HOYT: Is this primarily a protective mechanism: "I need to be on alert so it won't happen again"?

MEICHENBAUM: I think there are functional and adaptive values in such behavior. To become vigilant and to overrespond after exposure to a trauma can be adaptive initially. But what happens to the people who have difficulty recovering, who evidence maladjustment, is that they continue to behave in ways that may be no longer necessary. From my point of view, a central feature of individuals with PTSD can be characterized as a "stuckness" problem. That is, people get "stuck" using techniques such as dissociation that were at one time effective in order to deal with trauma such as incest, or dealing with the aftermath of rape, or dealing with combat. What happens is that some individuals continue to respond in the same fashion even when it is no longer needed. It is my task as a therapist to help clients understand and appreciate the adaptive value of how they responded. But I also help them appreciate what is the *impact*, what is the *toll*, what is the *price* to them and others of continuing to respond in this fashion when it is no longer needed. This approach helps clients reframe their reactions (their "symptoms") as adaptive strengths, rather than as signs of mental illness. In a collaborative fashion, this approach "inoculates" them, in some sense, to the impact of future stressors. We work together to help them not only change their behavior, but also to tell their "stories" differently.

HOYT: In your writing about stress inoculation training (SIT), you describe three phases: namely, education, skills acquisition and consolidation, and application training. The first phase, of education, sounds like you are having clients work to better understand the impact of their . . . [3]

---

[3]Meichenbaum (1993, 1994; Meichenbaum & Fitzpatrick, 1993; Meichenbaum & Fong, 1993) describes key features of SIT as including the following: (*continued*)

MEICHENBAUM: I even go beyond understanding, to nurturing the client's discovery process by using Socratic questioning. In the PTSD handbook [Meichenbaum, 1994], I have included the best Socratic questions you can ask in therapy. Moreover, I believe that I am at my "therapeutic best" when the client I am seeing is one step ahead of me, offering the advice that I would otherwise offer. I try to train clinicians how to emulate that fine inquirer of sorts—namely, Peter Falk playing the popular TV detective character, Columbo. I want clinicians, at times, to play "dumb." For some clinicians this is not a difficult nor challenging role. (*Laughter*) I encourage clinicians to use strategically their bemusement, their befuddlement; I want them to be collaborators. The goal is to help the client in the initial phase of stress inoculation to better understand what they have been through; how are things now; how would they like them to be; and what can *we* do, working together, to help them achieve their goals? The educational phase of SIT lays the groundwork whereby the client can come to say, "You know, I'm stuck." A related objective of this initial phase is to help clients move from global metaphorical accounts of their experience and reactions to behaviorally prescriptive descriptions that lead to change, and to nurture a sense of hope to undertake this change.

HOYT: In essence, I think you're saying that as clinicians we're trying to help clients reauthor their narratives, rather than us undertaking the role of correcting their accounts [see Simon, 1993, p.72]. We're there as sort of an amanuensis, as an assistant to take it down, rather than simply to correct their narratives or to tell them they're looking at it wrong.[4]

MEICHENBAUM: Correct. The metaphors that describe my therapeutic approach include "rescripting," "reauthoring," "helping clients generate a new narrative," and "being a coach." I don't just record the clients' accounts; rather, I help them alter their personal stories.

(*continued from p. 128*)

  a. Establishment of a nurturant, compassionate, nonjudgmental set of conditions in which distressed clients can tell their stories at their own pace.

  b. Normalization of distressed individuals' reactions.

  c. Reconceptualization of the distress process.

  d. Breaking down or disaggregating global descriptions of clients' stress into specific, concrete, behaviorally prescriptive stressful situations.

  e. Performance of personal experiments that produce experientially meaningful occur rences, in a gradual manner. These experiments should test the limits on how clients will respond to reentering the stressful situation, via imagery, via behavioral rehearsal, and eventually in real situations.

  f. Encouragement of taking credit for positive outcomes of coping efforts.

  g. Relapse prevention, including teaching ways to anticipate, accept, and cope with lapses so that they don't escalate into full-blown relapses.

Such change occurs as a result of my helping clients attend to and appreciate the strengths they possess, or what they have done to survive. A second way is to help them engage in "personal experiments" in the present that provide them with "data" that they can take as evidence to "unfreeze" the beliefs they hold about themselves and the world. The results of such ongoing experiments that occur both within and outside of the therapeutic setting provide the basis for the client to develop a new narrative. This co-constructive process is one that emerges out of experientially meaningful efforts by the client. In terms of strengths and coping efforts, I help people who have PTSD to appreciate that their intrusive thoughts, hypervigilance, denial, dissociation, dichotomous thinking, and moments of rage each represent coping efforts, and metaphorically reflect the "body's wisdom." For example, intrusive thoughts may reflect ways of making sense of what happened, as attempts to "finish the story," to answer "why" questions. Denial may be an attempt to "dose oneself," dealing with limited amounts of stress at a given time—a way to take a "time out." Hypervigilance may be seen as being on continual "sentry duty" when it is no longer needed.

In other words, it is not that people get anxious, angry, or depressed per se; those are natural human emotions. Rather, it is what people say to themselves about those conditions that is critical. The collaborative process of therapy is designed to help the client "say" different things to herself, as well as to others. A key element of cognitive-behavioral interventions is that an effective way of having people talk to themselves differently is to have them *behave* differently. Thus, a critical feature of cognitive-behavioral interventions such as stress inoculation training, is to encourage and even challenge clients to perform personal experiments *in vivo*, so, as I mentioned, they can collect data that will "unfreeze" their beliefs about themselves and about the world. Cognitive-behavioral therapy is *not* just a "talking cure." It is a proactive, enabling form of intervention that fits an "evidential" theory of behavior change (see Meichenbaum, 1977, 1994).

But such change is *not* enough. It is critical for clients to take credit for the changes that they have brought about. There is a need

---

[4]What's "right" is what works for the client. Again, to quote Meichenbaum and Fitzpatrick (1993, p. 698): "There are two important features to recognize about this reconceptualization or new narrative reconstruction process. First, the scientific validity of the specific healing theory that is developed is less important than is its plausibility or credibility to the client. Secondly, this entire 'narrative repair' effort is conducted in a collaborative inductive fashion and not imposed upon, nor didactically taught, to distressed individuals. The distressed client must come to develop and accept a reconceptualization of the distress that he or she has helped cocreate."

for the therapist to ensure that the clients take data resulting from personal experiments as evidence, and thus assume a greater sense of responsibility for the changes that they have brought about. This process of "ownership" is evident in the new narratives that clients relate. I listen carefully to the clients' stories. I listen for their spontaneous use of metacognitive self-regulatory verbs as part of their new accounts. Improvement is evident when clients use such verbs as "I noticed . . . caught myself . . . interrupted . . . used my plan . . . felt I had options . . . patted myself on the back . . . became my own coach . . . anticipated high risk-situations . . . tried my other options." When clients incorporate these expressions into their narratives, then they have become their own therapists, and truly have taken (appropriated) the clinician's "voice" with them.

HOYT: This is the power of new *experience*—not just explanation of what's wrong, but disconfirming the expectations with a new experience.[5]

MEICHENBAUM: But for meaningful change to occur, it has to be "affectively charged." I am referring to the time-honored concept of "corrective emotional experience" [Alexander & French, 1946]. People can readily dismiss, discount, dissuade themselves of the "data." They don't really accept data as "evidence," and it is critical therapeutically to work with clients in order to ensure that they take the data they have collected as evidence to unfreeze their beliefs—to get into the nature of the clients' belief system and to nurture an internal dialogue that they would find most adaptive, as compared to being "stuck" in maladaptive patterns of thinking and behaving.[6]

HOYT: Watching you work, I'm always impressed by how much caring and effort goes into developing a therapeutic alliance and a collaborative relationship with the client. It appears to be the vehicle that carries the rest of your work.

MEICHENBAUM: I agree. I think the therapeutic relationship is the glue that makes the various therapeutic procedures work. Some of the things that I try to highlight for a clinical audience

---

[5]As discussed in *The First Session in Brief Therapy* (Budman, Hoyt, & Friedman, 1992), the introduction of *novelty* is a key element across different therapeutic approaches. As the adage has it, "If we don't change directions, we'll wind up where we are heading!" (Hoyt, 1990, p. 128).

[6]Some of the ways people who have experienced traumas get "stuck" are catalogued by Meichenbaum and Fitzpatrick (1993, p. 697). These include the following:

a. making unfavorable comparisons between life as it is and as it might have been had the distressing event not occurred;

b. engaging in comparisons between aspects of life after the stressful event versus how it was before, and also continually pining for what was lost;

c. seeing themselves as "victims" with little expectation or hope that things will change or improve;

watching my videotapes is how often I "pluck" and reflect the client's key words, use Socratic questioning, and often over the course of the session, I let the client finish my sentences. The most valuable tool that a clinician has is the art of questioning. As Tomm [1987a, 1987b, 1988) has highlighted, the questions we ask clients have presuppositions, and as a result the clinician can use questions effectively and strategically to move clients towards self-generated solutions.

Let me also highlight, however, that in this movement toward solutions, a major clinical concern which is critical is that of timing. If the clinician only focuses on the positive, if you have clients move toward solutions too quickly, then the clients may *not* feel you have heard their emotional pain, nor appreciated the seriousness of their situations. You need to encourage clients to tell their stories, at their own pace, and to be in charge. But out of the telling of their stories, out of the narrative sharing—and there's a lot of therapeutic value in sharing one's story—new stories emerge that also reveal strengths and resources. As the radio commentator Paul Harvey highlights, there is a need to hear "the rest of the story." Clients come in and tell us their stories. Their stories are often filled with expressions of hopelessness and helplessness. They often convey a tale of having been victimized by individuals, by events, by their feelings and thoughts. It is my job, as the therapist, to not only hear their stories and empathize with them, but also to help them appreciate what they have done to survive and to cope with their feelings—namely, help them attend to "the rest of the story." For "the rest of the story" is often the tale of remarkable strengths.

Keep in mind that the story of how people cope with stressful events such as incest, rape, the Holocaust, war experiences, urban and domestic violence, [and] man-made and natural disasters is inherently the story of resilience and courage of human beings. That is, if you look at the impact of disasters, most people are going to "make it" and *not* evidence long-term debilitating effects. So even in the worst scenarios, people evidence remarkable strengths. As a

---

d. engaging in "undoing" counterfactual thinking of "only if"; "If I only had"; "I should have"; and continually trying to answer "Why" questions for which there are no satisfactory answers;

e. failing to find any meaning or significance in the stressful event;

f. dwelling on the negative implications of the stressful event;

g. seeing themselves as continually at risk or vulnerable to future stressful events;

h. feeling unable to control the symptoms of distress (i.e., viewing intrusive images, nightmares, ruminations, psychic numbing, avoidant behaviors, hyperarousal, and exaggerated startle reactions as being uncontrollable and unpredictable);

i. remaining vigilant to threats and obstacles.

therapist, I need clients to attend to that part of their stories. There are a number of clinical techniques designed to accomplish this goal and to incorporate these features into their personal narratives. Thus, the "bad things" that happened to people are only one chapter in their life stories. And, as Judith Herman [1992] indicates, it is *not* the most interesting chapter of their autobiographies.

HOYT: Oftentimes brief therapists (and others) rush past the painful material, trying to reframe or restructure so quickly that the person doesn't feel heard or validated. Do you think there's also—maybe following from Aristotle—a need for catharsis and abreaction? Is that part of the cure, or is it . . .

MEICHENBAUM: That is a challenging question. I can offer my clinical impressions, given the limited database that exists [see Meichenbaum, 1994]. The question about differential forms of treatment is complex. How one should proceed therapeutically is dependent upon which target group you are looking at. If you are treating people who have experienced traumas that are brief, sudden, yet life-threatening, such as automobile accidents, robberies, rape, and sudden disasters, or what have been characterized as "Type I stressors" [Terr, 1994] . . .

HOYT: You mean relatively discrete, sudden-onset stressors.

MEICHENBAUM: Yes. The data suggest that having clients go through reexperiencing procedures as a means of "coming to terms" with what happened is therapeutic and beneficial. Indeed, there are a variety of very creative clinical techniques, including direct therapy exposure, guided imagery procedures, graded *in vivo* procedures, and the like, that are helpful. They fit your Aristotelian catharsis model and provide a means of "working through" that can prove valuable.

HOYT: What about people with more prolonged trauma?

MEICHENBAUM: When, however, you are treating a different traumatized clinical group, where the PTSD is chronic and the traumatic events occurred many years ago, the treatment decision to undertake "memory work" of having clients "go back" may *not* be the most effective treatment strategy. Having clients recount and reexperience traumatic events, even in the area of incest, may not be the most therapeutic approach. Because in the attempt to conduct so-called "memory work," there is the danger that the therapist can inadvertently, unwittingly, and perhaps even unknowingly, help clients co-create memories. With such prolonged traumas that have a number of secondary sequelae, it is important to address the secondary consequences such as depression, interpersonal distrust, sexual difficulties, addictive behaviors, and the like that may accompany PTSD. The full cognitive-behavioral therapeutic armamentarium needs to be employed to address these signs of comorbidity. A "here-and-now" therapeutic focus, as compared to a "there-and-then" approach, may prove most helpful. Research is needed to determine how to blend the need for "memory work" with a coping skills model. But keep in mind that from a constructive narrative perspective, even when clients are doing so-called "memory work," they are not relating nor "uncovering" history, but rather they are co-constructing history in a mood-congruent fashion. As Donald Spence [1982] observes, it is the "narrative truthfulness," not the "historical truthfulness," of clients' accounts that needs to be the focus of therapeutic interventions.[7]

HOYT: You have worked clinically with many diverse groups, and you have taught and given workshops internationally. How do these guidelines vary across these diverse settings?

MEICHENBAUM: That question raises the important issue of how important it is to be culturally sensitive in formulating a treatment plan. Let me give you an example. As I review in the clinical handbook on PTSD [Meichenbaum, 1994], there are "testimony" procedures that are sometimes used in treating people who have been victims of torture. These procedures have individuals "go public" with what traumas they have experienced and what retribution should occur. For instance, one group of torture victims for whom this testimony procedure has been used came from Argentina, Chile, and other South American countries. Agger and Jensen [1990] have described how having these survivors write out testimonies, bear witness, go back and relive what happened, was highly therapeutic. On the other hand, there is another group of victims of torture who come from Southeast Asia—Cambodia and other countries—who have also received treatment. Therapists such as Mollica [1988] and Kinzie [1994] have indicated that a somewhat different therapeutic approach—one that is designed to deal with their "here-and-now" problems, their practical employment and living situations, rather than do "memory work"—is more effective. The torture victims' cultural orientation suggested that treatment should *not* encourage clients to go back and relive their victimization experiences per se.

Thus, being sensitive to cultural differences should influence the nature and form of the intervention. When I am in doubt, I spell out the treatment options and collaborate with the client in formu-

[7]For some additional discussions of the role of memory in therapeutic reconstruction, see Bonnano (1990), Bowers and Meichenbaum (1984), Rennie (1994), Russell and van den Broek (1992), Sarbin (1986), J. L. Singer (1990), and J. A. Singer and Salovey (1993).

lating, implementing, and evaluating the therapeutic options. This is especially important when the database for alternative treatments is so limited. For instance, Solomon and her colleagues [1992] reviewed some 255 studies on the treatment of PTSD. Out of those 255 studies, there were only 11 clinical trials that employed randomized control groups. Eleven! Five of these were in the area of psychopharmacology with PTSD clients. These five double-blind studies employed a total of 134 subjects, mostly combat veterans. There were only six well-controlled psychotherapy outcome studies. As you can see, we are at such a preliminary stage in the area of PTSD treatment that anyone who gets on a soapbox and says that "Memory work interventions are essential," or who claims that "This is the way to conduct intervention," should be received with a great deal of skepticism and caution, no matter what the therapeutic approach they advocate. It is critical for clinicians to appreciate the scope of our limited knowledge. I also think, however, that straightforward empiricism is *not* going to advance the field. We need a theoretical framework to explain therapeutic approaches. One such theoretical framework is that of a constructive narrative perspective.

HOYT: How would you distinguish the constructive narrative perspective from the other wing of cognitive therapy that sometimes is called "rationalist"?

MEICHENBAUM: I really take issue with the so-called "rationalist" perspective. It is *not* that people distort reality, nor make cognitive errors, that contributes to their difficulties. Instead of one reality that is distorted, as some "rationalists" would advocate, I believe that there are multiple potential "realities." Instead, the focus of therapy is to help the client appreciate how he or she has constructed his or her realities, and what is the impact, the toll, the price, of such constructions. Most importantly, what are the alternative (more adaptive) constructions? I am not alone in highlighting the distinction between the "rationalist" and "constructive" perspectives. For instance, see the ongoing debate between Michael Mahoney and Albert Ellis, and others.[8]

HOYT: How does this apply in the case of individuals who have been traumatized or victimized?

MEICHENBAUM: For instance, consider the client who has been victim-

---

[8]Summaries can be found in Guidano and Liotti (1985), Lyddon (1990), Mahoney (1991), Mahoney and Lyddon (1988), and Meichenbaum (1992a). Controversies abound, and readers interested in watching some of the recent jousting may want, in addition to these references, to look at Ellis (1990, 1992a, 1992b, 1993a, 1993b), Lyddon (1992), Meichenbaum (1992b), and Wessler (1992, 1993).

ized sexually. Envision the clinical impact of this individual characterizing herself as being "damaged goods" or as "soiled property." Such labels, such metaphors, may be culturally reinforced. Whatever the origins and influences of such labels, the consequences of such narrative constructions are likely to lead to dysphoric feelings and distressing behavior. In therapy, I would help the client share her story either in individual or group therapy; validate her feelings; but at the same time help the client appreciate the toll, impact, and price she pays if she goes around telling herself that she is "soiled goods," that she is "damaged property," that she is "useless." In this way, she can come to also appreciate that she speaks to herself in the same manner that the perpetrator spoke to her. She may inadvertently reproduce the "voice" of the perpetrator, as in the case of the victims of domestic violence. She needs to develop her own voice. One goal of treatment is to no longer let the perpetrator continue to victimize her when he is no longer present. Instead, what is the best revenge?

HOYT: Living well.

MEICHENBAUM: To live life well. In therapy, we need to explore with clients operationally what it means to live life well. Moreover, given the cognitive-behavioral approach, therapists also consider with clients what are the barriers, the obstacles, the potential reasons why clients may *not* do anything that they said they are going to do.[9] Thus, when clients say, "I need to live well," there is a need to help clients translate such general admonitions into behaviorally prescriptive statements such as "Between now and next time, how will that show up? What will you do differently?" There is also a need to build relapse prevention procedures into the treatment regimen—anticipating high-risk situations, as well as ways of handling possible setbacks, so lapses don't escalate into full-blown relapses.

HOYT: Some clients will get stuck in what I call a "persistent negative narrative," and oftentimes I think that a horrible stress event confirms for them some underlying schema, some assumptive thoughts they have. To use the example you were just giving, she says, "I *am* soiled property, useless; I *am* a piece of dirt; and this just proves it." How do we then get the person to move out of that belief about herself? Do we go back through the earlier assumptions?

MEICHENBAUM: I don't know the answer to your question, and I don't think the field knows either, but let me offer a clinical strategy that I would be prone to use in such a situation. When the client responds

---

[9]See Meichenbaum and Turk (1987) for a discussion of various clinical procedures designed to facilitate treatment adherence, reduce noncompliance, and enhance client motivation.

with "I'm soiled property," or "I'm useless," or words to that effect, it's usually said with a great deal of emotion. What I would be prone to do as a therapist is to not only attend to the client's words, but to the affect in which it is said. So I would say, "Soiled property? Tell me about that." I would pluck the key words and put them back in the client's lap, and encourage her to elaborate. I would also attend to the feelings with which this was said. The feelings might convey a sense of being overwhelmed, or feelings of being depressed, and the like. I want to learn about the circumstances that led to such self-perceptions and accompanying feelings.

Next, as part of my clinical approach, I "commend" the client for being depressed. After empathetically listening to their distress, I might say something like: "Given what you've been through (citing specific examples), if you were not depressed at times, if you did not feel at times like you were 'soiled property,' or at times as if you were 'useless,' then I think I would be really concerned and conclude that something was seriously wrong." In this fashion, I attempt to validate the client's experience. I am going to go beyond that and even compliment the client for the symptoms of being depressed. For instance, I might say to the client, "What does your being depressed say about what's going on? . . . Perhaps it conveys that you are in touch with your feelings, that you are reading your situation, that you're responsive to what you have experienced."

HOYT: The first step is to join with, to validate, to recognize . . .

MEICHENBAUM: And also to commend the client because her depression and the resultant withdrawal, the labeling of being "soiled property," at one time may have been adaptive. I need to help the client see that when she calls herself "soiled property," that maybe that self-attribution was an impression management stance and her way of trying to control the situation. So even if she says, "You know, I was a zombie with no emotions," I try to have her appreciate that the dissociative responses that she used were adaptive. The critical step in helping her to alter her view of herself is whether I can help her appreciate that what she is continuing to do now, even in "safe" relationships, is no longer her only option. The problem is that she is stuck. It is not that she is "deficient" nor "sick." I am helping her move away from a so-called "deficit model" where she continually questions her self-worth and even her sanity—"Am I losing my mind?" Instead, I want her to appreciate, I want to help her cognitively reframe her experiences as a form of "survival skills." The problem is that she is continuing to do what "worked" in the past, but it may no longer be necessary.

In order to facilitate this transition, I encourage the client to consider the question: What is the impact, toll, price she is paying for being stuck? The answer to this question is *not* discussed in the abstract, but rather the client is encouraged to experientially feel, in the session, the costs of being stuck. Moreover, if the client is stuck, I then ask, in my best Columbo-like style: "What, if anything, can you do to change your situation?" *If* I have laid the groundwork well—by means of

1. plucking key metaphorical terms;
2. validating the client's experience and the accompanying feelings;
3. commending the client for her presenting symptoms;
4. helping her cognitively reframe these symptoms as a form of coping and as a set of survival skills;
5. examining collaboratively how such survival skills worked in the past, but how she continues to do so now, even in situations in which the client is no longer in danger; and
6. considering the devastating impact, the emotional toll, and the interpersonal price of her being stuck—

it is *then* not a big step for the client to offer suggestions about possible ways that she can get unstuck. Remember, my therapeutic goal is to have the client come up with solutions about how to change. If she can come up with possible solutions that could be tried, then she will feel enabled and empowered, and moreover, since she came up with the ideas, there is a greater likelihood that she will follow through. Can I give you another example?

HOYT: Please.

MEICHENBAUM: In fact, I have two cases that come to mind. First, I wish to describe a challenging case of a woman who has experienced a disastrous accident. She was with her fiancé—the only man she had fallen in love with after several previous broken relationships. They were returning from a party and decided to take a shortcut and cross some train tracks. They were running along the train track to get to the other side where this woman lived, and a horrendous thing happened. As the train approached, she yelled out to her fiancé, "Let's beat it," and she darted in front of the oncoming train safely. Her fiancé tripped and did not make it. He was hit by the train and instantly killed. His body was severed.

HOYT: Oh, my gosh.

MEICHENBAUM: It was horrendous. In a dissociative state, she picked up his body parts. It was one of the most horrific stories that I have ever heard. She is suffering from PTSD, depression, and suicidal ideation, as she feels responsible and guilty about his death. Her intrusive thoughts are overwhelming.

I have another case of a mother who had a 10-year-old daughter. They were at home alone. In the middle of the night, she woke up thinking that someone had broken into her home. Since she had experienced such a robbery in the past year, she became fearful. In a state of panic, she reached into her night table to grab hold of a recently obtained pistol that her husband had given her. With gun in hand, she was running into her daughter's room when her bedroom door slammed open and hit her hand, and the gun discharged.

HOYT: Don't tell me.

MEICHENBAUM: Yes. It was her daughter. The mother shot her daughter and blew her daughter's brain away.

HOYT: That is terrible!

MEICHENBAUM: Michael, what are you going to say or do in therapy with these clients? In each instance, I listened sympathetically to the tale of the horrendous events. And eventually asked the mother, "What did you see in your daughter that made your relationship with her so special? Please share with me the nature of the loss." In fact, I asked the bereaved mother to bring to therapy a picture album of her daughter and to review with me the special qualities of her daughter. The picture album permitted the client to tell the story of her relationship with her daughter in some developmental (time-line) context, and thus not delimit her memories to only the time of the shooting—which she played over and over again, with the accompanying narrative of "If only . . . ," "Why didn't I tell my husband I didn't want to own a gun?", "Why my daughter?", "Tell me it is only a dream," "How could I have?", and so forth. Moreover, the review of the picture album provided the opportunity to query further what she saw in her daughter, and, in turn, what did her daughter see in her. Following this exchange, I asked the client, "If your daughter, whom you described as being 'wise beyond her years,' were here now, what advice, if any, might she have to help you get through this difficult period?" Fortunately, with some guidance I was able to help the client generate some suggestions that her daughter might have offered.[10] I then noted, "I can now understand why you described your daughter as being 'wise beyond her years.' She does sound special."

[10]Note that this line of "internalized other" questioning (White, 1988, 1989; Tomm, 1989; Nylund & Corsiglia, 1993) evokes the daughter as an ally rather than as a source of remorse (Hoyt, 1980, 1983).

Moreover, if the client followed through on her notion to commit suicide in order to stop the emotional pain, what would happen to the memory of her daughter? Did she feel that she owed her daughter more? Like many victims of traumatic events, this client found a mission in order to cope with her distress. She undertook the task of educating parents about the dangers of keeping guns in their homes.[11] She became an expert on the incidence of accidental homicides, and developed a foundation named after her daughter designed to decrease the likelihood that this could happen to other children. She felt that if she could save one other child, then her daughter would not have died in vain. Through her actions, she was writing a new script, fashioning a new more adaptive narrative. In therapy, we also addressed her feelings of guilt. I will have to refer you to my clinical manual on treating PTSD [Meichenbaum, 1994] to see the discussion of how such guilt reactions can be addressed therapeutically.

HOYT: I can see what you mean by arranging the conditions whereby clients come up with suggestions themselves, although you could have offered all of the advice that the daughter might have offered.

MEICHENBAUM: You're right, but there is a greater likelihood that clients will follow through if they come up with the ideas than if you, the therapist, give them the ideas. I use a phrase to caution therapists not to act as "surrogate frontal lobes" for their clients.

HOYT: (*Laughter*) I like that—"surrogate frontal lobes." It's better to support the client's own construction. What did you do with the client whose fiancé died in the train accident?

MEICHENBAUM: I used a similar therapeutic strategy, but I had to alter it somewhat. As in the case of the grieving mother, I asked the client who lost her fiancé to help me appreciate what happened exactly, and more importantly—"To help me understand what you saw in your fiancé, Jimmy. What was life like with him? What did you see in him that attracted you to him? . . . What do you think he saw that attracted him to you? . . . If Jimmy were here now, what advice, if any, would he have for you in this difficult time? . . . What do you think would be the best legacy, the best way to remember Jimmy—not only for yourself, but for others who knew him?"

Whereas this strategy worked with the bereaved mother, it did *not* work with this client. When I asked her to come up with advice that Jimmy might offer, she drew a blank. The image of Jimmy's grotesque death was so vivid and current (even some six months

[11]Each year there are approximately 1,400 such deaths in North America (Meichenbaum, 1994).

after the accident) that she could not assume any distance psychologically, to consider ways to handle her distress. So, instead, I pursued a somewhat different line of questioning. Since the image of Jimmy, her fiancé, was too emotionally laden to elicit suggestions about potential coping procedures, I asked her when else she might have experienced a personal loss. She described the loss of her grandmother, whom she loved a great deal. I then asked her what did she see in her grandmother that made the relationship so special. "What do you think your grandmother saw in you? . . . If your wise grandmother were here now, what words of support, what advice, if any, do you think your grandmother might have for you?" (Interestingly, this grandmother sounded like a good cognitive-behavioral therapist!) I then conveyed that "Now I understand why your grandmother was so special."

From my perspective, the "name of the game" is to use the art of questioning to enable and empower clients to come up with possible coping strategies.

HOYT: Thibaut and Kelley [1986], the social psychologists, wrote about "*bubbe* psychology," the native good sense of a wise grandmother.

MEICHENBAUM: But note that in this instance I could have told this client every single thing that the grandmother would have offered, but it would not have been as helpful. It is not just a case of giving information. There is data we review in the Meichenbaum and Turk [1987] book on facilitating treatment adherence that if people come up with ideas themselves and the accompanying reasons for behaving in this fashion, then, as the therapist, you have a greater likelihood of clients' following through than if you, the therapist, offer such advice. Whatever merit there is to our discussion, the readers should take away the notion that they should not be a "surrogate frontal lobe" for their clients. They should *not* do the thinking for them, nor put the words in their mouths; they should be respectful, collaborative, and remember that most people evidence the potential for a great deal of resilience and courage.

HOYT: What about the client who did not have the positive experience that they can draw from with the lost object? The person who says, "I've always had low self-esteem. I'm no good. I deserve what I got." It stimulates earlier relationships that were very negative; the family abused them. What would you have done if she had said, "My father told me I'd never be happy"?

MEICHENBAUM: In fact, that is what happened. Did you see the videotape of this case that I show in my workshop?

HOYT: No, I haven't.

MEICHENBAUM: Because you are right on target. One of the things she says is that her father called her up and conveyed that she is a "total screw-up" because she went down to the tracks. Not only that, but this guy, Jimmy, wasn't that good anyway, so the accident is a "blessing in disguise." Not very sympathetic, to say the least. In fact, she goes on to report a whole series of troubled parental interactions. During the course of therapy, the client came to realize that part of the reason she is so depressed is that she is talking to herself, reproducing the same narrative that her father said. Part of the reason that she is suicidal and depressed is not only due to this horrendous event, but she is playing the same "CD" she heard during her entire childhood. For the client who lacks positive developmental experiences, the therapist can help the client appreciate that she is reproducing someone else's script, that she is playing their narrative. The challenge or question is whether she can develop a voice of her own to write her own narrative.[12] Does she have the courage to do that? But a cognitive-behavioral approach goes further by ensuring that the client has the intra- and interpersonal skills to implement such a new script or construct a more adaptive narrative. Moreover, built into the treatment regimen are such therapeutic procedures as problem-solving training, cognitive restructuring techniques, "homework" assignments, relapse prevention, "personal experiments," and self-attributional procedures. It is *not* enough to have clients produce a new narrative, but this new narrative must be tied into behavioral acts that lead to "data" that is taken as "evidence" to alter the client's view of oneself and the world. While I advocate a constructive narrative perspective, it is important to appreciate that I also employ the full clinical array of cognitive-behavioral procedures that have been found to be so efficacious in treating clients with a number of psychiatric disorders.

HOYT: In psychodynamic terms, they might say that you try to help her "extroject the pathologic introject" in order to get the "voice" of her father out of her head [Hoyt, 1994].

MEICHENBAUM: As you know, mental health workers have their own metaphors to describe therapeutic interventions. There are innumerable potential metaphors. The bottom line is that people come

---

[12]See Gilligan (1982; Gilligan, Roger, & Tolman, 1991) for a discussion of the idea of claiming one's "voice," especially in the lives of women. The work of White and Epston (1990) is pertinent; for further application of the narrative therapeutic use of "voice" in the treatment of eating disorders, see Epston (1989) and Zimmerman and Dickerson (1994). Goulding (1985; Goulding & Goulding, 1979) also asks, "Who's been living in your head?", and describes many ways to take charge of those "voices." Related ideas of "voice" as internalized others include Firestone's (1988) "voice therapy" and Minuchin's (1987) discussion of his family therapy teachers and mentors as "the voices in my head."

into therapy with a "story," and you, the therapist, try to help them change their "stories." Now, clinical theorists can impose their metaphors to describe this process—for example, "extroject the introject." Other theorists use metaphors derived from learning theory, such as "deconditioning" and "habituation," or from information-processing theory in terms of "assimilating/accommodating," "schemas," etc. As I note in the PTSD handbook [Meichenbaum, 1994], there are many alternatives. My own approach is to remain much more phenomonologically oriented, using the client's metaphors. From my perspective, it is better to "unpack" the client's metaphor rather than to impose the therapist's metaphors. By "unpack," I mean help the client to appreciate the adaptive features of how he or she has constructed reality in the past, but to also consider anew what is the impact, toll, and price of continuing to view the world in such a fashion—moreover, to consider in some detail what exactly can be done to change his or her "construction," as well as the ways he or she behaves. From this perspective, the client's altered narrative becomes the "final common pathway" to behavioral change. (It seems that we can't get away from using metaphors when describing our own, as well as others', behavior.)

HOYT: Are you saying that it is better to find *their* central metaphor rather than having to first educate them to believing our system?[13]

MEICHENBAUM: Yes. You want to help "unpack" their metaphor, to have them appreciate the impact, the toll, the price of the stories they tell. Note that this joint exploration is *not* just something intellectual.[14] You need to have the client *feel* in therapy the impact, the toll, the price. And out of such discussions, you can then play your Columbo role. I'll give you an example. A client comes in and says that she "stuffs her feelings." I say, "Stuff feelings? Tell me about that." And we behaviorally and operationally define what "stuffed feelings" means. It's important to listen for such verbs as "stuffed."

HOYT: That is where the action's at, literally and figuratively.

[13]Since "the map is not the territory" (Korzybski, 1933), we can understand virtually all communication to be metaphor. Using clients' metaphors is a way of joining. Moreover, it appreciates their experience and allows it to unfold as they know it. Recognizing the validity of their reality avoids "resistance." They don't have to fight or defend against the therapist's incursion. It moves forward. Aristotle said, "The greatest thing by far is to have command of metaphor." (See Barker, 1985; Combs & Freedman, 1990; Kopp, 1995.)

[14]This same point—the power of experience in relearning—was emphasized by Freud (1914/1958) in his essay "Remembering, Repeating and Working-Through," and, as discussed above, is also central in the concept of the "corrective emotional experience" (Alexander & French, 1946). Cutting across different theoretical approaches, the induction of novelty requires a shift in narrative and thus generates change (Budman, Friedman, & Hoyt, 1992).

MEICHENBAUM: Right. I usually listen very attentively to how clients tell their stories. I especially listen for how clients use transitive verbs. When I hear such verbs being used such as "stuffed," or "noticed," "caught," "put myself down," etc., I pluck these from their narrative and reflect it back to them in an inquiring fashion: "Stuffed feelings?" I explore what she does. And then we consider what is the impact of such behavior. Once we do that, I say, "What could you do about it?" You don't have to be a rocket scientist for the client to then say, "Well, maybe I should not stuff the feelings." Then I say, "Not stuff the feelings. That's interesting. What did you have in mind?" Once again, I am laying the groundwork where the client is going to codefine the problem and collaboratively generate possible solutions. We are now collaborating in this constructive narrative process. Another example is when clients spontaneously offer an example of some strength, some successful coping effort, and I then use this "nugget" (as I perceive it) to ask: "Are you saying that *in spite of* all that you experienced (give specific examples), you were able to do (to try, to achieve—give specific examples)? How did you come to the decision that X? How did you manage to do X? Where did this courage come from?"

The strategy I employ to help clients "restory" their lives is (1) to solicit from the clients an example of their strengths; (2) ask an "in spite of" question, and (3) ask a "how" question. In turn, we can explore how clients can employ these coping skills and take credit for the change they bring about.

This is *not* just a "repair" process, as Schafer [1992] describes. The metaphor of "repair" implies that an individual's narrative is broken, like a tire, and one has to fix it. It conveys that the narrative one is using was "wrong"; it was "broken" and needs to be "fixed." Thus, I try to stay away from the term "narrative repair," but rather, talk about the "constructive narrative process" that clients are now engaged in. The client's narrative may have been adaptive at one time. It wasn't broken; it doesn't need fixing. I don't have to "fix the client's head." Instead, I help clients to become better observers and become their own therapist. As Tomm [1989] suggests, I ask the client, "Do you ever find yourself, out there, asking yourself the kind of questions that we ask each other right here in therapy?" I convey to clients that the treatment goal is to become your own therapist, your own coach. In this way, the clients can learn to take the therapist's voice with them[15] and appropriate, own, and internalize the suggested changes. They can now write their own stories. That is what the therapeutic process is all about.

---

[15]"My voice will go with you" was an expression Milton Erickson would use to encourage continued benefit (Rosen, 1982).

Our research task now is to demonstrate that doing all this makes a difference. The PTSD manual that I have spent the last two years writing [Meichenbaum, 1994] is designed to operationalize these procedures, so that investigators will be able to empirically validate what I have been describing. I thank you for the opportunity to share these ideas.

REFERENCES

Agger, I., & Jensen, S. B. (1990). Testimony as ritual and evidence in psychotherapy for political refugees. *Journal of Traumatic Stress, 3,* 115-130.

Alexander, F., & French, T. M. (1946). *Psychoanalytic Therapy: Principles and Application.* New York: Ronald Press.

Barker, P. (1985). *Using Metaphors in Psychotherapy.* New York: Brunner/Mazel.

Bonanno, G. (1990). Remembering and psychotherapy. *Psychotherapy, 27,* 175-186.

Bowers, K., & Meichenbaum, D. (Eds.). (1984). *The Unconscious Reconsidered.* New York: Wiley.

Budman, S. H., Friedman, S., & Hoyt, M. F. (1992). Last words on first sessions. In S. H. Budman, M. F. Hoyt, & S. Friedman (Eds.), *The First Session in Brief Therapy* (pp. 345–358). New York: Guilford Press.

Budman, S. H., Hoyt, M. F., & Friedman, S. (Eds.). (1992). *The First Session in Brief Therapy.* New York: Guilford Press.

Combs, G., & Freedman, J. (1990). *Symbol, Story and Ceremony: Using Metaphor Individual and Family Therapy.* New York: Norton.

Ellis, A. (1990). Is rational–emotive therapy (RET) "rationalist" or "constructivist"? In A. Ellis & W. Dryden (Eds.), *The Essential Albert Ellis.* New York: Springer.

Ellis, A. (1992a). Discussion. In J. K. Zeig (Ed.), *The Evolution of Psychotherapy: The Second Conference* (pp. 122–127). New York: Brunner/Mazel.

Ellis, A. (1992b). First-order and second-order change in rational–emotive therapy: A reply to Lyddon. *Journal of Counseling and Development, 70,* 449–451.

Ellis, A. (1993a). Constructivism and rational–emotive therapy: A critique of Richard Wessler's critique. *Psychotherapy, 30,* 531–532.

Ellis, A. (1993b). Another reply to Wessler's critique of rational–emotive therapy. *Psychotherapy, 30,* 535.

Epston, D. (1989). *Collected Papers.* Adelaide: Dulwich Centre Publications.

Firestone, R. W. (1988). *Voice Therapy: A Psychotherapeutic Approach to Self-Destructive Behavior.* New York: Human Sciences Press.

Freud, S. (1958). Remembering, repeating and working-through. In J. Strachey (Ed. and Trans.), *The Standard Edition of the Complete Psychological Works of Sigmund Freud* (Vol. 12, pp. 145–156). London: Hogarth Press. (Original work published 1914)

Gergen, K. J. (1991). *The Saturated Self.* New York: Basic Books.

Gilligan, C. (1982). *In a Different Voice.* Cambridge, MA: Harvard University Press.

Gilligan, C., Roger, A., & Tolman, D. (1991). *Women, Girls, and Psychotherapy.* Cambridge, MA: Harvard University Press.

Goulding, M. M. (1985). *Who's Been Living in Your Head?* (rev. ed.). Watsonville, CA: Western Institute for Group and Family Therapy Press.

Goulding, M. M., & Goulding, R. L. (1979). *Changing Lives through Redecision Therapy.* New York: Brunner/Mazel.

Guidano, V. F., & Liotti, G. A. (1985). A constructivist foundation for cognitive therapy. In M. J. Mahoney & A. Freeman (Eds.), *Cognition and Psychotherapy* (pp. 101–142). New York: Plenum Press.

Harvey, J. H., Weber, A. L., & Orbuch, T. L. (1990). *Interpersonal Accounts: A Social Psychological Perspective.* Oxford: Blackwell.

Herman, J. (1992). *Trauma and Recovery.* New York: Basic Books.

Hoyt, M. F. (1980). Clinical notes regarding the experience of "presences" during mourning. *Omega: Journal of Death and Dying, 11,* 105–111.

Hoyt, M. F. (1983). Concerning remorse: With special attention to its defensive function. *Journal of the American Academy of Psychoanalysis, 11,* 435–444.

Hoyt, M. F. (1990). On time in brief therapy. In R. A. Wells & V. J. Giannetti (Eds.), *Handbook of the Brief Psychotherapies* (pp. 115–143). New York: Plenum Press. (Reprinted in M. F. Hoyt, *Brief Therapy and Managed Care: Readings for Contemporary Practice* [pp. 69–104]. San Francisco: Jossey-Bass, 1995.)

Hoyt, M. F. (1994). Single-session solutions. In M. F. Hoyt (Ed.), *Constructive Therapies* (pp. 140–159). New York: Guilford Press. (Reprinted in M. F. Hoyt, *Brief Therapy and Managed Care: Readings for Contemporary Practice* [pp. 141–162]. San Francisco: Jossey-Bass, 1995.)

Janoff-Bulman, R. (1985). The aftermath of victimization: Rebuilding shattered assumptions. In C. R. Figley (Ed.), *Trauma and Its Wake.* New York: Brunner/Mazel.

Janoff-Bulman, R. (1990). Understanding people in terms of their assumptive worlds. In D. J. Ozer, J. M. Healy, & A. J. Stewart (Eds.), *Perspectives in Personality: Self and Emotion.* Greenwich, CT: JAI Press.

Kinzie, J. D. (1994). Countertransference in the treatment of Southeast Asian refugees. In J. P. Wilson & J. D. Lindy (Eds.), *Countertransference in the Treatment of PTSD.* New York: Guilford Press.

Kopp, R. R. (1995). *Metaphor Therapy: Using Client-Generated Metaphors in Psychotherapy.* New York: Brunner/Mazel.

Korzybski, A. (1933). *Science and Sanity* (4th ed.). Lakeville, CT: International Non-Aristotelian Library.

Lyddon, W. J. (1990). First- and second-order change: Implications for rationalist and constructivist cognitive therapies. *Journal of Counseling and Development, 69,* 122–127.

Lyddon, W. J. (1992). A rejoinder to Ellis: What is and is not RET? *Journal of Counseling and Development, 70,* 452–454.

Mahoney, M. J. (1991). *Human Change Processes.* New York: Basic Books.

Mahoney, M. J., & Lyddon, W. F. (1988). Recent developments in cognitive approaches to counseling and psychotherapy. *The Counseling Psychologist, 16,* 190–234.

McNamee, S., & Gergen, K. J. (Eds.). (1992). *Therapy as Social Construction.* Newbury Park, CA: Sage.

Meichenbaum, D. (1977). *Cognitive-Behavior Modification: An Integrative Approach.* New York: Plenum Press.

Meichenbaum, D. (1985). *Stress Inoculation Training: A Clinical Guidebook.* Elmsford, NY: Pergamon Press.

Meichenbaum, D. (1992a). Evolution of cognitive behavior therapy: Origins, tenets, and clinical examples. In J. K. Zeig (Ed.), *The Evolution of Psychotherapy: The Second Conference* (pp. 114–122). New York: Brunner/Mazel.

Meichenbaum, D. (1992b). Response: Dr. Meichenbaum. In J. K. Zeig (Ed.), *The Evolution of Psychotherapy: The Second Conference* (pp. 127–128). New York: Brunner/Mazel.

Meichenbaum, D. (1993). Stress inoculation training: A twenty-year update. In R. L. Woolfolk & P. M. Lehrer (Eds.), *Principles and Practice of Stress Management* (2nd ed., pp. 373–406). New York: Guilford Press.

Meichenbaum, D. (1994). *A Clinical Handbook/Practical Therapist Manual for Treating PTSD.* Waterloo, Ontario, Canada: Institute Press, University or Waterloo.

Meichenbaum, D., & Fitzpatrick, D. (1993). A constructive narrative perspective on stress and coping: Stress inoculation applications. In L. Goldberger & S. Breznitz (Eds.), *Handbook of Stress* (pp. 695–710). New York: Free Press.

Meichenbaum, D., & Fong, D. T. (1993). How individuals control their own minds: A constructive narrative perspective. In D. M. Wegner & J. W. Pennebaker (Eds.), *Handbook of Mental Control* (pp. 473–490). New York: Prentice Hall.

Meichenbaum, D., & Jaremko, M. E. (Eds.). (1983). *Stress Reduction and Prevention.* New York: Plenum Press.

Meichenbaum, D., & Turk, D. (1987). *Facilitating Treatment Adherence: A Practitioner's Guidebook.* New York: Plenum Press.

Minuchin, S. (1987). My many voices. In J. K. Zeig (Ed.), *The Evolution of Psychotherapy* (pp. 5–14). New York: Brunner/Mazel.

Mollica, R. F. (1988). The trauma story: The psychiatric case of refugee survivors of violence and torture. In R. Ochberg (Ed.), *Post-Traumatic Therapy and Victims of Violence.* New York: Brunner/Mazel.

Nylund, D., & Corsiglia, V. (1993). Internalized other questioning with men who are violent. *Dulwich Centre Newsletter,* No. 2, 30–35.

O'Hanlon, W. H., & Weiner-Davis, M. (1989). *In Search of Solutions: A New Direction in Psychotherapy.* New York: Norton.

Rennie, D. L. (1994). Storytelling in psychotherapy: The client's subjective experience. *Psychotherapy, 31,* 234–243.

Rosen, S. (1982). *My Voice Will Go with You: The Teaching Tales of Milton H. Erickson.* New York: Norton.

Russell, R. L., & van den Broek, P. (1992). Changing narrative schemas in psychotherapy. *Psychotherapy, 29,* 344–354.

Sarbin, T. (Ed.). (1986). *Narrative Psychology: The Storied Nature of Human Conduct.* New York: Praeger.

Schafer, R. (1992). *Retelling a Life.* New York: Basic Books.

Simon, R. (1988). Like a friendly editor: An interview with Lynn Hoffman. *Family Therapy Networker,* September/October. (Reprinted in L. Hoffman, *Exchanging Voices: A Collaborative Approach to Family Therapy* [pp. 69–79]. London: Karnac Books, 1993.)

Singer, J. A., & Salovey, P. (1993). *The Remembered Self: Emotion and Memory in Personality.* New York: Free Press/Macmillan.

Singer, J. L. (Ed.). (1990). *Repression and Dissociation*. Chicago: University of Chicago Press.

Solomon, S. D., Garrety, E. T., & Muff, A. M. (1992). Efficacy of treatments for posttraumatic stress disorder: An empirical review. *Journal of the American Medical Association, 268*, 633–638.

Spence, D. (1982). *Narrative Truth and Historical Truth: Meaning and Interpretation in Psychoanalysis*. New York: Norton.

Terr, L. C. (1994). *Unchained Memories: True Stories of Traumatic Memories, Lost and Found*. New York: Basic Books.

Thibaut, J. W., & Kelley, H. H. (1986). *The Social Psychology of Groups* (rev. ed.). New Brunswick, NJ: Transaction.

Tomm, K. (1987a). Interventive interviewing: Part I. Strategizing as a fourth guideline for the therapist. *Family Process, 26*, 3–13.

Tomm, K. (1987b). Interventive interviewing: Part II. Reflexive questioning as a means to enable self-healing. *Family Process, 26*, 167–183.

Tomm, K. (1988). Interventive interviewing: Part III. Intending to ask lineal, circular, strategic and reflexive questions. *Family Process, 27*, 1–16.

Tomm, K. (1989). Externalizing the problems and internalizing personal agency. *Journal of Strategic and Systemic Therapies, 8*, 54–59.

Turk, D., Meichenbaum, D., & Genest, M. (1983). *Pain and Behavioral Medicine: A Cognitive-Behavioral Perspective*. New York: Guilford Press.

van der Kolk, B. A. (1994). The body keeps the score: Memory and the evolving psychology of posttraumatic stress. *Harvard Review of Psychiatry, 1*, 253–265.

Wessler, R. L. (1992). Constructivism and rational–emotive therapy: A critique. *Psychotherapy, 29*, 620–625.

Wessler, R. L. (1993). A reply to Ellis's critique of Wessler's critique of rational–emotive therapy. *Psychotherapy, 30*, 533–534.

White, M. (1988). Saying hello again: The incorporation of the lost relationship in the resolution of grief. *Dulwich Centre Newsletter*, No. 1. (Reprinted in M. White, *Selected Papers* [pp. 29–36]. Adelaide: Dulwich Centre Publications, 1989.)

White, M. (1989). *Selected Papers*. Adelaide: Dulwich Centre Publications.

White, M., & Epston, D. (1990). *Narrative Means to Therapeutic Ends*. New York: Norton.

Zimmerman, J. L., & Dickerson, V. C. (1994). Tales of the body thief: Externalizing and deconstructing eating problems. In M. F. Hoyt (Ed.), *Constructive Therapies* (pp. 295–318). New York: Guilford Press.

CHAPTER 6

Consulting the Problem about the Problematic Relationship

An Exercise for Experiencing a Relationship with an Externalized Problem

SALLYANN ROTH
DAVID EPSTON

Externalizing conversations, introduced by Michael White and David Epston and developed and expanded by them and other practitioners, depict problems as external to people (White, 1989, 1991/1992, 1995; Epston & White, 1992; White & Epston, 1990). In this way of working, problem-externalizing questions replace and exclude problem-internalizing questions. By *problem-internalizing questions,* we mean questions that address the person and problem as one and the same. For example, typical questions from a perspective that views the problem as within the person might be phrased like this: "How long have you been depressed?" and "When you are less depressed, how does your relationship with Sue change?" Or like this: "Have you been a fearful person for much of your life, or is this new?" Such problem-internalizing questions effectively join the problem with the person, so that they are represented as indivisibly

Note. This exercise derives partly from the standard psychodramatic practice of interviewing "parts of people" as "other" than themselves—as particular feelings, ideas, angst, and so on—in order to develop more complex relationships with these "parts." It most immediately draws on David Epston's practice of engaging in clinical dialogues initiated by such invitations as "Do you mind being The Problem and I'll be you?" or "Do you mind being you and I'll be The Problem?" The exercise was partly inspired by a paper by Chris Kinman (1994) and was revised following extensive suggestions by Michael White (personal communication). A variation of this exercise focused on language (Roth & Epston, 1996) has been published in the *Journal of Systemic Therapies.*

We are equal contributors to this chapter. We thank Carole Samworth and Richard Chasin for their generous and generative comments on earlier drafts of this chapter.

unified. Seeing oneself as one with a problem implies that one's identity is the problem or includes the problem, and therefore that change requires the alteration of one's very being (White, 1989, 1991/1992, 1995; White & Epston, 1990).

Problem-externalizing conversations address the person as separate from the problem, and hence as in a relationship with it. For example, in a problem-externalizing conversation, we might ask, "What has Demoralization talked you into about yourself?" and "What has Demoralization talked you into about your partner?"[1] Or we might ask, "As you tell it, Fears have really been pushing you around for the last year or so. Have there been times when you've pushed them back? Even a bit?" Or "Have there been times when you have insisted that Fears stop taking charge of the little things and confine themselves to the big ones?" A key realignment of the person and The Problem thus occurs through problem-externalizing questions: Seeing oneself as in a relationship with a problem (through its objectification or personification), rather than as having a problem or being a problem, immediately opens possibilities for renegotiating that relationship. Moreover, the prescriptions of many cultures induct us into thinking of emotional or behavioral problems as inside ourselves, into blaming ourselves, feeling guilty or ashamed for having these problems, and into experiencing ourselves as helpless to act against our problems without acting against ourselves. In this way, externalizing problems can even be seen as a kind of revolutionary, counter-culture, or counteroppressive act.

We do not see externalizing as a technical operation or as a method (Combs & Freedman, 1994; Freedman & Combs, 1996; Neal, 1996). It is a language practice that shows, invites, and evokes generative and respectful ways of thinking about and being with people who are struggling to develop the kinds of relationships they would prefer to have with the problems that discomfort them (Epston, 1993; Roth & Epston, 1996a; Tomm, 1989; White, 1989, 1991/1992, 1995; White & Epston, 1990). We believe that engaging the people who consult us in problem-externalizing conversations can encourage their capacity to act for themselves in relation to problems; to act upon whatever relational context most immediately supports their problems; and to notice and actively respond to the many ways that their self-stories have been shaped by cultural prescriptions and proscriptions laid down by communities of people in our present, our recalled past, and even the past that came long before our time.

This chapter and the exercise it includes do not describe or teach every aspect of the actual use of externalization in narrative therapies.

---

[1]These kinds of questions were developed by Michael White as a means of "externalizing the internalized problem discourse."

Rather, the exercise gives clinicians who have little or no hands-on experience with this approach a sense of what engaging in an independent relationship with an externalized problem is like, and thus enables them to experience the resulting perceptual shift in thinking about a problem and the person it besets. It is this experience of the power of problem externalization that the exercise is designed to demonstrate, not the complexities of conducting externalizing conversations. These complexities include, for example, ways of assuring that any language introduced by the therapist feels accurate and familiar, as well as new, to those consulting with the therapist. They also include ways of being guided by the person's unique language and descriptions, and ways of assuring that externalizing conversations develop as joint enterprises and are not impositions of the therapist's ideas. These complexities include the ways that problem-externalizing conversations are introduced and coproduced, so that they are not experienced as trivializing of people's pain or as bypassing of their experience. The practitioner attends to the subtle and important differences between working with externalizations of the problem and externalizations of the internalized problem discourse.

Beyond the dimensions we have already mentioned, there is also the particularly effective trajectory of problem-externalizing questions developed by Michael White—those questions that track the problem's "effects on . . . [people's] emotional states, familial and peer relationships, social and work spheres . . . [or the ways] it has affected their view of themselves and of their relationships, [and the ways they have been] . . . recruited into these views" (White, 1991/1992, p. 126). We elaborate none of these points in this chapter.

The rich resources for those who want to consult well-explicated material about the clinical use of externalizing practices include key writings by White and Epston (Epston, 1993; Epston & White, 1992; White, 1989, 1991/1992, 1993, 1995; White & Epston, 1990), as well as recent articles and books by other practitioners that discuss these practices though description and example (Adams-Westcott, Dafforn, & Sterne, 1993; Adams-Westcott & Isenbart, 1996; Combs & Freedman, 1994; Dickerson & Zimmerman, 1993, 1996; The Families, 1995; Freeman & Lobovits, 1993; Freedman & Combs, 1996; Jenkins, 1990; Kamsler, 1990; Linnell & Cora, 1993; Madigan, 1996; O'Neill & Stockell, 1991; Roth & Epston, 1996; Zimmerman & Dickerson, 1996).

SOME COMMON MISUNDERSTANDINGS ABOUT EXTERNALIZING PRACTICES[2]

A common misunderstanding of work that relies on externalizing conversations is the belief that it aims to eliminate, conquer, or kill off problems. It does not,[3] although it can seem to have a divide-and-conquer aspect. Rather, it aims to create linguistic and relational contexts in which people experiencing themselves as burdened, crushed, or taken over by problems can imagine and activate alternative and preferred relationships with these problems.

Can problems be kept in their place? Can they be resisted? Can they be flirted with but not married? Can a problem be an old friend, one a person may have grown past? Can a problem be left behind or put on the shelf? Can a problem learn not to speak unless it's called upon? Can a problem be given enough space to stay healthy and stick around for any good it might do, but not be given so much room that it takes over more territory than the person wants to give it? For example, one would never choose to be taken over by Perfection to the point of becoming immobile, anorectic, or obsessive in behavior; however, one may wish to retain a good enough relationship with Perfection to hand in papers that are not filled with misspellings or to get to work on time. It's not the person who is the problem; it's not even fully The Problem that is the problem. It is, to go the whole way, the relationship of the person with The Problem that is the problem!

Why not try to kill off The Problem? Why do we favor going the whole way—viewing the relationship of the person and The Problem as the problem? First, The Problem may not be only a problem. It may, in some fashion, be a partly a friend. Second, even if it is of no help at all, a long-time associate cannot be retired or sidelined without paying respect to it. And if a person frees himself or herself of a problem, and it returns and tries to reassert itself at some later time, the person is less likely to be humiliated or deeply demoralized if The Problem can be seen as having been set aside, grown past, risen above, or the like, rather than as not having been effectively conquered or killed off.

Another common misunderstanding is the belief that only one problem is externalized in this work, but that is not the case. What is externalized may shift during a single meeting, and shift again and again over the course of several meetings. And often what gets externalized is not the problem the person names at the outset. We may experiment with externalizing anything that a person experiences as a deleterious and intrinsic part of himself or herself. The possibilities are numerous[4]:

---

[2]Zimmerman and Dickerson (1996) discuss common misconceptions about narrative therapy at the broader, theoretical level.

[3]Freeman and Lobovits (1993) propose the utility of a variety of relational metaphors for externalizing conversation. In particular, they question the use of metaphors that denote "power over."

[4]One proviso is not to externalize abuse or other catastrophic events that have actually occurred. Kamsler (1990) and Linnell and Cora (1993) warn of the futility if not danger of externalizing "Abuse" or other such catastrophic events, since the fact of abuse cannot be altered. Rather, one externalizes and works with the effects of the abuse on the identity and abilities of the person, as these effects are subject to change.

They include affect states (e.g., Despair, Hopelessness, Excitement), an internalized problem discourse (e.g., Self-Blame, Self-Negation), a behavior (e.g., Weepiness, Inertia, Mischief), the armor of self-protection that often follows abuse by another (e.g., Silence, Secrecy, Isolation, Numbness), and oppressive social arrangements that have been internalized (e.g., Male Superiority, Racial Disqualification, Standards of Physical Beauty).

Crucial to the effectiveness of a problem-externalizing conversation, whatever its content, is the degree to which people experience it as experience-near and refreshing. Does the conversation leave people feeling that their unique experience in living is being fully, complexly, faithfully, and poignantly described? Do they feel that the conversation is bringing forth descriptions, observations, feelings, and perspectives that seem very close to their experience as they live it? Does the conversation illuminate the obscure and overshadowed; that is, does it go just a step beyond what has previously registered in their consciousness? Do people feel that they are sharing an experience—not a theory—of what is, what has been, and what might be? Are their lived experiences being storied rather than deduced and explicated?

We do not want to support inadvertently the limited and limiting view that externalization is merely a technique, by presenting the exercise that follows in isolation from the larger body of theory that supports the use of externalizing practices in the context of narrative work. For this reason, we will say just a bit about narrative work and the way that these practices fit with it.

NARRATIVE THERAPIES
AND PROBLEM-ACCOMMODATING STORY LINES

Narrative work is based on the belief that the stories we hold about our lives are mined from our relationships and experiences (both past and present), and that these stories shape our present experience and future possibilities. They shape what we see ourselves as being able to do, as well as the ways that we interpret what we and others do. Here we refer to the full panoply of individual, couple, family, institution, culture, and gender stories. When we are in a problem place (troubling predicament), the story lines we draw on and draw forward—those that shape and are shaped by our present meanings and actions—are, not surprisingly, generally those that accommodate the problem place and that accommodate us to the problem place. These problem-accommodating stories limit or even block our access to the full vein of resources available to us. The narrative work we discuss here aims to open access to a greater range of story-line choices for people at those times when the stories they currently live are limited and dominated by meanings that restrict their current lives and foreclose future possibilities (White, 1989, 1991/1992, 1995; White & Epston, 1990).

EMERGING NARRATIVES OF CONTRARY EXPERIENCE

We try to develop clinical and training contexts that cultivate attention to those less noticed—even previously unnoticed—experiences that can be instrumental in countering the dominant, limiting story while promoting stories and actions the person prefers (Epston & White, 1992; White, 1989, 1991/1992; White & Epston, 1990). We focus on aspects of people's experience that are contrary to their problem-accommodating and discouraging way of seeing and describing themselves—and on the generation from that contrary experience of at least one encouraging additional story that has coherence across time. That is, we work with emerging narratives of contrary experience.

The work of drawing forth narratives of contrary experience is often initiated by attention to what White and Epston have called "unique outcomes" (White, 1989; White & Epston, 1990): times when the problem could have prevailed but did not, or when it could have influenced the person more than it actually did. These events are likely to become cornerstones in constructing novel and contradictive narratives—that is, full, historically situated, forward-projected narratives of experience (and identity) that are contrary to the usual story (White, 1993).

Crucial to the emergence of enriched narratives and the new thinking and behavior that they generate is the creation of a context that encourages these narratives of contrary experience. Such a context is more important than the person's recall of individual events or specific acts by the therapist. We foster such a context largely, but not solely (Roth & Chasin, 1994), through the use of externalizing questions. An externalizing conversation is rich in powerful linguistic descriptions that are so at odds with many conventional ways of thinking, talking, acting, wishing, needing, wanting, and evaluating in relation to problems that they often catalyze a swift and fluid transit into new meanings, new observations, and fresh storying. In other words, these descriptions are alternative constructions of reality that enrich the future possibilities available to the person.

A WORD ABOUT THE TRAINING EXERCISE

Next, we present a training exercise we have found to be a lively and potent introduction to the transformative power of engaging in problem-externalizing conversations. We have designed other, related exercises—one emphasizing the use of metaphoric language practices in problem-externalizing conversations (Roth & Epston, 1996a), and another addressing some interviewing structures that encourage the description of people's relationships with problems in experience-near detail and some specific language practices that potentiate the work (Roth & Epston, 1996b).

We invite readers to approach problem-externalizing conversation in this exercise by acting *as if* the statements "The problem is neither the person nor inside the person," and "The problem is the person's relationship with The Problem," were literally true. The aim of the exercise is to provide learners with an experience of a relationship with The Problem so immediate and unusual that it is likely to shift and expand the meanings, questions, and positions available to them as listeners, as inquirers, and as side-by-side allies when they hear clients speak about the challenges in their lives.

Finally, a suggestion: Reading this exercise will not provide the same experience that doing it will. We strongly recommend that learners find some colleagues and do it with them, even if learners have some familiarity with this kind of work.

Whose Life Is It Anyway? A Training Exercise for Therapists to Explore the Relationship of a Person and a Problem from The Problem's Perspective

I. SETTING UP THE EXERCISE

A. Form small groups of four to six people. Each group selects a single, nameable problem familiar to most, such as fear, self-hatred, insecurity, distrust, self-harm, self-negation, nightmares, unwanted habits, intimidation, etc. (3–5 minutes)

B. In each group, one person takes the role of The Problem as it might be experienced by a particular person and/or the person's family. We know that problems often tailor themselves to specific people and contexts, even though they have a great deal in common with other problems of their general type. (1 minute)

C. The person who takes the role of The Problem tells something about the context in which it is operating—one of the stories that situates its activities. For example: "I am Jack's Fear-of-the-Unknown and I have confined him to his house, and even to his bed, for much of his 35 years on this earth. He's epileptic, so he needs me to keep him safe. The doctors say the medication is enough to keep him safe, but I know better. I've also kept him from making a really stupid move—from marrying Judy. He's been talking about getting a job, but I'm working on convincing him that that's really out of the question. Sometimes he thinks that his world is so small he should kill himself, but I tell him if he moves into the larger world it will kill him for sure." (2–5 minutes)

II. INTRODUCTION TO INTERVIEWING THE PROBLEM

Group members who are not enroled as The Problem take the roles of investigative reporters and inquire with great curiosity and interest into its modus operandi. In this sample case, they would interview Jack's Fear-of-the-Unknown about how it established, how it maintains, and how it tries to extend its influential relationship with Jack, his family, his friends, his potential workmates, and others important in Jack's life. Every question to The Problem should be addressed to it as "Jack's Fear-of-the-Unknown," or "Bill's Perfection," or "Amy's Temper," or the like.

III. SUGGESTIONS FOR INTERVIEWING THE PROBLEM ABOUT ITS INFLUENCE ON PERSONS

Instructions for The Problem: Remain fully enroled as The Problem throughout the exercise, and don't slip into being the person, even for a minute. If reporters address you as the person and not as The Problem, tell them you don't know who they are talking to, and remind them of who you are. If the reporter asks anything that you feel is an attempt to be therapeutic, say suspiciously, "You're not a therapist, are you? I thought you were a reporter! If you're a therapist, I'm gone!"

Instructions for reporters: Ask The Problem questions that invite a highly detailed description of its intentions and practices. Your goal is to develop enough material in this interview to write a ground-breaking exposé that will reveal to all just how The Problem operates, and to what purpose. To do this, you need to find out what The Problem does that it considers accomplishments of influence. In other words, what does it do that serves its purposes, and by what means does it go about making sure it can do it? Inquire as fully as you know how to; do not be shy. Problems are often arrogant as well as boastful, and when asked directly, they will talk about things you would imagine they would keep to themselves. You may be surprised at how easy it can be for you to get them to spill the beans. Go for high degrees of specificity!

A special warning to reporters: It can be hard to move away from the traditional therapist role. You might find yourself tempted to be helpful to The Problem, to "cure" it, to get it to see the error of its ways, to reform it, or to rehabilitate it. Only by refusing this temptation will you get The Problem to clarify the following:

A. Its purposes.
B. Its hopes and dreams for the person's life.
C. The myriad techniques it uses to get its way.
D. The voice, tone, and content that it finds most persuasive.
E. Who stands beside it—that is, what people and what forces are in league with it.

Use your questions to bring out The Problem's description of its relationship with the person it is tormenting. If you get really curious about The Problem's means of going about achieving its goals and follow its lead, questions are likely to come easily to you. To follow The Problem's lead in forming your own questions, listen to The Problem with great precision and openness. There are no one-size-fits-all questions for such interviews. Just to warm you up to the task, however, here are some sample questions. Use them to stimulate your own imagination about what kind of interview this can be.

The sample questions below contain more information than the reader was given. We assume that each question develops from The Problem's Responses to the prior questions; subsequent questions are, in a sense, responses to responses. For this reason, the sample questions "flesh out" as we hope your questions will.

IV. CONDUCTING THE ACTUAL INTERVIEW, PART ONE: THE PROBLEM'S WAYS AND MEANS OF ACHIEVING INFLUENCE

Instructions for reporters: Conduct the first parts of the interview with The Problem. Remember, the aim of the first part of the interview is to elicit from The Problem its ways and means of achieving influence over the person. (15 minutes)

Sample questions for part one

- Jack's Fear-of-the-Unknown, did you enter his life as a friend? If so, do you think you are still a friend? Or have you gotten turned around in some way? Are you the legacy of his epilepsy, from the days when he was required to stay close to home and plan ahead for each and every eventuality? The days before he found the right medication?

- Is it your intention to keep him young? As he puts it, "I feel like a three-year-old child, not a 35-year-old man."
- Are you exploiting his controlled medical condition for reasons of your own? What are they? How come you warn him about danger just about every time he gets close to someone? Have you warned him away from each and every one of his friends? How have you convinced him to follow your instructions?
- Jack's Fear-of-the-Unknown, does his reluctance to leave his own neighborhood have anything to do with your insisting that he can only be safe and sound in bed? If so, how does your insistence on this fit with your future plans for Jack? What *are* your plans for Jack, anyway?
- What did you tell him that got him to break off with Judy? How did you persuade him to listen to you instead of to his heart's desires? By what means did you chip away at his confidence?
- Did Pessimism come onto the scene at your invitation? Did you invite Pessimism to join you because you thought you were getting your way and wanted Pessimism to let loose the final blows? Or did you invite Pessimism in because you thought your influence might be slipping?
- How did you win him over to your opinions about what to do with his life? How did you win him away from the opinions of others who know and respect him? And away from his own opinions and feelings about what gives him satisfaction?
- Are you always whispering, "Watch out!", "Be careful!", and so on? Or do you have other things you say to him to convince him to slow down or to stop altogether in following his own dreams? What are they?
- Do you sometimes issue threats like "If you drive over the bridge to town, something will go wrong"? If you do issue threats, which ones have been effective for your purposes? By what means have you gotten Jack to listen to you when you have been threatening him?
- How do you decide when to use threats and when to use whispers? Do you threaten and whisper suggestions to his family members, too? To Judy? Which of them, if any, have you been able to enlist to support you in your efforts to keep Jack jailed in his own home?
- What did you convince him about himself that has made him so susceptible to your whispers and threats?

- Is it your wish to keep Jack holed up in his house with no company except you, Pessimism, and Jim Beam?[5] Is Jim Beam a buddy of yours? What does Jim Beam do to Jack might show me that he's your buddy?
- Are you and Pessimism hoping that Jack's collapse in the face of your restrictions will become so complete that he will do what he has been threatening to do, and take his own life? If he did, would he be taking his own life, or would you have stolen it from him?

V. CONDUCTING THE ACTUAL INTERVIEW, PART TWO: THE PROBLEM'S FAILURE TO ACHIEVE INFLUENCE (or, from The Problem's perspective, the effect of the person on The Problem)

Instructions for reporters: Now conduct the second of the two interviews with The Problem. The aim of this second interview is to elicit from The Problem material about its experiences of failure to influence the person and The Problem's demoralization. In other words, here you want to find out what kinds of encounters The Problem considers as allowing it little or no influence, and what plans it has to reassert its influence. (15 minutes)

Suggestions for interviewing The Problem about its influence on persons: To develop information for part two of your expos, ask The Problem about the following.

A. Times the person has frustrated The Problem's plans, schemes, and dreams.
B. What the person has done to keep some of his or her territory safe from The Problem's grasp or to defy The Problem.
C. What plans The Problem has to reassert itself in the face of such resistance or defiance.
D. What voice, tone, and language The Problem plans to use to reassert itself, to regain influence in the person's life.

Sample questions for part two

- Jack's Fear-of-the-Unknown, has Jack ever been able to resist your smooth-talking, terror-inducing voice? Even a bit? If not in action, has he defied you in his thoughts? Has he ever tricked you into silence for a time? When has he managed to savor his own purposes and dreams, despite your persuasive silver tongue? How do you account for his

[5]A whiskey brand name.

giving you the slip on that occasion? Did he divert your attention? Or did he just plunge ahead as if you weren't even there?

- What conditions set the scene for his closing his ears and his mind to your plans and dreams for his life and opening his ears, mind, and heart to his own plans and dreams for his life? What was your first clue that he was doing this?

- Do you think that when he decided to come to therapy—even to drive across a bridge to do so—this was a sign that he might be growing such a strong voice of his own that it might drown out your whispers and threats?

- Jack's Fear-of-the-Unknown, have you been chagrined not only by Jack's determination to seek therapy but by his drive over the long bridge into town to get it? Has it been unnerving for you that he hasn't had one seizure in five years? Were you taken back by his jogging all the way to the sea last week and not just around the block, as you have always instructed? Has he done other things that have startled, shocked, or frightened you? What are they? Do you feel that you might be losing your grip on him?

- Is it growing harder for you to keep Jack under your thumb? Are you finding him difficult to discipline? To discourage? Is it harder for you to get him to comply? What was your response to his ignoring your dire warnings and engaging in such daredevilish activities last week as driving 200 miles south and then 200 miles back on one weekend to see a football game? Does any of this put you in mind to oppose his opposition to you, Jack's Fear-of-the-Unknown? Have you already opposed his opposition to you? If so, how? Did he see through you when you did this? What were the clues?

- If he keeps on securing himself by his policy of "becoming more secure by being insecure," might he become immune to your policy of "becoming secure by being secure"?

- Might *you* become demoralized if Jack continues to assert that he has "put a dent in Pessimism" by taking his life into his own hands for the first time since he was seven years old? And by his continued feeling that he's ready to "get a life"?

- How will you ever talk him out of listening to Judy, who told him the first time she met him, "I think you are a confident person"? How will you try to talk him back into your idea that bed is safe and sound, when he has started referring to it as a "trap"? Now that Jack has started to see a "daring" future ahead of him, do you think you can still forbid him to dream with your threats and your whispers?

- What will you try to slip in to replace Pessimism and Jim Beam, now that Jack says he won't let either of them continue to cloud his vision or to interfere with his plans?
- Do you think if he continues to ignore you that you'll end up going off in a snit, or do you think you might stick around in the wings just to keep him on his toes? How will you decide?

VI. REFLECTING ON WHAT HAS HAPPENED

All members of the group become themselves and discuss their experience of doing this exercise. *Because The Problem is likely to be quite demoralized, the person enrolled as The Problem must make sure to de-role completely.* (10 minutes)

- What was it like to be The Problem? To be a reporter?
- How was your experience different from, or similar to, the experiences you have had in other professional conversations?
- How do you account for any differences you noticed?
- What surprised you as The Problem or as a reporter?
- How might anything you noticed influence you with your colleagues and clients in the future?

VII. REFLECTING ON WAYS OUR OWN PRACTICES CAN INADVERTENTLY SUPPORT PROBLEMS

The goal of the following question is to stimulate reflection on, and to increase awareness of, the ways that many of our everyday, taken-for-granted ways of speaking and being with people may serve to maintain an internalizing problem discourse: (8 minutes)

- How could we, as therapists, have supported or coached The Problem to be successful in achieving its aims?

CLOSING

As you, our readers, use this exercise to guide you in a conversation with The Problem, we hope that you will feel the cognitive and emotional differences between this kind of conversation and other professional conversations in which you have engaged. We further hope that the exercise provides an experience of the differences between problem externalizing as a technique and problem externalizing as a principled language practice that generates alternative constructions of reality.

People who have participated in this exercise have told us that it was fun. They were surprised to find their imagination and their sense of play engaged even in regard to very serious matters. Many have told us that doing the exercise precipitated a kaleidoscopic shift in their own thinking. We hope that this was also your experience, and we welcome feedback about your use of this exercise and your ideas about other exercises that this one may stimulate you to develop.

REFERENCES

Adams-Westcott, J., Dafforn, T. A., & Sterne, P. (1993). Escaping victim life stories and co-constructing personal agency. In S. G. Gilligan & R. Price (Eds.), *Therapeutic Conversations* (pp. 258–271). New York: Norton.

Adams-Westcott, J., & Isenbart, D. (1996). Creating preferred relationships: The politics of recovery from child sexual abuse. *Journal of Systemic Therapies, 15*(1) 13–28.

Combs, G., & Freedman, J. (1994). Narrative intentions. In M. F. Hoyt (Ed.), *Constructive Therapies* (pp. 67–91). New York: Guilford Press.

Dickerson, V. C., & Zimmerman, J. L. (1993). A narrative approach to families with adolescents. In S. Friedman (Ed.), *The New Language of Change: Constructive Collaboration in Psychotherapy* (pp. 256–250). New York: Guilford Press.

Dickerson, V. C., & Zimmerman, J. L. (1996). Myths, misconceptions, and a word or two about politics. *Journal of Systemic Therapies, 15*(1), 79–88.

Epston, D. (1993). Internalizing discourses versus externalizing discourses. In S. G. Gilligan & R. Price (Eds.), *Therapeutic Conversations* (pp. 161–177). New York: Norton.

Epston, D., & White, M. (1992). *Experience, Contradiction, Narrative and Imagination: Selected Papers of David Epston and Michael White, 1989–1991.* Adelaide: Dulwich Centre Publications.

The Families. (1995). Reclaiming our stories, reclaiming our lives, *Dulwich Centre Newsletter,* 1.

Freedman, J., & Combs, G. (1996). *Narrative Therapy: The Social Construction of Preferred Realities.* New York: Norton.

Freeman, J. C., & Lobovits, D. (1993). The turtle with wings. In S. Friedman (Ed.), *The New Language of Change: Constructive Collaboration in Psychotherapy* (pp. 188–225) New York: Guilford Press.

Jenkins, A. (1990). *Invitations to Responsibility: The Therapeutic Engagement of Men Who Are Violent and Abusive.* Adelaide: Dulwich Centre Publications.

Kamsler, A. (1990). Her-story in the making: Therapy with women who were sexually abused in childhood. In M. Durrant & C. White (Eds.), *Ideas for Therapy with Sexual Abuse* (pp. 9–36). Adelaide: Dulwich Centre Publications.

Kinman, C. (1994). If you were a problem . . . : Consulting those who know about the tactics of a problem. In C. J. Kinman & C. Sanders (Eds.), *Unravelling Addiction Mythologies: A Postmodern Conversation about Substance Misuse Discourse and Therapeutic Interactions* (pp. 32–45). Abbotsford, BC: Fraser Valley Education and Therapy Services.

Linnell, S., & Cora, D. (1993). *Discoveries: A Group Resource Guide for Women Who Have Been Sexually Abused in Childhood.* Haberfield, Australia: Dympna House.

Madigan, S. (1996). The politics of identity: Considering community discourse in the externalizing of internalized problem conversations. *Journal of Systemic Therapies, 15*(1), 47–61.

Neal, J. H. (1996). Narrative training and supervision. *Journal of Systemic Therapies, 15*(1), 63–77.

O'Neill, M., & Stockell, G. (1991). Worthy of discussion: Collaborative group therapy. *Australian and New Zealand Journal of Family Therapy, 12*(4), 201–206.

Roth, S., & Chasin, R. (1994). Entering one another's worlds of meaning and imagination: Dramatic enactment and narrative couple therapy. In M. F. Hoyt (Ed.), *Constructive Therapies* (pp. 189–216). New York: Guilford Press.

Roth, S., & Epston, D. (1996a). Developing externalizing conversations: An exercise. *Journal of Systemic Therapies, 15*(1), 5–12.

Roth, S., & Epston, D. (1996b). *Language Charged with Meaning.* Manuscript in preparation.

Tomm, K. (1989). Externalizing the problem and internalizing personal agency. *Journal of Strategic and Systemic Therapies, 8*(1), 54–59.

White, M. (1989). The externalizing of the problem and the re-authoring of lives and relationships. In M. White, *Selected Papers* (pp. 5–28). Adelaide: Dulwich Centre Publications.

White, M. (1992). Deconstruction and therapy. In D. Epston & M. White, *Experience, Contradiction, Narrative and Imagination: Selected Papers of David Epston and Michael White, 1989–1991* (pp. 109–152). Adelaide: Dulwich Centre Publications. (Original work published in the *Dulwich Centre Newsletter,* 1991, No. 3, 1–21. Also reprinted in S. G. Gilligan & R. Price [Eds.], *Therapeutic Conversations* [pp. 22–61]. New York: Norton, 1993.)

White, M. (1993). The histories of the present. In S. G. Gilligan & R. Price (Eds.), *Therapeutic Conversations* (pp. 121–132). New York: Norton.

White, M. (1995). *Re-Authoring Lives: Interviews and Essays.* Adelaide: Dulwich Centre Publications.

White, M., & Epston, D. (1990). *Narrative Means to Therapeutic Ends.* New York: Norton.

Zimmerman, J. L., & Dickerson, V. C. (1996). *If Problems Talked: Adventures in Narrative Therapy.* New York: Guilford Press.

CHAPTER 7

From Deficits to Special Abilities
Working Narratively
with Children Labeled "ADHD"

DAVID NYLUND
VICTOR CORSIGLIA

Attention-deficit/hyperactivity disorder (ADHD) is being diagnosed in epidemic proportions.[1] The *Diagnostic and Statistical Manual of Mental Disorders*, fourth edition (DSM-IV; American Psychiatric Association, 1994) describes ADHD as a clinical disorder characterized by problems with inattention, hyperactivity, and impulsivity. According to conventional psychiatry, ADHD is a neurological condition that requires assessment, medication, and/or behavior therapy to alleviate or control the symptoms (Barkley, 1990). This chapter presents a narrative approach to children who are labeled "ADHD." The theoretical ideas that underlie this approach are discussed. Two clinical case examples from our work are then presented to illustrate these concepts.

THE TRADITIONAL PSYCHIATRIC APPROACH

As therapists who are informed by the narrative metaphor, we take an approach in our work with these children that is very different from the traditional psychiatric approach. Rather than viewing ADHD as an essential biological condition, we understand ADHD as a social construct that exists in discourse (Law, 1995; Nylund & Corsiglia, 1994a;

[1]Although this is not the focus of this chapter, we have speculated about the pandemic numbers of children diagnosed as having ADHD. Although it has been estimated that 3–10% of children are diagnosed with ADHD, a recent study stated that 50% of school-age boys are described as "hyperactive" and referred to mental health agencies (Crook, 1994). A recent *Time* article (Wallis, 1994) claimed that the use of Ritalin, the drug of choice
(continued)

Weaver, 1994). From this social constructionist perspective (McNamee & Gergen, 1992), we conceive of the traditional psychiatric approach to ADHD as a discourse that has influence in the lives of families and children. We question the taken-for-granted "truths" of the traditional ADHD discourse, which characterizes the young person in pathological terms, privileges "expert" knowledge, and restrains alternative discourses that may be more empowering.

Instead of totally dismissing the traditional ADHD discourse, we contend that it should coexist along with other discourses. This positioning allows us to recognize the value of the dominant discourse. Many families we have worked with state that practices associated with the traditional ADHD discourse can be useful. For instance, once a child has been diagnosed as having ADHD, many educational services are made available to him or her. Second, the ADHD diagnosis helps reduce parent and teacher blaming. Relatedly, the child who is diagnosed with ADHD may no longer be scapegoated and described as "lazy" (Buchanan & Stayton, 1994; Kelly & Ramundo, 1994). Lastly, medication can help some young persons improve their attention (Zametkin et al., 1990; Griffith & Griffith, 1994).

Although we acknowledge these possible merits of the established psychiatric approach to ADHD, we believe that the diagnosis may have a totalizing and narrowing effect on a child's life. From a narrative perspective (White, 1991; White & Epston, 1990), the child's ADHD diagnosis may invite parents and professionals to develop a deficit-saturated story about the young person. Past, present, and future events can be interpreted through the lens of that problem story. The parents and/or teacher may then only notice events that fit with the dominant, problem story; experiences that do not fit with the dominant story are edited out. Thus, the dominant story of "My child has ADHD" may restrain parents from noticing times when their child was, is, or may be more focused and less distracted.

The deficit-saturated story is supported by restraints that prevent parents, professionals, and/or the child from noticing exceptions to the problem. These restraints can include certain "essentialist" or "expert" ideas about ADHD. For example, essentialist ideas of ADHD may invite

---

(*continued from p. 163*) for ADHD, has increased significantly; prescriptions are up more than 390% since 1990. We wonder to what extent the increased numbers are a reflection of (1) overwhelming classroom sizes, which make it impossible for teachers to attend to the unique needs of children (thus, children who require a stimulating educational experience may be bored in these classrooms and, hence, become vulnerable to being diagnosed with ADHD); and (2) the recent flurry of media exposure and self-help literature on ADHD (Hallowell, 1994; Wallis, 1994). We also wonder whether marginalized ethnic groups will be particularly vulnerable to being labeled "ADHD" through the lens of the dominant (white) culture.

parents to assume a one-down position in relationship to the profession-als' expert knowledge. One of the more common ways that parents (and the child) assume a one-down position is through the psychological testing technologies. There are an increasing number of assessment tools and measurements to determine whether a child "has ADHD" (such as the widely used Conners rating scales; see Barkley, 1990). Therapists who embrace expert language and expert knowledge can become convinced that their psychological assessment tools are "real," "true," and objective. Such therapists may not take into account how their assessment proce-dures and assumptions influence the data that are being obtained. Hubble and O'Hanlon (1992) refer to this phenomenon as "delusions of certainty" and "hardening of the categories."

Other commonly accepted therapy practices, such as behavior modification and psychoeducation, may also undermine a young per-son's local and unique knowledge. Traditional behavior therapy and psychoeducation can be highly prescriptive, instead of being collabora-tive endeavors: The clinician, from an authoritative stance, instructs the child and family as to what will be helpful. Although behavior therapy techniques and information may be useful, the family and young person can be rendered passive objects by the therapist's expertise. From the expert position, the therapist may suggest parenting management tech-niques that, instead of being experienced as helpful, reinforce parent blaming. Parents have told us that teachers, therapists, and/or physicians often offer unsolicited advice from a very judgmental stance (e.g., "Johnny needs a parent who can stay on top of him"). Moreover, if the parents do not follow through with the therapist's directives, they are labeled as "resistant." This one-way therapy process preserves hierarchies of knowledge, while possibly discouraging the unique solution knowl-edges that the young person and family may possess.

Other ideas (such as advising parents that their expectations need to be lowered) invite despair and self-blame. We agree with Cade (1990), who states: "It is my opinion that using a diagnosis such as 'hyperactive' is largely unhelpful (unless you manufacture Ritalin, or some other similar medication) and often leads to pessimism and resignation on the part of parents (and therapists)" (p. 45). These reduced expectations and resultant pessimism can recruit both the child and his or her parents into reciprocal patterns of interaction that support the problem.[2] As the parents' expectations are lowered, their child is inadvertently invited to act in less age-appropriate ways. The child may blame certain problem

---

[2]See Dickerson and Zimmerman (1992) for discussion of reciprocal patterns of invitation. For example, a young boy may neglect his homework, which may, in turn invite his parents to do his homework for him, which may inadvertently cooperate with the problem (the boy's not initiating and doing his own homework).

behaviors on ADHD that are under his or her control, and thus abdicate personal responsibility. Parents, particularly if they place ADHD exclusively within the domain of their child's biochemistry, can also surrender responsibility for aspects of the problem(s) that they could manage and change.

Traditional ADHD discourse is deficit-based and objectifies the person (Foucault, 1980; Gergen, 1994; Stewart & Nodrick, 1990). Hubble and O'Hanlon (1992) state that labels stick to persons like "crazy glue" and may have a disempowering effect; one has to be careful not to create a "self-unfulfilling prophecy," as Hoyt (1994) has put it. In summary, traditional ADHD therapy ideas and practices limit the discourse of alternative knowledges and descriptions, and may disqualify children and families from bringing forth more empowering alternatives.

AN ALTERNATIVE MODEL: NARRATIVE THERAPY

There have been attempts by educators and family therapists to address the reductionism associated with the medical/psychiatric discourse on ADHD (O'Callaghan, 1993; Kohn, 1989; Schachar, 1986; Schrag & Divoky, 1975). These professionals contend that the environment causes the behaviors traditionally described as aspects of ADHD. Most of these arguments replace a reductionistic biological model with an equally simplistic environmental model. Most ADHD discourse is reduced to a "pejorative dualism" (Buchanan & Stayton, 1994), a simplistic "either–or" position. Instead, narrative ideas are situated in therapeutic practices that encourage multiple perspectives ("both–and"; Lipchik, 1993), deconstruct expert knowledge, and generate alternative and local knowledges. Instead of a preoccupation with the etiology of ADHD, the narrative therapist is interested in what ADHD *means* to the child and the family. Through a conversational domain, family stories about ADHD, the child, and medication are explored. Preferred and healing stories are coconstructed, with the therapist adopting a therapeutic stance of curiosity and uncertainty. We outline the process of therapy and then provide clinical examples.

After joining with the family, we ask each member of the family about the problem. Usually, the parent(s) state that their child "is hyperactive" or "may have ADHD." In a majority of the cases, a previous professional (teacher, pediatrician) has told the parents that their son or daughter is hyperactive and may require stimulant medication and therapy. We ask each family member to tell his or her story without interruption. Very carefully, a description of the problem that everyone agrees with is coconstructed. This may be difficult, because one or both parents may invite us to confirm the diagnosis by asking questions such as "Is Johnny

ADHD?" We decline such invitations by stating, "I don't know; I need to ask more questions." Of particular interest is the family's language about the problem. From the onset, we use nontechnical language rather than clinical language to describe the problem. We encourage the parents to describe the problem in such a way that is "experience-near" to the child (White, 1992a). This may include the child's and parents own descriptions, such as "the fidgities," "the inattention," or "the hyper monster." Most adolescents we have worked with prefer to call the externalized problem by its clinical name, "ADHD." In addition, we inquire about problems that "team up" with ADHD, such as "trouble" or "temper."

Many traditional approaches privilege verbal therapy and focus primarily on working with the parents. As narrative therapists, we are interested in entering the worlds of children in addition to working with the parents. Although our therapy can be highly verbal, we also value young persons' unique ways of expressing themselves. This is referred to as a "child-focused family therapy" (Freeman & Lobovits, 1993; Epston, 1995). Therapy that relies solely on the spoken word can exclude and marginalize children in the therapeutic process (Stacey, 1994). Sometimes, particularly with children who are artistic, we invite them to draw or paint the externalized problem. Artwork helps to personify and further separate the problem from the young person. Drawings are particularly useful with children who prefer nonverbal methods of communication. Other alternative modes of therapeutic conversation may include puppets or role playing (Dunne, 1992; Freeman & Lobovits, 1993). Many children labeled "ADHD" prefer these more active ways of expressing themselves. These more artistic modes tend to bring forth a young person's imagination and solution knowledges.

After coconstructing a description of the problem, questions are asked to determine the effects of the problem in the lives and relationships of the family members.

Through an externalizing conversation about the problem, the dominant, problem-saturated story is separated from the child. Complementary questions may be asked to invite family members to consider their inadvertent participation in reciprocal patterns that collude with the problem (Stewart & Nodrick, 1990). Further questions are asked to deconstruct the parents' ideas and understandings about ADHD. These deconstructing questions may also invite the parents to explore restraining ideas that support the problem. Critical to this process is to determine the meanings that the parents and child have constructed for ADHD.

We encourage young persons to describe their experiences with ADHD. John, age 15, described ADHD as "being able to watch two TV channels at the same time . . . I pick up something from each channel." With the child's and parent's consent, these novel descriptions are passed on to others affected by ADHD, so that we and they can appraise whether their experience is similar or not. The purpose is to replace psychiatric and medical ideas on ADHD with alternative ideas that are generated by the families we work with.

Often the child referred to us has already has been diagnosed with ADHD, and the parents and child are very comfortable with the diagnosis. The child may have already started taking medication. Instead of attempting to argue them out of their construction of the problem, we take up a stance of curiosity. We may ask questions such as these:

- How has the diagnosis been helpful?
- What are the limitations of the diagnosis?
- How has the medication helped, and what behaviors does it seem not to help?
- What are some qualities your child possesses that are separate or have nothing to do with ADHD?

These deconstructing questions are intended to invite the parents and the young person to separate from some of the taken-for-granted views on ADHD. They suggest that the current psychiatric discourse on ADHD may not fully account for their experience.

Early in therapy, parents will typically furnish us with written reports from their child's teacher. This report usually describes the young person's learning deficits (e.g., problems with concentration, difficulty in reading or writing for long periods of time, problems with sitting still and not talking). Such a focus on the young person's deficits may reinforce the idea that he or she is "dumb" or "stupid." We invite young persons labeled "ADHD" to reconsider the idea that they are incompetent; we suggest instead that they are much more intelligent then they have believed, but according to different standards than those privileged in our society. Many of these young persons possess many creative talents (e.g., capacities for music, sports, dance, spatial awareness) that fall outside the narrow band of skills our society most values. Engaging families in a deconstructing conversation about the effects of the Western educational system assists both parents and children in recognizing the extent to which our schools privilege certain abilities such as logic, repetitive tasks, and mathematical capacities, and overlook creative skills such as art, music, athletics, and dance.

During the deconstructive stage in therapy, we may inquire about the effects of the traditional school system. We may ask parents such questions such as the following:

- Do you think our schools are set up to meet the unique and creative needs of your child? Or does your child's school favor students who sit still and perform repetitive tasks?

- Should children who learn in different ways be seen as having a deficit?
- Do you think the recent epidemic of ADHD has more to do with better clinical measurements that are objective? Or are more children being labeled "ADHD" because of our schools' being placed under the burden of underfunding and teacher overload?

After this deconstruction process, the cultural conditions that shape traditional ADHD discourse are more visible to parents and families. Often parents begin to hold society and the Western school system accountable for problems associated with ADHD, and cease pathologizing their children. Deconstruction also makes it more possible for young persons to discover and appreciate their special gifts that have been undervalued in the dominant culture. Many times, we encourage these young persons to view themselves as "weirdly abled" (Epston, 1993).

Next, we encourage the child to "reclaim" the gifts and talents that have been "hijacked" by the problem, and use them for his or her advantage. At this point, many children begin to view their so-called "deficits" (distractibility, short attention span, hyperactivity, impulsivity) as special abilities, such as flexibility, being able to monitor their environment, being independent, and/or being tireless. Once young persons have accessed their own unique skills, they are more likely to generate their own solutions to problems (Epston, 1991).

We are particularly interested in the metaphors a child and family use in relation to the externalized problem. Rather than suggest and impose our metaphors, we encourage the family and child to choose their preferred ways of relating to the problem. Sometimes the child prefers to "defeat" or "beat" the externalized problem. Other times, the child may favor a metaphor of power in relation to the problem (Freeman & Lobovits, 1993; Stacey, 1994). Such metaphors may include coexistence and compromise with the problem rather than fighting against the problem. With problems such as distractibility, a coexistence metaphor may be more useful than a defeat metaphor. A coexistence metaphor invites the young person to redefine his or her relationship with the externalized problem. For example, a young person we worked with, Jimmy, used "mental aikido" to help him rechannel his "brain energy" to improve his concentration (he was taking an aikido course at the time). Many of the metaphors associated with martial arts—self-discipline, self-control, centering one's focus—fit nicely with the idea of coexistence.

Once the metaphor is chosen for how to relate to the problem, and the ideas surrounding the problem are deconstructed, space is opened to notice "unique outcomes"—those aspects of a young person's life that are free from the influence of the ADHD. These "unique outcomes" serve as entry points to an alternative, preferred story.[3] Reauthoring questions are then asked, to make meaning of the unique outcomes (White, 1991). In addition, tapes or letters sent to the child and/or parents can contribute, reinforce, and expand the new story (Nylund & Thomas, 1994; Epston, 1991, 1994; White & Epston, 1990).

To sustain the new story, recruiting an audience to authenticate the solution knowledges is helpful. Letters sent to teachers or treatment reports (letters of reference) to physicians can be very valuable, along with the follow-up letters sent to families (Nylund & Thomas, 1994; White & Epston, 1990). Reflecting teams (Andersen, 1991; White, 1991), in which observers provide their multiple perspectives, can also be valuable in highlighting the new story. Lastly, "consulting your consultant" interviews (Epston & White, 1990) and certificates that document the young person's changes (White & Epston, 1990) can be used to celebrate and acknowledge the new story. We feel that "consulting your consultant" interviews (documented on videotape, on audiotape, or in writing) are invaluable in generating local knowledges with families affected by ADHD.[4] When young persons or parents seek our advice on a particular problem related to ADHD (e.g., how to improve one's concentration), we refer them to our "anti-ADHD league" archives.

Medication is a central issue with children who are labeled "ADHD." Either a child is already on stimulant medication (such as Ritalin), or the parents or professionals want the child placed on medication. We agree with White (1992b), who states that he is not opposed to medication if it is "enabling of people." However, we are concerned about the negative effects and limitations of pharmacological treatment. For instance, the hierarchical power imbalance between the physician who prescribes the medication and the child/family may marginalize the parent's and child's concerns, experience, and own knowledges of solutions. It has been our experience that many children labeled "ADHD" are given simplistic and deficit-saturated explanations about the problem(s) from their psychiatrist or pediatrician (often the prescribing physician does not even explain to the child why he or she is taking medication). One such explanation is that ADHD is solely a biochemical deficiency. This explanation invites children and families to depend too much on the drug for the entire solution. Similarly, families and children affected by ADHD may have

---

[3]We think that it is important for the young person and family to evaluate the unique outcome as significant, rather than for the therapist to attempt to convince the family that the unique outcome is meaningful. When the therapist enters a convincing position, he or she may be conducting "solution-forced" therapy (Nylund & Corsiglia, 1994b).

[4]"Consulting your consultant" (Epston & White, 1990) refers to a practice of interviewing the young person on tape as an expert on overcoming the problem. The tapes are collected and make up antiproblem archives that others can view to gain knowledge and inspiration.

unrealistic expectations about what the medication can accomplish because of clinicians' "promising too much" (Griffith & Griffith, 1994, p. 202). These unrealistic expectations may lead to disappointment.

A loss of a sense of personal agency may be another effect of overemphasis on pharmacological therapy. As Griffith and Griffith (1994) state:

> For many, taking a medication evokes images of weakness, loss of responsibility, and submission to medical authorities. Historically, these are attributions that have closely accompanied the sick role in Western culture. These associations can invite an emotional posture of submission that obscures a patient's awareness of life choices, to the patient's detriment. (p. 199)

We have found that on many occasions a young person describes the medication as the sole reason for his or her success, while undermining his or her personal strengths and characteristics, imagination, creativity, and motivation.

Our reservations about stimulant drugs notwithstanding, we will, under certain circumstances, refer a child for a medication evaluation. We feel more comfortable in making the referral when conditions of *true informed consent* are respected. These include the following:

1. The family has a good understanding of the medication, its side effects, and what the medication can and cannot do (with special emphasis on its limitations).
2. The outcome measures for what the medication may accomplish are coconstructed by the family, child, and psychiatrist.
3. The family is in control of when and whether a trial of medication is started (as opposed to a professional's heavily urging the child and parents to start the child on medication).
4. The psychiatrist who is prescribing the medication uses nonclinical language that the child can understand.
5. The child's concerns and meanings about taking medication are taken into account, explored, clarified, and destigmatized.

When a young person is labeled "ADHD," many systems may become involved (teachers, counselors and psychologists, pediatricians, psychiatrists, probation officers, other therapists, etc.), all with their own ideas, constructions, and concerns. Anderson and Goolishian (1988) refer to these systems as "problem-organizing, problem-dissolving" systems. Many of the systems can develop rather adversarial relationships, with each system blaming another part of the system for the problem (it is particularly easy for tension and reciprocal blaming to arise between the school and parents). Usually, the family and young person are left out of this dialogue and may easily be blamed or pathologized. To address this potential problem, we prefer to have ongoing, collaborative relationships with the school and physicians. Ideally, it is helpful to have a joint meeting with the teacher and other school officials, the parents, and the young person to discuss everybody's concerns. In this meeting, we ask for specific, behavioral descriptions of these concerns; these help to forestall the tendency for people to use clinical, vague, and pathologizing descriptions. Once everyone has given a specific description of the problem(s), we co-create a common goal that all can agree upon. Through the therapy process, we bring the school and other systems up to date with preferred developments via letters or phone dialogue. The family and young person are made aware of these discussions, so as to not feel "out of the loop." This ongoing communication with the school and other professionals helps to circulate and authenticate the alternative story.

CLINICAL VIGNETTES[5]

The first example illustrates an initial session with Nicole, a very bright 8-year-old. In this first session, we demonstrate questions we use in deconstructing and externalizing ADHD. We also include transcript from a follow-up session. The second example portrays a "consulting your consultant" interview with 12-year-old Shawn and his mother, as they shared their solution knowledges that might be passed on to others affected by ADHD.

Nicole

Nicole was referred to our clinic by the school because of her teacher's concern that she might be "ADHD." Attending the appointment were both her parents, who were concerned with some of the reports they had been receiving from Nicole's teacher. According to the school reports, Nicole had difficulty with sitting still in class and paying attention. The teacher had recommended a medication evaluation.

THERAPIST: What's your understanding of ADHD?

MOM: Well, I think it has to do with problems paying attention.

THERAPIST: So that's what you've heard from the teacher?

---

[5]David Nylund was the therapist in both cases.

MOM: Yes, she [the teacher] seems real concerned and think Nicole needs Ritalin. We're concerned, too.

THERAPIST: How have you expressed your concerns to Nicole? Have you talked with her about it?

MOM: Yes, Nicole said it's hard for her to listen to the teacher and sit still.

THERAPIST: It's tough sometimes, Nicole, to listen to the teacher?

NICOLE: Yes.

THERAPIST: So you have a lot of energy?

NICOLE: Yes.

THERAPIST: Do you have fun with your energy? What kind of things do you do with your energy?

NICOLE: I like to play outside.

MOM: She's good at soccer and other sports.

THERAPIST: Really! So using her energy is one of her best talents?

DAD: Yes, she can be a lot of fun. She's very social.

THERAPIST: Does your energy, Nicole, make it tough sometimes to listen to the teacher?

NICOLE: Yes.

[Later in the session:]

THERAPIST: Is school fun or boring to you?

NICOLE: Boring . . . my mind wanders.

THERAPIST: Your teacher wonders if that is ADHD. You know, when it's hard to sit still and listen to the teacher. . . . What would you call it?

NICOLE: (*Ponders*) Tickles.

THERAPIST: Tickles! That's a great name! (*Family laughs*) So what do the Tickles get you to do?

NICOLE: They make my feet tired because I go like this (*she demonstrates by swinging legs back and forth*). My hands hurt too after a while, because I move them around too.

THERAPIST: What else do the Tickles do?

NICOLE: I can't sit still in my chair.

THERAPIST: Do the Tickles lead to trouble?

NICOLE: Sometimes the teacher has to remind me to get back in my seat.

MOM: Before she would get in trouble, but now the teacher is more understanding. She lets Nicole get out of her seat and let some of her energy out from time to time.

THERAPIST: So has that helped keep Trouble away?

NICOLE: Yes.

THERAPIST: What happens when the teacher is talking to the class or writing on the board? Could you show me? How about I play your teacher and you act as if you're in class. [Because of Nicole's playfulness and energy, the therapist decided to utilize a more active way of discussing the problem. In the role play, he played her teacher talking and writing on the board, while Nicole sat in a chair moving her legs back and forth and looking around the room.]

THERAPIST: That was good. I get a good sense of what happens when the Tickles are in charge. Do you see the Tickles as your friend or enemy?

NICOLE: They're a friend when I am playing.

THERAPIST: How about when you're in class?

NICOLE: An enemy, I guess.

THERAPIST: What would you like to do about these Tickles in class?

NICOLE: I'd like to listen to the teacher.

THERAPIST: How could you do that even when the Tickles are around?

NICOLE: Ignore them and pay attention to the teacher.

THERAPIST: That's a good idea! Have you found any way to ignore them?

MOM: Lately when I read to her, she looks all around the room at everything. I notice her head is going all over . . .

DAD: Yes, her head goes all over, but when her mom asks her what the book was about, she can tell her mom in detail the whole book.

THERAPIST: How do you do that? That's quite a skill! You pay attention while looking all around. Can you teach me your skill? Because when I don't make eye contact with the person, I don't hear what they say. How do you do that?

NICOLE: I look at everything. I like to look around and listen at the same time.

THERAPIST: So you're real curious and real observant? You can pay attention to many things at one time? Is that when you turn the Tickles into your friend?

DAD: Do you think that the Tickles have something to do with me? Because when I was a kid, I couldn't pay attention and learn sitting still. I have to learn practically hands-on.

MOM: Yes, he has to work with his hands.

DAD: Yeah, I work with appliances. When I went to school to learn this, I couldn't understand it by the book, but when we went to the shop to learn hands-on, I learned real fast.

THERAPIST: So you're good at your "hands thinking" [a term borrowed from Kathleen Stacey, 1994]. You've been able to utilize your best skills to your advantage. I wonder if Nicole can learn from you?

DAD: Yes, she's real good at working with her hands. She builds things, loves to do the dishes!

THERAPIST: So, Nicole, you're talented at hands thinking? It seems the Tickles have left your "ears thinking" a bit behind your hands thinking. What I mean by ears thinking is listening to the teacher ["ears thinking" is another term invented by Stacey, 1994]. It seem our schools downplay hands thinking and only recognize kids who are good at ears thinking. Do you agree, Dad? Was that your experience? [This is an attempt at deconstructing the culture's preference for learning by sitting still and reading while discounting other ways of learning.]

DAD: Yes, I thought I was dumb in school. But I'm pretty smart at working with appliances.

THERAPIST: So, Nicole, you're good with your hands; you're good at paying attention at many things at once. What else are you talented at?

MOM: Well, the teacher says she's really been trying lately. The teacher catches Nicole sitting on her hands to keep them still and really trying to pay attention.

THERAPIST: Wow, can you show me how you do that? (*Nicole sits on her hands*) Was that your own idea? (*Nicole nods yes*) Can I pass that on to other people who struggle with listening to the teacher? (*She again nods yes*) You have many abilities. Did you know that? Do the Tickles know it?

NICOLE: I don't know.

THERAPIST: So you're going to work on ignoring the Tickles and using them as your friend at the right times—like during recess. What does it tell you about Nicole that's she's coming up with her own techniques in ignoring the Tickles?

MOM: We think she's trying. We hope she can deal with this without medication.

DAD: Yes, we don't like the idea of medication.

MOM: Yes, I have heard some negatives about the medication. I have a friend who is in her 30s and when she was 8 she was put on Ritalin, and she hated it because it made her feel drugged and feel not in control of her body. So we would prefer her not taking medication.

THERAPIST: Okay, why don't we reschedule, and we won't schedule you with a doctor for medication due to your concerns.

[The therapist listens to their concerns and does not assume that this means "resistance" or that medication is necessary for solution. The session continues for a while longer; all parties review the discussion and make plans for the next meeting.]

Nicole and her family were seen for two more sessions over a two-month period. Her attention continued to improve, according to her teacher's reports. We then did not meet for six months. The following conversation took place at our fourth meeting, which occurred eight months after our initial visit.

THERAPIST: Well, it's been a while since we've seen each other. I'd like to catch up with you and see how things are going. How are you doing, Nicole? How are the Tickles?

NICOLE: Okay. I don't feel the Tickles as much.

DAD: She's been changing a lot.

THERAPIST: She has? How so?

DAD: She's paying attention and listening better, and her reading skills have improved.

THERAPIST: So Nicole has strengthened her concentration?

MOM: Yes, we're real proud of her. She's trying real hard to control the Tickles.

THERAPIST: Really! How are you taking your thinking back from the Tickles?

NICOLE: I just try not to be looking around the room.

MOM: What else? What else works, Nicole? Share your secrets.

NICOLE: I put my hands in my lap.

MOM: Show me. (*Nicole puts her hands in her lap to demonstrate her technique*)

THERAPIST: So that helps control her hands moving around.

NICOLE: Yes.

THERAPIST: And you've done this without any medication?

MOM: Yes. The teacher said she's doing great. She gives Nicole a lot of freedom to do the work in her own way. She's a very good teacher. She uses Nicole's energy in a positive way.

THERAPIST: You know, I was thinking: Nicole has a great deal of creativity and energy. Do you think if Nicole was a boy that her energy would be seen as so problematic by her second-grade teacher? Do you think boys are allowed more freedom to be active than girls—that if girls are energetic, they are seen as problematic or ADHD?

MOM: Yeah, maybe so. Maybe there's a double standard.

[Later in the session:]

THERAPIST: What about the way I worked was helpful or not helpful?

MOM: Nicole felt very comfortable with you and understood what you were explaining to her. It helped her understand the problem of staying still. I liked the way you talked about the problem as the Tickles.

DAD: Yes, you made things very clear and fun.

THERAPIST: How about you, Nicole? What did you think of coming in here and talking about the Tickles?

NICOLE: You're fun!

[Later in the session:]

THERAPIST: How has your experience with Nicole proved different from the traditional understanding of ADHD?

MOM: The teacher's explanation of ADHD was that Nicole needed to be checked by a doctor and be put on medication to help her control her behavior. I felt Nicole was strong enough to control her own behaviors without any prescriptions.

[The conversation continues highlighting and supporting Nicole's changes. This is the family's last meeting with the therapist.]

Shawn

The following transcript is a segment from a "consulting your consultant" interview with Shawn (age 12) and his mother. The therapist had seen Shawn six times over a five-month period because of problems with distractibility, particularly around homework time. The consulting psychiatrist had diagnosed him as having attention-deficit/disorder without hyperactivity[6] and prescribed Ritalin. Shawn's attention span improved, as did his grades. The interview was taped (with the permission of Shawn and his mother) so that other families affected by ADHD could gain knowledge from their expertise.

MOM: They always said you can't get an attention-deficit student to get the homework assignments done, but you can if someone sits down and helps him.

THERAPIST: So you have proven the experts wrong. Shawn, do you call the problem "attention-deficit," or do you want to call it what we named it before—"Distraction"?

SHAWN: Distraction.

THERAPIST: Okay, so what's helped with the ADHD or the Distraction?

MOM: After school, to make sure he has done his homework assignment and making sure he has whatever he needs to do the assignment.

THERAPIST: Making sure he has . . .

MOM: Almost like a homework assignment sheet every day. The teacher writes down all his assignments.

THERAPIST: So how does that help?

MOM: Well, it helps him remember.

THERAPIST: What else has been helpful?

MOM: Of course, the medication he has been on, but that's been the same—a constant throughout.

THERAPIST: So is it safe to say the medication is not the sole reason for the changes?

MOM: Oh, yeah. If I were to look at it on a scale, the medication was just one point of what we had to do. There was a lot of things we had to do. Does that make sense? I would say 25% medication and 75% effort.

SHAWN: Actually, probably only 5% medication.

THERAPIST: Wow, only 5%!

SHAWN: Yeah, 95% effort!

MOM: (Laughs) That's interesting. I think medication gets us to the point where we can start doing the effort. Like a jump-off.

THERAPIST: You say 25% medication and you, Shawn, say only 5%. I guess the key point is both of you are not giving medication the entire credit.

---

[6]By DSM-III-R criteria. The DSM-IV equivalent would be ADHD, predominantly inattentive type.

MOM: Right. Maybe it's close to only 15%!

THERAPIST: This must suggest that Shawn possesses some real special abilities, since the changes were more effort than medication. Shawn, what skills do you have that helped improve concentration?

SHAWN: I don't know.

THERAPIST: Hm . . . you don't like to brag about your talents? Do you mind if I say I'm impressed? I imagine your mother is, too.

MOM: Oh, yeah! Shawn, I think, is very smart and he never gives up.

THERAPIST: So perseverance . . . never giving up is an antidistraction technique?

SHAWN: Yeah, I guess so.

THERAPIST: I'm just thinking that a lot of young people take Ritalin but don't put the effort in as you have. I think it must say something about your capabilities. Are you proud of yourself?

SHAWN: Yes.

THERAPIST: Why?

SHAWN: Because I keep on trying, and I'm doing better in school.

THERAPIST: I also imagine that your mother was helpful in having success with the Distractions. How was your mother helpful?

SHAWN: Well, she always helped me with my homework.

THERAPIST: Have you learned anything about how a parent can help? Any advice you'd give parents who have a young person who's affected by Distractions?

MOM: I think the main thing is patience. Also, to encourage your child and praise him for any small success. It's important to have a good relationship with the school, the teacher.

THERAPIST: You (*to Mom*) have put in a great deal of time and effort in helping Shawn. You have such a busy life. What might it say about you as a mother that you can appreciate?

MOM: I think I'm a good mom!

THERAPIST: Getting back to medication, did you believe at first that medication would be the complete answer?

MOM: Oh, yeah. We thought it would be the key. But now we know the medication was just a launch-off to the other areas.

THERAPIST: So the effort part, the assignment sheet was a good idea. So whose idea was that?

MOM: All three of us: Shawn and I and the teacher. That's another key, having a good teacher.

THERAPIST: So having an understanding teacher helps.

MOM: Another helpful thing was having a joint meeting with the teacher and the school psychologist to come up with an individualized program for Shawn. You don't know that these resources exist unless you ask, so I'd recommend that parents become assertive. The school psychologist is helping him become better organized.

[Later in the interview:]

THERAPIST: Any other ideas you'd like to pass on, Shawn?

SHAWN: It's good to sit next to a kid who gets straight A's!

THERAPIST: So how does that help you with the Distraction?

SHAWN: Well, there is still Distraction all around me, but I just look at the good student's behavior and study habits.

MOM: Well, it's working. He's been getting all A's on his tests.

THERAPIST: Excellent! In spite of the Distraction, you're getting all A's. What does this say about Shawn?

MOM: Well, he definitely has the ability. I help him a lot, but I can't take his tests for him.

THERAPIST: So what are his best abilities, Mom?

MOM: He has the knowledge. He's very smart.

THERAPIST: So the Distraction has not stolen your smarts?

[Later in the session:]

THERAPIST: I have seen a lot of kids pushed around by the Distraction, particularly around homework time at home. What did you do there, Shawn?

SHAWN: It has to be quiet . . . but I like to be in the family room rather than in my room.

MOM: Yeah, he does worse in a quiet room alone. But that's what the experts say—that you have to do homework in a quiet room with no distraction.

THERAPIST: That's why I'm interested in what works for you, not what the experts say.

MOM: He stands up at the kitchen counter with all the distraction and does his homework because he feels a part of the family. [There are six family members.]

THERAPIST: That's amazing! In spite of all the distractions, you're able to do your homework and concentrate. You must have a strong mind.

How do you keep your mind on your homework and distract the Distractions away?

SHAWN: I just block them out of my mind. I know I take a little longer to do my homework this way, but it works for me!

CONCLUSION

The case examples exemplify how narrative ideas can transform traditional approaches to ADHD and open alternative therapeutic possibilities. When a therapy that enters the imaginary is conducted, the special abilities and local knowledges of children labeled "ADHD" are articulated. Novel ideas and solutions emerge when therapists enter the worlds of children. Erin, a young person we were working with recently, said the following when asked her ideas about ADHD: "Therapists should not make ADHD sound like a disease or a medical condition. It should be treated as a situation, something that can be helped—not something that needs to be cured."

REFERENCES

American Psychiatric Association. (1994). *Diagnostic and Statistical Manual of Mental Disorders* (4th ed.). Washington, DC: Author.

Andersen, T. (Ed.). (1991). *The Reflecting Team: Dialogues and Dialogues about the Dialogues.* New York: Norton.

Anderson, H., & Goolishian, H. (1988). Human systems as linguistic systems: Evolving ideas about the implications for theory and practice. *Family Process, 27,* 371–393.

Barkley, R. A. (1990). *Attention-Deficit Hyperactivity Disorder: A Handbook for Diagnosis and Treatment.* New York: Guilford Press.

Buchanan, B., & Stayton, C. (1994). *The Hype about Hyperactivity.* Paper presented at the 17th Annual Family Therapy Network Symposium, Chicago.

Cade, B. (1990). The mini-tornado: Turning "hyperactivity" into energy. *Family Therapy Case Studies, 5*(1), 45–50.

Crook, C. (1994). ADHD: Disorder or symptom? *White Rock Journal of Family Therapy, 2*(1), 17–20.

Dickerson, V., & Zimmerman, J. (1992). Families with adolescents: Escaping problem lifestyles. *Family Process, 31*(4), 341–353.

Dunne, P. (1992). *The Narrative Therapist and the Arts.* Los Angeles: Possibilities Press.

Epston, D. (1991). "I am a bear": Discovering discoveries. *Family Therapy Case Studies, 6*(1), 11–20.

Epston, D. (1993). *Narrative Therapy with Children.* Workshop held in Cupertino, CA.

Epston, D. (1994). Extending the conversation. *Family Therapy Networker, 18*(6), 31–37, 62–63.

Epston, D. (1995). Towards a Child-Focussed Family Therapy: Narrative, Play and Imagination. Workshop held in San Rafael, CA.

Epston, D., & White, M. (1990). Consulting your consultants: The documentation of alternative knowledges. *Dulwich Centre Newsletter,* No. 4, 25–35.

Foucault, M. (1980). *Power/Knowledge: Selected Interviews and Other Writings.* New York: Norton.

Freeman, J., & Lobovits, D. (1993). The turtle with wings. In S. Friedman (Ed.), *The New Language of Change: Constructive Collaboration in Psychotherapy* (pp. 188–225). New York: Guilford Press.

Gergen, K. J. (1994). *Realities and Relationships.* Cambridge, MA: Harvard University Press.

Griffith, J., & Griffith, M. (1994). *The Body Speaks.* New York: Basic Books.

Hallowell, E. (1994). *Driven to Distraction.* New York: Random House/Simon & Schuster.

Hoyt, M. F. (1994). Is being "in recovery" self-limiting? *Transactional Analysis Journal, 24,* 222–223. (Reprinted in M. F. Hoyt, *Brief Therapy and Managed Care: Readings for Contemporary Practice* [pp. 213–215]. San Francisco: Jossey-Bass, 1995.)

Hubble, M., & O'Hanlon, W. H. (1992) Theory countertransference. *Dulwich Centre Newsletter,* No. 1, 25–30.

Kelly, K., & Ramundo, P. (1994). *You Mean I'm Not Lazy, Stupid or Crazy?! A Self-Help Book for Adults with Attention Deficit Disorder.* New York: Scribner's/Simon & Schuster.

Kohn, A. (1989, November). Suffer the restless children. *Atlantic Monthly,* pp. 90–100.

Law, I. (1995). *ADHD and ADD: Attending to Deficit-Based Discourses. Workshop presented at the 3rd Annual Narrative Ideas and Therapeutic Practices Conference, Vancouver, British Columbia, Canada.*

Lipchik, E. (1993). "Both/and" solutions. In S. Friedman (Ed.), *The New Language of Change: Constructive Collaboration in Psychotherapy* (pp. 25–49). New York: Guilford Press.

McNamee, S., & Gergen, K. J. (Eds.). (1992). *Therapy as Social Construction.* Newbury Park, CA: Sage.

Nylund, D., & Corsiglia, V. (1994a). Attention to the deficits in attention-deficit disorder: Deconstructing the diagnosis and bringing forth children's special abilities. *Journal of Collaborative Therapies, 2*(2), 7–17.

Nylund, D., & Corsiglia, V. (1994b). Becoming solution-focused forced in brief therapy: Remembering something important we already knew. *Journal of Systemic Therapies, 13*(1), 1–8.

Nylund, D., & Thomas, J. (1994). The economics of narrative. *Family Therapy Networker, 18*(6), 38–39.

O'Callaghan, J. B. (1993). *School Based Collaboration with Families.* San Francisco: Jossey-Bass.

Schachar, R. J. (1986). Hyperkinetic syndrome: Historical development of the concept. In E. Taylor (Ed.), *The Overactive Child* (pp. 19–40). Philadelphia: J. B. Lippincott.

Schrag, P., & Divoky, D. (1975). *The Myth of the Hyperactive Child: And Other Means of Child Control.* New York: Pantheon.

Stacey, K. (1994). *Language as an Exclusive or Inclusive Concept: Reaching beyond the Verbal.* Paper presented at the 1st annual California Narrative Participants Conference, Santa Barbara, CA.

Stewart, B., & Nodrick, B. (1990). The learning disabled lifestyle: From reification to liberation. *Family Therapy Case Studies,* 5(1), 61–73.

Wallis, C. (1994, July 18). Life in overdrive: An epidemic of attention deficit disorder. *Time,* pp. 42–50.

Weaver, C. (1994). Understanding and educating students with attention deficit hyperactivity disorders: Toward a system-theory and whole language perspective. In C. Weaver (Ed.), *Success at Last!: Helping Students with ADHD Achieve Their Potential* (pp. 1–23). Portsmouth, NH: Heinemann.

White, M. (1991). Deconstruction and therapy. *Dulwich Centre Newsletter,* No. 3, 1–22. (Reprinted in S. Gilligan & R. Price [Eds.], *Therapeutic Conversations* [pp. 22–61]. New York: Norton, 1993.)

White, M. (1992a). *Recent Developments in Narrative Therapy.* Workshop presented at the annual conference of the American Association of Marriage and Family Therapists, Fort Lauderdale, FL.

White, M. (1992b). *The Narrative Approach.* Workshop presented at the Mental Research Institute, Palo Alto, CA.

White, M., & Epston, D. (1990). *Narrative Means to Therapeutic Ends.* New York: Norton.

Zametkin, A., Nordahl, T., Gross, M., King, A., Semple, W., Rumsey, J., Hamburger, S., & Cohen, R. (1990). Cerebral glucose metabolism in adults with hyperactivity of childhood onset. *New England Journal of Medicine, 323,* 1361–1366.

CHAPTER 8

Taking Safety Home
A Solution-Focused Approach with Domestic Violence

CHARLES E. JOHNSON
JEFFREY GOLDMAN

Solution-focused therapy (de Shazer, 1985, 1988; de Shazer et al., 1986) can be used effectively to help clients suffering from domestic violence. Since 1987, we have used solution-focused treatment principles to actively engage abusive and abused clients in identifying, believing in, and succeeding at living a future that is violence-free. This chapter describes our approach.

THE CONTROVERSY

In the last decade and a half the family systems literature has begun to raise serious questions about the wisdom and the ethics of doing therapy with couples involved in domestic violence. Some feminist therapists (Adams, 1988; Avis, 1992; Bograd, 1984, 1992; Goldner, Penn, Sheinberg, & Walker, 1990; Kaufman, 1992; Pressman, 1989) contend that concepts of neutrality and circular causality can function as a screen that allows the batterer to escape the responsibility for his violent acts,[1] blurring the distinction between violent and nonviolent behavior, and further endangering the victim. They note that seeing a couple conjointly could imply that the woman has some responsibility for her partner's

---

[1]Although the commonest most injurious forms of domestic violence occur when men batter women (Gelles & Straus, 1988; Kruz, 1993), we acknowledge that men can be battered as well (Straus, 1993), and that battering can occur in same-sex couples (Renzetti, 1993). The concepts and methods that we describe herein are general and applicable, regardless of gender or sexual orientation.

actions—an indirect form of "blaming the victim" (Hansen, 1993). In addition, there is an apprehension that couple therapy fails to address the imbalance of power that exists in the culture, while perpetuating traditional sex roles (Goldner et al., 1990). Finally, some therapists, in view of feminist concerns, have proposed that couple therapy could actually become a dangerous and coercive instrument, with the therapist functionally colluding with the batterer, obliquely communicating that violence is an understandable though unfortunate response to the victim's behavior (Adams, 1988; Kaufman, 1992; Lindsay, McBride, & Platt, 1993).

Currently in North America, treatment programs for batterers are influenced primarily by state and local authorities' legal and political responses to the domestic violence in their communities (Sherman, 1992). The goal of these interventions is often separation of the partners, insurance of the victim's safety (frequently through shelters), and the containment and rehabilitation of the abuser's behavior (routinely through group therapy)(Adams, Rosenbaum, & Stewart, 1994; Lipchik, 1991).

Critics of a family systems approach recommend that couple therapy begin *only* after the batterer accepts responsibility for the violence, has not committed any more violent acts (usually for six months or more), and has completed a substantial amount of group or individual therapy. They suggest that these interventions be part of an integrated approach that would also provide group or individual therapy for the victim and her children if necessary (Edleson & Tolman, 1992; Lindsay et al., 1993; Pressman, 1989).

More recently, some family therapists (Erickson, 1992; Lipchik, 1991) have questioned the therapeutic usefulness of this political and clinical debate, lamenting its polarizing effect on the field. Goldner (1992, pp. 59–60) notes that conflicting therapeutic and political injunctions sometimes result in a woman's being "caught in the middle between two incompatible characterizations" of her relationship with the abuser, leaving her stigmatized and isolated.

TAKING SAFETY HOME

We share these authors' concern about the importance of safety in the family, and have found the solution-focused approach to be one of the most effective ways to achieve that goal. The couples we see come from all income levels and cultural strata. In some cases, they may be involved in the legal system. The state in which we practice, Colorado, has a mandatory arrest provision in its domestic violence statutes.

For the purpose of distinguishing our work from that of others, we begin by describing some of the things we do *not* do. One of the most significant things that we don't do is demand a confession from the batterer. Nor do we deconstruct the moments of violence in the couple's relationship, repetitively examining the descriptions and sequences of the abuse in the hope of bringing new meanings to the experience (Goldner et al., 1990). We don't engage in protocols of psychological education, sociopolitical indoctrination, or examination of the ideas about masculinity or femininity that the couple may possess (Gardiner & McGrath, 1995; Jenkins, 1990). We do not require that the couple be engaged in any other type of individual or group treatment; however, in the course of therapy, we may recommend it. We don't inquire about the role of violence in the partners' families of origin. Finally, we rarely separate the couple to inquire about the violence that has occurred in the past, although we will do separate interviews if either member requests it.

Instead, we attempt to discover the different ways in which a couple might become "customers" (Berg, 1989; Berg & Miller, 1992; de Shazer, 1988) for safety. We do this by emphasizing hopefulness, goal setting, future orientation, and the strengths the couple identifies in the relationship. When we determine that the partners are committed to achieving safety, we assume that it is our job to help them co-construct goals and skills that they can take home with them. Essential to this task is eliciting the couple's answers to questions contained in the solution-focused interview, with its emphasis on "miracles," exceptions, and scaling questions (Berg & Miller, 1992; de Shazer, 1985, 1988).

CLINICAL EXAMPLE[2]

Sometimes the family's presenting problem is not domestic violence. For example, Melinda brought her older daughter, Joleen, to therapy and presented a straightforward complaint: "Joleen won't go to school and won't follow the rules." Joleen acknowledged this, but complained that her parents were unfair and had too many rules. The therapist gave Melinda an observational task (Berg & Miller, 1992; de Shazer, 1988), suggesting that she notice "the times that Joleen observed the rules," and asked her to bring any other family members whom she thought would be helpful to the next session.

---

[2]This case and the following two cases were seen by a solution-focused therapy team (de Shazer, 1985; de Shazer et al., 1986), which utilized an intrasession consultation break along with suggestions and questions phoned in from behind the one-way mirror. Goldman was the therapist in front of the mirror. Behind the mirror, in addition to Johnson, were Evelyn Braithwaite, Marty Waters, and Denise Webster.

Two weeks later Melinda returned with her husband, John, and her younger daughter, Linda, but without Joleen, who had run away. During the session, we learned that John was attending an alcohol treatment program that had a family therapy component. Clearly he believed that our sessions were superfluous and that he was thus not a "customer" of ours. We also learned that John had been in prison some years ago for armed robbery and was a recovering heroin addict. We complimented John on "doing what was necessary" to help himself and his family, and let them all know that we were always available as a resource.

Three months after this, we were mildly surprised to hear again from John. He called because he'd abused alcohol and become physically violent with Melinda (not for the first time). The police were called, and he was arrested and court-ordered into domestic violence therapy.

When we saw them again, we asked the family members how we might be helpful, given this new situation. Melinda, from her almost fetal position on the couch, said that she wanted the violence to end, John to stop drinking, and Joleen to return home. John, his voice just above a whisper, said that he just wanted to get his family back; he added that Melinda wouldn't talk to him and that Linda wouldn't come out of her room. Linda said that she was "going crazy from listening to all the arguments."

When the family members were asked to rate (Berg & de Shazer, 1993; de Shazer, 1988) how safe they felt in their household, with a 10 on the "safety scale" being completely safe and a 1 representing a complete lack of safety, Melinda said that she was at 1, John said that he was at 2, and Linda said that she was at 3. When John was asked whether he was surprised at the other members' scores, he said "No," and added that he was amazed that they were willing to come to the session.

We asked the family members what would allow them to move up 1 point on the safety scale. Melinda clearly stated that there was considerably more safety in the house when John was sober. John and Linda agreed that this was true. When asked to expand on this, Melinda explained that when John was sober, she didn't have to look over her shoulder all the time or worry about his explosiveness. Likewise, she didn't feel that she had to hide from him as she did when he was drinking.

We like to emphasize the *presence* of desired changes (Berg & Miller, 1992), rather than the *absence* of undesirable behaviors. We told Melinda that we were curious about what she might experience instead of the fear and isolation. She responded that she would feel freer to walk around the house and that she would be able to experience some of the things that she and her husband enjoyed when they were first married. When asked what difference this would make, she said that she would be much more able to relate to John as a husband rather than as someone to be feared. When John was asked whether he knew what Melinda was talking about, he enthusiastically answered "Yes!" He described the activities and adventures that they had had when they were younger, commenting that he missed "being a husband and father." He also sadly described his own history of abandonment by his parents, his subsequent placement in foster care at the age of 13, and his seven-year stint in prison for armed robbery. (The children, were four and two years old at the time of his imprisonment.) When John was asked what differences that he might notice in Linda when the family had moved up on the safety scale, he said that he would notice her leaving her room more and perhaps participating in some family activities.

As the interchange continued, with John, Melinda, and Linda all participating, the therapist and the family continued to co-construct a vessel of safety, exploring the differences that the above-mentioned exceptions made and speculating hopefully on a future without violence. Every exception was linked back to John's sobriety, and thus to safety. We complimented the family members' honesty, their understanding of the importance of safety, and the fact that they had a good sense of what to do to take safety home with them. The family was given the assignment of noticing the things that John did to increase the amount of safety in the family. John was given the assignment of noticing the differences that it made when he was able to raise the level of safety in the family.

The first interview session in solution-focused therapy is not unlike the opening night of a Broadway play, with critics in the audience who can ensure that the endeavor continues or falls flat. In the case of therapy, the critics are the clients (*not* the therapists!), and it is essential in the first session to introduce them to a clinical model that will develop a level of customership that will prove beneficial to the solution of their problem. In this second "first" session (the first after this family's return to treatment), we and the family were able to cover an enormous amount of ground—developing customership for safety, and punctuating and expanding upon exceptions, while continually steering around recriminations (which would be contrary to positive treatment outcomes). The family brought in the problem of violence and took home the solution of safety.

When the family members returned a week later for the next session, they appeared decidedly different. Melinda spoke with confidence, John looked less ashamed, and Linda participated actively in the session. All three of them were able to use humor and joke with one another. Melinda reported that John had stayed sober, allowing her to feel more secure and open to attending a picnic that he suggested. John commented that he had noticed her openness and that it allowed him to feel more a part of the family. Linda commented that she now had a reason to come out of her room, and her parents approvingly noted her increased level of participation in the family. As in the previous session, we continued to explore these "differences that make a difference" (de Shazer, 1988, 1991), with the continual link to safety. In response to our safety-scaling question, Melinda reported that she was at 5, John said that he was at 6, and Linda said that she was at 8. After noting the differences from the last session and complimenting the family members on their achievements, the therapist asked them to rate their confidence in their ability to maintain these changes, with a 1 indicating a complete lack of confidence and a 10 representing a level so high that they would never have to think about the problem again. Interestingly, they all answered 5. Acknowledging this realistic number, we asked what would allow them to be confident at a level of 6. They unanimously answered, "Time."

We have found that clients' confidence after a change almost always increases with the passage of time. Asking about confidence is important, especially in cases where change is experienced quickly. Simply waiting is not enough. Rather, our emphasis, particularly in cases of domestic violence, is on what specific things clients do during that time to nurture, encourage, and further strengthen the changes that they desire (Walter & Peller, 1994). This way clients' participation is dynamically engaged; they are proactively constructing the reality that they seek.

In addition to reinforcing change and confidence, we often find it helpful to ask clients questions about the distant future, which may help maintain changes in the present and near future (Penn, 1985). In this case, we asked John what he would like his children to remember about his and Melinda's relationship when they reached their parents' age. He became very serious and again recalled the violence in his own family. "I sure don't want them to go through what I went through," he said. He talked eloquently about how important it was to live in a safe household, again noting, along with Melinda and Linda, the differences they had achieved to ensure safety.

At this point, safety was linked to John's sobriety, and his sobriety was linked to his knowing of his family's desire to talk to and be with him. After complimenting the family members on the changes that they had made, as well as their realistic view of confidence, we gave them the assignment of celebrating sobriety at least once a week. We also encouraged them to develop a set of family rituals that would continually remind them of the importance of safety. This assignment reinforces and ritualizes the family members' developing relationship to their desired goal—in this case, safety (Dolan, 1994). This intervention, along with the constructive interviewing techniques previously mentioned, serves to "externalize" and personalize the solution (Dolan, 1991), encouraging the family members to embrace a recent addition to their household. This differs from narrative therapy's notion of "externalization" (White & Epston, 1990), with its emphasis on objectification and personification of the problem. Instead of fighting against the oppressive effects of the problem, our approach encourages development of new "solution states of consciousness" (Dolan, 1994) that clients can identify, utilize, and incorporate into their daily routines.

When John, Melinda, and Linda were seen a month later, they reported that each week they had celebrated by taking a family trip to various sites around Colorado. Once again, we asked them to rate their confidence in their new-found safety. Melinda and Linda reported that they were at 9, and John reported that he was at 8. The therapist asked, "What else needs to be different for therapy to end?" John and Melinda couldn't answer the question, but both stated that they would like to schedule one more visit in six weeks, to make sure that they were still "on track" (Walter & Peller, 1994).

They kept the appointment. The first thing John told us, before the family members had even taken their seats, was that he had gotten drunk. This time, however, Melinda had locked him out and told him that should he try to come in, she would call the police. John said he believed her, and "instead of breaking down the door like I would have before, I slept it off in the car." We asked Melinda, "How did you do that?" She answered, "I knew what I needed to do to keep Linda and me safe, and I'll do the same thing again if I have to."

The family members indicated that there had been no other problems, and agreed that John's relapse was handled in "the best way possible." We congratulated them on their achievements and reminded them to continue with their celebrations. As with all clients, we encouraged them to call in the future if they thought that we could be of help.

Melinda did indeed call six months later. She reported that although things were still "safe and sober," their older daughter, Joleen, was now in the custody of social services after being a runaway for almost six months. Social services was requiring family therapy to integrate Joleen back into the home. We met with the family members for three more sessions before they acknowledged that they had become successfully reunited. When we asked at the last session what was different, they agreed that Joleen was now following the rules and going to school. Joleen told us, "It is a lot easier to follow the rules when my parents aren't fighting."

UTILIZING SELF-DETERMINATION
TO SUPPORT LEAVING AN ABUSIVE RELATIONSHIP

A perhaps unexpected benefit of solution-focused treatment with cases of domestic violence is the influence it can have in supporting a victim of abuse to end the abusive relationship safely and expediently. There is an inaccurate perception among many clinicians working with abused women that couple treatment will, like some evil potion, have the effect of forcing an unwilling woman to override her own better judgment and continue in a relationship that is dangerous and unchanging. In many cases, we see just the opposite occur.

TWO CLINICAL EXAMPLES

Case 1

Oliver and Judy had been married three years when we saw them for the first time. In answer to our first session question about how they would each know that therapy had been useful, Judy said, "There won't be any more yelling and screaming and fighting." When we then asked her how she would know the relationship was safer, she quickly responded, "He'll show me he respects my opinion." Oliver stated that he'd know therapy was helpful if "Judy would stop complaining all the time." In answer to our question about safety, he acknowledged that "mutual respect was important" and indicated on our scaling question that he was at 10 in his efforts to make it happen. At the end of this first session, we gave the couple a variation of the "first-session formula task" (de Shazer, 1985) relating to safety. Specifically, we asked both Oliver and Judy to pay attention to those times when safety was present, and to think about how that made a difference for their relationship.

When the couple returned two weeks later, we asked both spouses what they had learned from their homework. Oliver looked over to Judy and asked, "What was the homework?" Judy opened her purse and brought out a list of "all the times safety was present." We engaged both members in conversation about what differences it made when either or both felt safe. We asked about who did what and how they did it. We asked them who else would be noticing. At the end of this session we gave them a observational homework assignment, suggesting that they notice the times when mutual respect and safety were present.

We saw them again two weeks later. At this third appointment, Oliver said he'd been busy and "forgot to do the homework." Judy, however, was again expansive in her discussion about what was different and how she appreciated "mutual respect and safety." We apologized to Oliver for giving him a "forgettable" homework assignment, and continued to ask him questions about what he thought was important that they do differently. He talked about her "keeping the house clean," but was less clear about what he could do "to show respect."

The fourth session went much the same as the previous three. Oliver had forgotten to do his homework (of noticing how he expressed respect to Judy), while she had conscientiously cleaned the house. At this point we had a clear sense that Oliver was not a customer for a "respectful relationship" (at least not in the way that Judy appeared to think about respect). We had an equally clear sense that Judy was a customer for a "respectful relationship," which, by her definition, had to include safety.

After this fourth session, we decided that during our next appointment we would invite Judy to a session individually, and at the same time apologized to both spouses for not having helped them. That very week Judy called us to cancel the next appointment, stating that Oliver would be out of town for the scheduled date and that she would call back to reschedule. She never did.

We spent some time reviewing videotapes (which had been made with the clients' written consent) to reexamine our interventions, but, frankly, we were perplexed. We assumed this to be one of our "failure cases," and discussed among ourselves how perhaps it might have made a difference if we had ended therapy sooner, while acknowledging our incompetence to the couple. Interestingly, we received a letter from Judy six months later. In it she enclosed a release of information so that we could talk with her current therapist. She also thanked us profusely for helping her resolve to get a divorce: "I realized that he wasn't going to change. I understood that if he wasn't going to pay attention to professionals, he was never going to pay attention to me."

This letter reinforced for us the power of the solution-focused model in encouraging "self-determination." It is our belief that had we told either member of the couple what to do, we would have failed them by telling them the wrong thing. ("Judy, it's obvious that Oliver is not willing to do the homework. What do you think you should do?" or "Oliver, you need to take responsibility for your abusive behavior.") Because a solution-focused approach demands only that we find out from the clients what they think they should do, the failure—at least for this particular woman—became her husband's, not ours or hers. We speculate that Judy's ability to act on her own construct ("he wasn't going to change") was supported by a process that takes clients at face value. As in this case, when clients contradict themselves, we presume that their partners and/or children will draw their own conclusions without our well-intended advice.

Case 2

A couple was referred to us by the therapist at a domestic violence program where the abusive husband was receiving his court-mandated treatment. The husband, Richard, called asking us to see him and his wife, Sylvia, from whom he had been separated for two years. At our initial session with the couple, Richard responded to the first question, "What will be different when therapy is over?", by glaring at the therapist and saying, "How the fuck should I know? You're the therapist." The therapist immediately apologized for asking a dumb question. As the session progressed, the husband became somewhat more responsive. Sylvia indicated that her goal was "to make up her mind about the divorce," and she was forthright in her answers. When we asked each of them what would be "a small step in the right direction," he said, "She'll tell me where she lives." Sylvia said, "He'll be less angry." We ended the session by giving them the standard first-session formula task: "Notice what is there in your relationship you wish to continue."

Several days later, Richard called and tearfully told us by phone, "We might as well cancel the next appointment." When asked what he meant, he replied, "She's going through with the divorce." After two years of separation, his wife had made up her mind. It is our view that although she would have done this sooner or later, our single interview with the couple helped her to end the relationship at that time. Although we never told either of them what to do, our questions assumed that each was paying attention to the other's answers. Like Judy in the preceding case, this woman may well have thought, "If he acts this way with a therapist who is only asking questions, he's probably going to continue to act this way with me."

COMMENT

We believe the reasons why the women in both of these latter cases were able to make a decision to end an abusive relationship (after four conjoint sessions and one such session, respectively) are related to the principle of self-determination that solution-focused and other constructive therapies so strongly emphasize. A solution-focused approach can fortify a battered woman to make decisions more readily in her own best interest—decisions that can, as noted, include separating from or ending a relationship.

Miller and Rollnick (1991) address the importance of self-determination in the context of their discussion about ambivalence. They state in reference to clients with substance abuse problems that interviewing techniques must allow clients to consider both sides of their ambivalence open. Obviously, both Judy and Sylvia had mixed feelings about continuing their relationships. Solution-focused interviewing implicitly supported these women to consider the possibilities of both staying and leaving.

Again, our work with these couples was distinguished by what we did not do. For all of us as human beings (including us therapists as a subset), it seems that our "natural" tendency when we see someone in danger—or at least acting against their own self-interest—is to advise them, warn them, and even attempt to protect them from the consequences of their actions. We acknowledge an urge to have separated each of these two couples in the session and to have given the abused woman heartfelt advice.[3] But we overcame these urges to "advise" because we know that advice doesn't work. Those working in shelters for battered women also know how often their well-intended advice is ignored (McKeel & Sporakowski, 1993).

Intimate relationships encompass conflicting values. Most relationships value respect and safety between partners. But so, too, do they value loyalty within the relationship. When shelter staff, victim advocates, district attorneys, and friends and family of a battered woman advise her to leave her partner—telling her, "He's dangerous and will never change," and "You're crazy to stay"—she is confronted with this question of loyalty. As evidence suggests, to her detriment, she often chooses in favor of loyalty. This same dynamic is experienced by those police officers who, intervening in domestic violence disputes, report being attacked by a battered woman when they attempt to take the man to jail (Sherman, 1992).

Solution-focused interviewing provides individual partners the opportunity to make use of their own immediate experience (given the here-and-now orientation of solution-focused therapy). This immediacy of experience, in combination with an emphasis on active construction or "doing"—for example, homework assignments such as "Notice when safety is present," or "Celebrate sobriety"—provides an environment in which clients can choose safety, *either as a couple or individually.*

CONCLUSION

We maintain that solution-focused therapy enhances safety rather than diminishing it. This occurs either when clients create new, safer relationships or when they choose to end relationships in which they have lost the hope for safety. As the case material we have provided illustrates, when clients are treated with respect, given hope, and supported to establish their own criteria for success, they can bring safety home (either together or individually) and include it as a valued member of the family.

[3]This does not obviate any legal or ethical obligations therapists may have to warn potential victims or to take protective action in imminently life-threatening circumstances. The spirit of our position is to respect clients' ability to exercise their own judgment.

REFERENCES

Adams, D.(1988). Treatment models for men who batter: A profeminist analysis. In K. Ylló & M. Bograd (Eds.), *Feminist Perspectives on Wife Abuse* (pp. 176–199). Newbury Park, CA: Sage.

Adams, D., Rosenbaum, A., & Stewart, T. P. (1994). Treatment standards for abuse programs. *Violence Update, 5*(1), 5–9.

Aldarondo, E., & Straus, M. A. (1994). Screening for physical violence in couple therapy: Methodological, practical, and ethical considerations. *Family Process, 33,* 425–440.

Avis, J. M. (1992). Where are all the family therapists? Abuse and violence within families and family therapy's response. *Journal of Marital and Family Therapy, 18*(3), 225–232.

Berg, I. K. (1989). Of visitors, complainants, and customers: Is there any such thing as resistance? *Family Therapy Networker, 13*(1), 21.

Berg, I. K., & de Shazer, S. (1993). Making numbers talk: Language in therapy. In S. Friedman (Ed.), *The New Language of Change: Constructive Collaboration in Psychotherapy* (pp. 5–24). New York: Guilford Press.

Berg, I. K., & Miller, S. (1992). *Working with the Problem Drinker,* New York: Norton.

Bograd, M. (1984). Family systems approaches to wife battering: A feminist critique. *American Journal of Orthopsychiatry, 54*(4), 558–568.

Bograd, M. (1992). Values in conflict: Challenges to family therapists' thinking. *Journal of Marital and Family Therapy, 18*(3), 245–256.

de Shazer, S. (1985). *Keys to Solution in Brief Therapy.* New York: Norton.

de Shazer, S., Berg, I. K., Lipchik, E., Nunnally, E., Molnar, A., Gingerick, W., & Weiner-Davis, M. (1986). Brief therapy: Focused solution development. *Family Process, 25*(2), 207–223.

de Shazer, S. (1988). *Clues: Investigating Solutions in Brief Family Therapy.* New York: Norton.

de Shazer, S. (1991). *Putting Difference to Work.* New York: Norton.

Dolan, Y. M. (1991). *Resolving Sexual Abuse: Solution Focused Therapy and Ericksonian Hypnosis with Adult Survivors.* New York: Norton.

Dolan, Y. M. (1994). Solution-focused therapy with a case of severe abuse. In M. F. Hoyt (Ed.), *Constructive Therapies* (pp. 276–294). New York: Guilford Press.

Edleson, J. L., & Tolman, R. M. (1992). *Intervention for Men Who Batter: An Ecological Approach.* Newbury Park, CA: Sage.

Erickson, B. M. (1992). Feminist fundamentalism: Reaction to Avis, Kaufman, and Bograd. *Journal of Marital and Family Therapy, 18*(3), 263–267.

Gardiner, S., & McGrath, F. (1995). Wife assault: A systemic approach that minimizes risk and maximizes responsibility. *Journal of Systemic Therapies, 14*(1), 20–32.

Gelles, R. J., & Straus, M. (1988). *Intimate Violence: The Causes and Consequences of Abuse in the American Family.* New York: Touchstone.

Goldner, V. (1992). Making room for both/and. *Family Therapy Networker, 16*(2), 54–61.

Goldner, V., Penn, P., Sheinberg, M., & Walker, G. (1990). Love and violence: Gender paradoxes in volatile attachments. *Family Process, 29*(4), 343–364.

Hansen, M. (1993). Feminism and family therapy: A review of feminist critiques of approaches to family violence. In M. Hansen & M. Harway (Eds.), *Battering and Family Therapy: A Feminist Perspective* (pp. 69–81). Newbury Park, CA: Sage.

Jenkins, A. (1990). *Invitations to Responsibility: The Therapeutic Engagement of Men Who Are Violent and Abusive.* Adelaide: Dulwich Centre Publications.

Kaufman, G. (1992). The mysterious disappearance of battered women in family therapists' offices: Male privilege colluding with male violence. *Journal of Marital and Family Therapy, 18*(3), 233–243.

Kurz, D. (1993). Physical assaults by husbands: A major social problem. In R. J. Gelles & D. R. Loseke (Eds.), *Current Controversies on Family Violence* (pp. 88–101). Newbury Park, CA: Sage.

Lindsay, M., McBride, R. W., & Platt, C. M. (1993). *Ammend: Philosophy and Curriculum for Treating Batterers.* Littleton, CO: Gylantic.

Lipchik, E. (1991). Spouse abuse: Challenging the party line. *Family Therapy Networker, 15*(3), 59–63.

McKeel, A. J., & Sporakowski, M. J. (1993). How shelter counselors' views about responsibility for wife abuse relate to services they provide to battered women. *Journal of Family Violence, 8*(2), 101–112.

Miller, W. R., & Rollnick, S. (1991). *Motivational Interviewing: Preparing People to Change Addictive Behavior.* New York: Guilford Press.

Penn, P. (1985). Feed forward: Future questions, future maps. *Family Process, 24,* 299–310.

Pressman, B. (1989). Wife abused couples: The need for comprehensive theoretical perspectives and integrated treatment models. *Journal of Feminist Family Therapy, 1*(1), 23–43.

Renzetti, C. A. (1993). Violence in lesbian relationships. In M. Hansen & M. Harway (Eds.), *Battering and Family Therapy: A Feminist Perspective* (pp. 188–199). Newbury Park, CA: Sage.

Sherman, L. (1992). *Policing Domestic Violence: Experiments and Dilemmas.* New York: Free Press.

Straus, M. A. (1993). Physical assaults by wives: A major social problem. In R. J. Gelles & D. R. Loseke (Eds.), *Current Controversies on Family Violence* (pp. 67–87). Newbury Park, CA: Sage.

Walter, J. L., & Peller, J. E. (1994). "On track" in solution-focused brief therapy. In M. F. Hoyt (Ed.), *Constructive Therapies* (pp. 111–125). New York: Guilford Press.

White, M., & Epston, D. (1990). *Narrative Means to Therapeutic Ends.* New York: Norton.

CHAPTER 9

When the Past Is Present
A Conversation about EMDR
and the MRI Interactional Approach

CLIFFORD LEVIN
FRANCINE SHAPIRO
JOHN H. WEAKLAND

The kind of brief therapy practiced at the Mental Research Institute (MRI) in Palo Alto, California, would seem at first glance to have little in common with eye movement desensitization and reprocessing (EMDR). The MRI method of brief strategic therapy focuses on the present, not on history or memory, with the goal of treatment being to alter the interactional patterns maintaining the problems that clients present (Fisch, 1994; Fisch, Weakland, & Segal, 1982; Watzlawick, Weakland, & Fisch, 1974; Weakland & Fisch, 1992; Weakland, Fisch, Watzlawick, & Bodin, 1972). EMDR, originated by Shapiro (1989, 1991, 1995), is based on an intrapsychic rather than an interpersonal model of change; it concentrates on the effects of past experiences on people's current lives. EMDR, which was developed as a treatment for the aftereffects of trauma, locates the problem in the brain and body of the individual client. It is assumed that traumas have left unprocessed memories, feelings, and thoughts that can be "metabolized" during the application of the EMDR method, one of the major components of which involves having the client engage in patterned (back-and-forth) eye movements. Although further research is needed and is underway, detailed procedures and protocols have been described and evidence has begun to mount that EMDR can yield powerful and enduring results. Indeed, there are more empirical studies supporting the efficacy of

EMDR in the treatment of the aftereffects of trauma than there are for all other methods combined (see Shapiro, 1995).[1]

We joined together to further explore these seemingly disparate practices, with the intention of considering possible common factors and connections between the ways in which "past" and "present" might be understood and approached therapeutically within each respective method. Shapiro agreed to speak about what she thought was going on in EMDR, and Weakland agreed to respond with a condensed version of his interactional view of central parts of the procedure. Levin, who had previously published a case report (Levin, 1993) describing the combined use of EMDR and MRI brief therapy, served as moderator. Although further trialogue was precluded by John Weakland's death, the following edited transcript invites consideration about the processes of change.

SHAPIRO: The original population I worked with was suffering from posttraumatic stress disorder (PTSD) because their earlier experiences were causing nightmares, flashbacks, and intrusive thoughts. The victim's perceptions seemed locked in the nervous system in the form that they were input, so all the disturbances held. In most instances, when a less disturbing experience would occur, what we'd see in everyone is a natural, inherited, hard-wired information-processing system that is physically geared to take the information to a place of nondisturbance. We'd learn what was necessary, we'd integrate what was useful, we'd let go of the negative affect, etc., and it would get stored in a way that was useful and could guide us in the future. But something about the trauma experience itself would cause an imbalance in that information-processing system, so the perceptions would basically be locked up in that original form. In EMDR, the person concentrates on these earlier traumas—be it a Vietnam experience or a rape experience—through the picture of the event and the negative statement that they might be saying to themselves about the event. Accessing that target and then adding in the eye movements or other kinds of stimulation activates that information-processing system. It rebalances the system and allows the information to be digested from this state and to be taken to a place where it is resolved.

[1]The advent of new treatment paradigms and methodologies usually engenders countermovement or "resistance," regardless of (or perhaps because of) their efficacy. This response is often based on some combination of preference for the familiar, theoretical obligation, and a desire to protect status quo financial arrangements (Fisch, 1965; Hoyt, 1985; Kuhn, 1970). It may be noted that MRI has encountered such opposition as it has advanced brief therapy, and that there have been parallels in the early response to EMDR (although more than 10,000 clinicians worldwide have been taught the approach since its introduction in 1989). Indicative of its broad scope of interest is the fact that MRI serves as an institutional "home" for both interactional brief therapy and EMDR.

WEAKLAND: Even though there was—am I correct—a perception at the time that this is a terribly difficult or almost impossible problem to work with?

SHAPIRO: Yes, at that point the view of PTSD was that we could easily get Vietnam vets that were still hot after 25 years, or molestation victims after years and years of therapy and they weren't getting resolved, but it seemed comparatively easy to deal with using EMDR—and very rapidly. Then it became clear that it didn't have to stop there, because any dysfunctional present disturbance is clearly based on an earlier life experience. If the person was not reacting appropriately at the present time, and was feeling unwarranted anger and shame or guilt or anxiety, it had to be based on earlier associations that were there. So we started to look for the earlier experiences that set the groundwork for that type of reaction. When we targeted those associated experiences, then we'd get the same type of resolution. So with the client who had been badly abused or beaten, we might concentrate on that memory in childhood. And with EMDR it would resolve with the client saying, "I'm fine, Dad really had a problem," and the negative feelings, feelings of power-lessness, and all the attributions would change. The essence of the memory and associations would be different and simply reside in the nervous system in a different way, so the negative aspects would no longer be triggered. Basically, it was the equivalent of being digested, in that what was helpful was integrated; what wasn't useful was let go. It became clear that this applied to a wide range of pathology.

WEAKLAND: Okay, let me raise this other question with you: Is there any sort of thing that you think this would not be applicable to, or at least it wouldn't be your number one choice to solve the problem?

SHAPIRO: I think anything that you would say is biochemical. If it turned out that bipolar response was purely biochemical, that schizophrenia was purely biochemical, then this would not be the treatment of choice. But if people were given a diagnosis of endogenous depression because it's been there their whole life, and you investigated and found out that in childhood they were consistently being given messages of not being good enough or of not being in control, then EMDR would be a treatment of choice—because if we go in and reprocess those earlier memories, then those feelings would go away in present time. I look at EMDR as a way of changing the experiences that are driving the person to react in a certain way, and then you have to reprocess or tend to how they are in present time. Their reaction to their boss, or reaction to their spouse, has to be targeted along with addressing new behaviors by teaching them new ways of being, so that all of the system issues are taken into account. EMDR is used to help the learning process. However, if a system, a situation is problematic—if a person was responding for a good reason in present time to someone else, and there wasn't any dysfunction that was coming up, they were just reacting appropriately to a present situation—then it wouldn't be EMDR that would be called for.

WEAKLAND: So it still might be reprocessing.

SHAPIRO: It's always reprocessing. Reprocessing is always there.

WEAKLAND: The end of what you've been describing is more the reprocessing part of your program, which I understand is something that has become clearer since the beginning of the time you've been working with this.

SHAPIRO: Yeah, I was thinking of it initially as desensitization of something, and then it became clear the desensitization was just a byproduct of the information itself resolving.

LEVIN: As a point of clarification, it seems that you, Francine, put an emphasis on the past, whereas John would not put an emphasis on the past. I find myself somewhere in between. For example, I worked with a male a couple of years ago who had been raped. The rape had happened when he was in college and now he was in his mid-30s, and yet when a situation came up that was reminiscent of something in the rape scene from 15 years ago, what he experiences in the here and now is very real and very with him. We're not talking about what happened to him 15 years ago; we're talking about what he is experiencing at that moment in real time. What is past and what is present, in terms of how human beings carry information and process information?

SHAPIRO: I think it's part of the paradigm, that "digestion" or "metabolism" basically hasn't taken place. The event hasn't taken its appropriate place in the past. Any past experience is part of us, like any food we have eaten becomes part of ourselves, so it's always going to be a question of how is the person reacting in present time. Whenever we look at the past events, it's because they impinge upon the present; things that happened in the past that don't impinge upon the present aren't of interest in the EMDR. Just those things that are making a person dysfunctional or unhappy in the present. The reason for going in and directly targeting the past experiences first is that when I first started using the method and viewed it from a behavioral vantage point, I would go in only on the present reactions, so instead of dealing with his rape I would have dealt with his present interaction. What I found in most people is that they automatically flipped back into their earlier experiences, and that's how I really discovered how strong those linkages were. For other people they would not flip back into earlier experiences, and the method wouldn't work. In other words, they would get more upset, they would get more disturbed, and nothing would happen. It didn't change until I deliberately asked them to go back and search for an early experience and targeted that and resolved it. Then when I retargeted the present, the disturbance was much decreased and was easier to deal with. So going into the earlier experiences first became a way of making sure that the client had good, effective treatment and good success experiences, and was also prepared for the type of material that might emerge. But it is all present.

WEAKLAND: That last word would be the key in my answer. It *is* all present. The present is all you ever have while you are working, but the present may include present memories of past—present ways that you could preserve the past in anything from your thinking to your neurology, which could include even your imagination. But even if it is about what somebody sees as being about the past, you are working with it now.

LEVIN: Yet in terms of trauma situations, Vietnam veterans, rape survivors, and people like that, it seems like—as you often put it—a tragic case of "the same damn thing over and over again" for a very long time.

WEAKLAND: That is what I and my colleagues think we are always working on. The difference between a current problem and a chronic problem is that someone has been stuck in the same thing, attempting to resolve it in ways that don't work, for a longer time. Even when you're dealing with the present, you are not dealing with the present in terms of what is clear and concrete; you are dealing with somebody's construction of the present, which includes construction about things in the past. Also, perhaps, constructions about the future.

SHAPIRO: Actually, I'd assume that within five minutes what you're dealing with is your memory of the experience, which is . . .

WEAKLAND: . . . but your memory is not really that different from what's going on right this minute. In any case, you're dealing with the way you construct and construe it in your mind.

SHAPIRO: Well, with trauma, though, we'll go back and find people that keep reliving it in a certain way and are blaming themselves for certain things. When you go back in and process it, they get more of the associations coming up, and they recognize that they've forgotten details about it. So a vet who has been blaming himself for 25 years for having killed three men and has been beating himself up for that—the processing remembers that that happened to him right after they killed his buddy, and that explains it to him. So part of that grief and part of that guilt is able to resolve. That information was there; it just wasn't accessible. So I think part of what we're looking for in EMDR is to associate more of the experience together, so that the person is able to take a different view of it or have it fit in differently.

WEAKLAND: "Take a different view" is the key phrase there to me.

LEVIN: So you would see it as a reframing?

WEAKLAND: I would see it essentially as a reframing.

SHAPIRO: And I see reframing as a byproduct of that reprocessing, just the way the desensitization is—that the information gets less disturbing, and the restructuring, the reframing is a byproduct, in that it's a more therapeutic or better-enhanced or more constructive way of viewing it. But that happens automatically as the processing occurs and it's not . . .

WEAKLAND: . . . it's not happening automatically. It's happening in relation to what you're doing.

SHAPIRO: In that if you set in motion the processing system within the person, that it also will be coming up with these new ways of viewing it that aren't necessarily imposed or offered by the clinician.

WEAKLAND: No, not proposed or offered, but the context is set to milk that sort of reprocessing that I'm terming "reframing." Two other points: That is also what is happening when one is reframing a present or recent experience; and, in addition, I'm sure that you found that some of your therapists can screw this up even if they get it started, depending on how they continue to deal with what is being produced by the client.

SHAPIRO: Yeah, the most important thing that I always caution the clinicians is to stay out of the way. (*Laughter*)

WEAKLAND: Yeah . . .

LEVIN: For a further point of clarification, if we were to take an example of a Vietnam vet who has PTSD and he were to come to each of you—if I have this right, John, you would more typically say, "What are you trying to do about these problems now?" and Francine, if I have this right, you would be more interested in "What memories do you have that may have contributed to this problem forming?" Is there a different emphasis in what you're looking for at the point of contact with the client?

WEAKLAND: That's not quite what I would do, but that's part of it. Probably the first thing that I would do would be to ask, more or less directly, "Okay, something happened to you that was a terrible experience. How is it relevant to you today?" Then I might bother to go on to how you've been trying to deal with whatever social problem it's still presenting you right now.

LEVIN: Okay. So, first, "How is it a problem for you?" And, second, "What are you doing about it?"

WEAKLAND: Yeah.

SHAPIRO: That would be similar to my first question: "What's the problem that brings you in here?"

WEAKLAND: Yeah.

SHAPIRO: And then define what the overall picture looks like for them in the present, and how they are presently affected by it. What are their beliefs that might be inherent in it now, and then get a clear picture of what the present looks like: alternative problems or complaints; how are they affected; the frequency of his flashbacks, and whatever might bring them on in present time; and a clinical understanding of the whole present situation. Then I would target the original event that set it in motion.

LEVIN: So the initial inquiry might look very similar between the two of you. It's very much "What is the problem you're bringing to us now?"

WEAKLAND: Yeah.

SHAPIRO: Right.

WEAKLAND: There would be one possible difference. In asking, "How is it relevant to you now?", I think that I would hope to do that in such a way that is to imply that things in the past do not necessarily control your behavior today, and I would carefully at the same time . . . the implication, crudely put, would be "Christ, that was a long time ago. Why didn't you forget it?"

LEVIN: Are you borrowing from Ericksonian thought there?

WEAKLAND: Well, I'd have to give that a lot of thought, because while I haven't particularly thought about it in those terms, I'm probably borrowing from Ericksonian thought a lot of the time automatically now, without even giving it a second thought. Because I've just been changed because of contact with Erickson.

SHAPIRO: Even if the experience is just locked in the nervous system and continues impacting on the present, I'm still going to see if there are contributing factors in the present that are keeping it going. So are they in a chaotic situation that keeps on triggering it, or are they with the same type of individuals that keep bringing it on? And then that would tell me what different things would have to be addressed, in addition to that initial experience that started it.

WEAKLAND: Well, we've already gotten to, I think, a point which is perhaps the major point of difference between the way you look at things and the way I look at them. And that is—I think I oversimplify it a little, but not much—my tendency is to think things only get locked in the nervous system, if they are, by means of being locked into the way people behave in the present. You can behave in certain ways that make you continue to respond, react, think, feel, in ways you've done for a long time, but that only occurs when you continue to behave in a certain way with yourself and with other people.

SHAPIRO: Well, we could look at a behavioral description of PTSD. They talk about a two-factor theory [Mowrer, 1960; see Shapiro, 1995, pp. 19–20]. One is the classical conditioning, when the person had the impact of the event; and what maintains it is the operant conditioning, that a person keeps avoiding exposure to it. Because they keep avoiding situations of prolonged exposure to similar situations, that keeps it from going away. So in that way you may be right.

WEAKLAND: I think that avoidance is a central factor in the way we think about things. There is an alternative that I think has much the same effect, probably less important in PTSD, but in other situations involving other types of problems and involving anxiety. I think that there are at least a portion, maybe a minority, of people who as an alternative to avoiding try its opposite, apparent opposite—which is "I'm going to charge the wall and break through it this time." And they bounce off the wall, and you get the same result as you do from avoidance: You reinforce "I can't possibly face up to that."

SHAPIRO: I just see a lot of it going on below the conscious threshold, so that it becomes out of the person's real control. And some of the experiences of people with PTSD are so horrific they really can't maintain control. The person may go back into flashback situations automatically when exposed to auditory stimuli, so people can be triggered into a flashback every time they hear a plane go overhead. And they've heard planes going overhead a whole lot of times, and that still isn't allowing it to extinguish. The difference would be that with the EMDR, there is the holding of that exposure to the event and then accelerating the processing of it in a way that stays manageable for them by going in and out of the experience. Because one of the hallmarks of EMDR is keeping them in the present as they are noticing the memory. They are noticing the experience of the memory or the event, but it's the maintaining of the connection to the present that I think is really crucial for dealing with the event.

WEAKLAND: Okay.

LEVIN: John, what do you make of the idea of stimulating the brain via the eye movements, and that the brain has its own natural process of moving information to being held in a completed state? Francine is saying that by having a person hold certain ideas and then adding in the eye movements or other forms of stimulation, we bring the brain along a course of processing this information, which has been sitting there unprocessed for a long time. What would you make of that physiological view?

WEAKLAND: It's a physiological view, but it is also something more. Just from Francine's description (at least as I hear it), because of what you said talking about getting it wrong, it's a combination of returning more fully to the traumatic situation, but at the same time maintaining oneself to some extent in the present, which I would see as maintaining a particular kind of contact with the therapist. That combination makes a great deal of sense to me. There are two things going on at the same time, although my immediate colleagues and I would probably describe it in somewhat different terms. That is, when we deal with problems of anxiety, we avoid two things and we do a third thing, the third thing being somewhat double. We avoid letting people escape into avoidance; we [also] avoid people saying, "I'm going to lick the thing this time." Instead, essentially we push people toward what they're afraid of and hold them back at the same time. I see that as very similar to what Francine just said about coming to the traumatic situation more fully, but yet at the same time maintaining a contact in the present with the therapist.

LEVIN: Any thoughts about what combination of stimuli that the client experiences, how that might help the . . .

WEAKLAND: I think you're moving in the direction of "*Why* does it work?", but I prefer to stick to "*How* does it work?" Again, you find an alternative to the two things that we have elicited a great deal of information showing that they don't work. One is the more or less complete avoidance or attempt at avoidance, and the other is the attempt to break through the wall by main force—that I'm going to be determined that this time I'm going to do it, regardless of all. You find something that is—that sounds different from both of those.

SHAPIRO: Well, the paradigm that we're using involves the concept of dual focus. Don't deliberately do anything except follow my finger; with everything else essentially just notice what occurs, don't make it significant, don't try to grab a hold of it—and, at the same time, stay with me. You go through it, then just let it go and to talk to me." That juxtaposition is going on through the entire 90 minutes. They need to maintain the two together. So you could come up with the theory that following the finger is stimulating information processing in the present time. Now that you have that information-processing system functioning, at the same time when you ask the person to attend to the trauma, it kicks in the processing of that trauma because you're keeping that information-processing system moving in the present just by following the finger. So what was locked up before and wasn't touchable before is now moved into the system that's already functioning.

WEAKLAND: I would like to hear a little more from you about how you get people ready and willing to participate in this, because I am quite sure from things I've heard you say before that it takes some doing. It probably always takes some doing. Particularly, I've heard you mention cases in which people were very leery about getting to the point of actually trying the procedure, and you have dealt with them in a way that has brought them past often considerable reluctance to touch anything. I think that can be very important. How do you lead them up to that point?

SHAPIRO: I think at this point I don't necessarily meet them when they are leery and difficult (*laughter*). They're usually coming in asking for it.

WEAKLAND: Well, somebody can come in for something and still be leery and reluctant after they get in the door.

SHAPIRO: I think that part of it is really laying out a picture for both of us of how they're being affected right now—so they really get an understanding of how pervasive it is in their relationships, and maybe in their work setting, and in the way they enjoy life or don't enjoy life, and all the different triggers that are there, connections to the old—as well as identifying the negative beliefs they have about themselves. They may say something and describe an event, and I might offer, "Does it sound like you're saying this?" or give them suggestions of what the negative thoughts might be or negative cognitive assessments might be, if they don't come out with it on their own. They very often do; it's just part of the language that they use as they are describing the way they are in the present. So I'll either pull out that language and offer it back to them, or I'll formulate something and offer it back to them. And they—to the point they are able, they accept it, or see it as something that is really impinging on them. Often isolating these negative thoughts that they've had about themselves that they really haven't looked at before gets them to see how badly they've been affected by it, and then it's framing it in a way . . .

WEAKLAND: Okay.

SHAPIRO: . . . in a way that it's not their fault that they've been affected, by basically explaining the whole theory of the method that it's information that's been locked in their nervous system before they had any choice in the matter. As children they had no choice in the matter, or as a combat vet they had no choice in the matter, and so the onus goes off of them.

WEAKLAND: Okay, so there's two things. One is, together with them you make clear the seriousness of the problem, clearer and more specific—express the seriousness of this problem and its effects on their current daily lives. And the other is, you begin to take the tack that "It's not your fault."

SHAPIRO: Yes.

WEAKLAND: I also think you have a certain ability to urge people without urging them directly to go forward, and also a willingness to back off when it looks like you're going a bit faster than they're prepared to go, so that there is a matter of pacing here that I think can be very subtle and that you're very good at.

SHAPIRO: Thank you.

WEAKLAND: But you may be doing it automatically, for all I know.

LEVIN: It doesn't sound all that dissimilar to the concept of restraint that has been practiced as part of the MRI brief therapy model.

WEAKLAND: I would agree with that.

SHAPIRO: Well, it's always trying to get clients to develop their view of it, in their own language and in their own way. And in that way you really have to be hooked up with the clients and get a sense when they're with you and walking along beside you, and the point that they're not ready or they back off or they don't understand it, or they've gone off on a tangent and you have to follow where they're going for a while and try to get them back on the course . . .

WEAKLAND: But a lot of therapists don't see it when a client is giving the therapist a sign: "Slow down." Yet you do see it, and you do respond to it. I don't think I'm being unfair to the profession as a whole, but that is not a common talent—to be able to combine a way of urging and an ability to draw back. I think that it mostly tends to be one or the other, and I think one or the other does not work.

LEVIN: In the beginning of your interviews, Francine, you elicit the negative thoughts and then, before you even begin the actual EMDR eye movements, you also elicit the positive thoughts. In other words, you hang out there an essential reframe for them. You are providing them both frames and saying, "We're going to start here and we're going to get to there, and in between we're going to do a lot of this eye movement stuff."

SHAPIRO: I've always viewed this new cognition as the light at the end of the tunnel. First of all, it's motivating when there is something to go towards and some sense of maybe there can be an alternative, but it's not necessarily a high probability for the client when they start that they're actually going to get exactly there.

LEVIN: That's the restraint aspect of it.

SHAPIRO: Most often, or very, very often, they'll come up with an even better positive thought along the way that will automatically emerge, so I think that all of the components that are in the method have more than one reason and more than one use. Each of the components is there in order to help in accessing the material or help in moving the material along. A lot of it is for the client's comfort and maintaining the state where the client is able to comfortably go from one place to another. In accessing some of the earlier material, for instance, there can be a great deal of disturbance that emerges. So a lot of the parameters of the EMDR are placed to make the client feel safe in present time and to make sure that nothing in the present is being made more disturbing, so that they can safely concentrate on the material that's come up.

WEAKLAND: I want to comment on that. There is something else I think that you didn't make too much of, but you're probably good at it, and I think it's something that is seldom discussed but it can be very important. You give people confidence because you can at the same time be prepared to hear how terrible their experience has been and is, without yourself getting threatened and lost, and I think sometimes this can be very important. I think there are a lot of people that are very poor at that.

SHAPIRO: I think that part of that is a product of knowing that it will be gone. I think part of the problem with a lot of clinicians out there is that they get lost in the stuff, because they don't have confidence themselves that the client is going to be able to emerge from it. I see it just as a starting point, and even as we get into the processing and they are experiencing the terror of the old moment, for me the experience that they are going through at that moment is a stage in their getting rid of it, so it's a lot easier to keep a detached compassion.

WEAKLAND: Yes. But that confidence and that detached compassion are very different from, let's say, overt reassurance.

SHAPIRO: Yes.

LEVIN: John, you were talking about how the two things you avoid are having them go into total avoidance or total confrontation with an anxiety. And Francine described, in her own language, much the same thing. You don't tell them not to think about it; you don't tell them to charge headlong; you find a comfort range in which they can encounter it with a therapist who has a therapeutic distance and can offer restraint as is needed.

WEAKLAND: Yeah, I agree. There is a lot of similarity. There are certain ways to get them up to the more active and specific part of your therapy. You were doing something similar from the word go, even just discussing "What is your situation? What are you here about? What might we be doing?"

SHAPIRO: Yes. In a lot of ways I think some of it is a bird's-eye view of the problem, and it allows them also to get an understanding of the complexity or the significance and, at the same time, seeing it in perspective—which means it's only a beginning and there is an end, there's an alternative, and this is not an interminable process or problem. For me a lot of it, and a lot of the components of the EMDR, is to give clients the understanding that they are larger than the pathology.

WEAKLAND: Yes. And in a sense you're also modeling, implicitly, the sort of stance that you wish them to take. I'm particularly interested in this, because over the course of the years I have heard I don't know how many statements about how the essence of things is a good therapeutic relationship; and practically without exception, people leave it at that and don't go on to define what does a therapist do that constitutes establishing a good therapeutic relationship. I think that's what we are now talking about. Establishing a good therapeutic relationship—how is someone supposed to go out and do that, if they know that's the important thing? We're talking about what is the form or pattern of the therapist's behavior and the relationship to the client, and the more we talk about it, the more it seems to be things to carry through from the very beginning to the specifics of the actual procedure.

LEVIN: It may not be the eye movements alone, and it may not be those other factors alone. This might be a synergistic phenomenon.

SHAPIRO: It's always a problem when you're trying to view one thing, or view one answer, in any form of therapy. I think that the relationship, the way we've set out the protocols that we have, and the procedures that we have, in and of themselves, without the eye movement, are really very good. And I think that the eye movement in isolation with certain people would be sufficient, but that's not a large group of people. I think that in order to enhance the eye movement, these other things are really necessary. That's why they all came about.

WEAKLAND: I would agree that people keep looking for things that are too single-factor or too highly specific.

REFERENCES

Fisch, R. (1965). Resistance to change in the psychiatric community. *Archives of General Psychiatry, 13,* 359–366.

Fisch, R. (1994). Basic elements in the brief therapies. In M. F. Hoyt (Ed.), *Constructive Therapies* (pp. 126–139). New York: Guilford Press.

Fisch, R., Weakland, J. H., & Segal, L. (1982). *The Tactics of Change: Doing Therapy Briefly.* San Francisco: Jossey-Bass.

Hoyt, M. F. (1985). Therapist resistances to short-term dynamic psychotherapy. *Journal of the American Academy of Psychoanalysis, 13,* 93–112. (Reprinted in M. F. Hoyt, *Brief Therapy and Managed Care: Readings for Contemporary Practice* [pp. 219–235]. San Francisco: Jossey-Bass, 1995.)

Kuhn, T. S. (1970). *The Structure of Scientific Revolutions* (2nd ed.). Chicago: University of Chicago Press.

Levin, C. (1993). Case studies: The enigma of EMDR. *Family Therapy Networker, 17*(4), 75–83. (With commentaries by Francine Shapiro and David Waters.)

Mowrer, O. H. (1960). *Learning Theory and Behavior.* New York: Wiley.

Shapiro, F. (1989). Efficacy of eye movement desensitization procedure in the treatment of traumatic memories. *Journal of Traumatic Stress Studies, 2,* 199–233.

Shapiro, F. (1991, May). Eye movement desensitization and reprocessing procedure: From EMD to EMD/R—a new treatment model for anxiety and related traumata. *The Behavior Therapist, 14,* 133–135.

Shapiro, F. (1995). *Eye Movement Desensitization and Reprocessing: Basic Principles, Protocols, and Procedures.* New York: Guilford Press.

Watzlawick, P., Weakland, J. H., & Fisch, R. (1974). *Change: Principles of Problem Formation and Problem Resolution.* New York: Norton.

Weakland, J. H., & Fisch, R. (1992). Brief therapy—MRI style. In S. H. Budman, M. F. Hoyt, & S. Friedman (Eds.), *The First Session in Brief Therapy* (pp. 306–323). New York: Guilford Press.

Weakland, J. H., Fisch. R., Watzlawick, P., & Bodin, A. (1972). Brief therapy: Focused problem resolution. *Family Process, 13,* 141–168.

CHAPTER 10

The Relational Self
The Expanding of Love beyond Desire

STEPHEN G. GILLIGAN

And the priestess spoke again and said: Speak to us of Reason and Passion.

And he answered, saying:

Your soul is oftentimes a battlefield, upon which your reason and your judgment wage war against your passion and your appetite.

Would that I could be the peacemaker in your soul, that I might turn the discord and the rivalry of your elements into oneness and melody.

But how shall I, unless you yourselves be also the peacemakers, nay, the lovers of all your elements?

—KAHLIL GIBRAN, *The Prophet* (1923, p. 51)

The experience of Self is always a defeat for the ego.

—CARL G. JUNG (1957/1970, par. 778)

Growing up in an Irish Catholic alcoholic family in San Francisco, I used to get into big trouble. Such rascality would typically earn me a face-to-face encounter with my drunken father, who would demand to know, "Who the hell do you think you are, anyway?" The question arrested my attention, so it is not surprising that I have continued to ponder it over the years. How we ask and answer this question of psychological identity seems crucial to how we experience and express ourselves in the world.

Of course, much of the time the inquiry is straightforward. When I go into a store, I am in the identity of a customer, with all my understandings and associations of that role identity. At the same time, still in a rather straightforward way, I may sense the clerk as a bully, and respond by identifying myself as assertive. If the clerk speaks with a heavy foreign accent, I may additionally think of myself as a native-born American.

Although the identity question is straightforward and not so interesting in some contexts, it is of central relevance in others, especially that of psychotherapy. In fact, we might say that people become psychotherapy clients precisely because the ways they are answering identity questions don't allow a fit to the social context or a connection to an inner sense of self, and thereby generate inappropriate behavior or painful experience. For example, when a depressed person locks into the singular self-truth of "I am worthless," all other self-descriptions are functionally dissociated, and the person's response to the outside world and connection to the inside world are lost. In this sense, a goal of psychotherapy is to support the fixed identity a client may be stuck in, while expanding the field of consciousness to activate and connect additional identities.

This is what the therapeutic approach of *self-relations* seeks to do. As we will see, self-relations sees therapy problems in terms of a position's, truth's, or identity's becoming isolated from its larger field, and sees solutions developing when relational processes are reactivated and cooperative processes developed. For example, say a client is espousing the position of "Life sucks and you can't trust anybody." (Such a person usually receives the diagnosis of adolescence.) Is this good or bad? Self-relations suggests that it is neither. It is one of the great "truths" of the world, whose value and meaning depends in large part on whether the person also has access to other, especially complementary truths, such as "Life is beautiful." In other words, *the problem is not the problem; the problem is that what is pointed to as the problem is isolated from other positions, persons, experiences, or truths*. As the existentialists used to say, the study of psychopathology is precisely the study of loneliness. The idea of a *relational self* is that every person is a conversation between positions, the holder of differences, the integrator of opposites. The person is relationship itself—figure, field, and form.

How that idea plays out in psychotherapy is the focus of this chapter. I begin by describing two different psychological approaches to experience, fundamentalism and aesthetics. I show how fundamentalism is a succinct formula for violence, and how the alternative of an aesthetic approach gives rise to the basic premises of self-relations. I next discuss how these premises suggest a psychological model of symptoms based on the alienation of a social/cognitive self from an experiential/soulful/archetypal self, and then explore a prototype structure for renewing the spirit of relatedness within the relational self.

FUNDAMENTALISM VERSUS AESTHETICS

One can approach the question of identity or meaning in different ways. Some ways lead to limited answers, violence, and symptoms; others lead to growth and solutions. In the view of self-relations, the two most relevant approaches are fundamentalism and aesthetics.

Fundamentalism is the more common approach. It is not tied to a particular content or ideology. It may be used by the right wing as well as the left, in secular contexts as well as religious, in artistic domains as in scientific ones. It may be applied equally to the Bible, to the DSM-IV, to the lyrics of the Grateful Dead, to the work of Milton Erickson, to a memory, or to any other experience or view of life.

Fundamentalism starts with the premise that identity is defined according to allegiance to some single truth. This truth is revealed in a special text. I use the term *text* loosely here, meaning any frame of words, images, and feelings. The therapist's theory is a text; so is each memory, experience, or story of the client. In fundamentalism, a particular text is assumed to reveal *the* truth rather than *a* truth, and identity is based on strict adherence to that truth. The text is more important than experience itself, so in fundamentalism the primary relationship of a person is with the unchanging, single text, rather than with the organic here and now of life itself. Needless to say, this makes learning difficult if not impossible.

Fundamentalism further requires that the text be read literally; it is not to be sensed poetically, metaphorically, or with a sense of humor. (Is it not rare to hear of hilariously funny fundamentalist comics or poignant fundamentalist artists?) In fundamentalism, psychological identity is expressed by fixating on the text, rather than seeing or feeling through it to a deeper, aesthetic meaning. Thus, the metaphor of an inner child, the idea of an unconscious mind, a depression, or a solution is taken literally, rather than as a process description that points beyond itself to something more ineffable, something more primary. In the words of William Blake (quoted by Yeats, 1905/1979, p. xxxii), "Satan has many names, Opacity being the most common."

In positing that one way is correct and all others are wrong, fundamentalism sees the relationship between differences as irreconcilable opposites. A person is either an insider or an outsider in relation to the truth, and the possibility of relatedness across the boundaries is forbidden. If intimacy involves the holding of two different "truths"—the "I" and the "thou," "self" and "other"—in relationship, then intimacy is disallowed. If creative activity—whether it be humor, art, or scientific discovery—involves the holding of two different frames simultaneously, then creative activity and aesthetic experience are forbidden.[1] If altered states of consciousness such as hypnosis are developed by assuming that a person has two different selves, then trance is to be feared.

The idea that differences are irreconcilable spells trouble when opposites meet, as they have a habit of doing. (As Bateson [1970/1972] emphasized, difference is the basic unit of mental process.) In fact, the "I–it" relationship given to one person's position and another's different position is, I suggest here, a formula for violence. The position of the "other" is deemed invalid in a way that legitimizes attempts to eliminate it, by any means necessary. The thinking is, "There's only room in this here self for one of us, so you better be destroyed." This gives rise to a series of "final solutions" that seek, in the name of freedom, purity, mental health, justice, or God, to eradicate the bad, sick, crazy, or evil "other." Our image of the "other" is degraded, as Sam Keen (1986) has brilliantly illustrated, into the archetypal face of the enemy. Once the image of the enemy is locked into neuromuscular freeze, any "freedom-loving" person may feel not only justified but obligated to engage in violence to eradicate it.

In the clinical context, a client struggling with a symptom is a person struggling with, among other things, fundamentalism. For example, say a person has experienced a sexual trauma. In an almost unavoidable way, the memories or images of the trauma become imprinted as the text (or frame) by which future sexual or intimate relationships are understood. The traumatic memory becomes the fundamentalistic text that says, "All relationships are like this; you can't trust anybody." Furthermore, the text of the memory is regarded as an "it" that the person may try to keep out of his or her self, though it keeps coming back (via flashbacks, etc.).

As therapists, we need to have compassionate understanding for how fundamentalism develops. *The "break in relatedness" between self and other occurs via violence, and requires violence (against self and/or others) to maintain.* We need to appreciate how the consequent reduction of identity to an image or an "-ism," rather than to the consciousness of being, is a recipe for suffering and violence. At the same time, we are committed to exploring how the chain of violence may be ended, rather than perpetuated. Thus, we engage in what T. S. Eliot

---

[1]This idea of holding double frames simultaneously as the basis for the distinctly human experiences of humor, love, mythology, intimacy, craziness, play, and so on, has been suggested by a variety of writers. Bateson's (1979) idea of "double description" as a minimal requirement for an ecological view, stemming from his earlier work on the double bind hypothesis, was central to his later work. Jung (1916/1971) suggested the idea of the transcendent function, involving the capacity to hold opposite truths simultaneously, as the basic means of individuation. And Arthur Koestler (1964), in his opus *The Act of Creation*, suggested the idea of bisociation—involving the holding and integrating of two disparate matrices—as the essential mechanism of creative activity.

(1943/1952) in *Four Quartets* has called the "expanding/Of love beyond desire" (p. 142), or the expanding of identity beyond the fixed frame of a single text. We may be helped in this process by the epistemological approach of aesthetics, which constitutes a different approach to identity.

In an aesthetic approach, the image is not primary. God has many faces. *The relational self can be imaged in many ways, but this self is no image.* It is not a position or an image, but a context and a relational process. The consciousness that feels and sees (and is felt and seen) through images and descriptions, to a deeper pattern that connects, is more basic. Thus, the identity question is answered not in terms of "I am the follower of orthodox images," but rather "I am (with you) the consciousness that experiences multiple truths." (In this way, the poetic is a more grounded, primary, direct language than the literal.)

As Bateson (1955/1972) pointed out, the simultaneous holding of multiple frames or truths underlies many distinctly human contexts, such as intimacy, play, hypnosis, mythology, and psychopathology. Stated simply, to generate a nonrational state of consciousness (love, intimacy, humor, pathology, trance, symptoms, play, etc.), one must activate two seemingly contradictory truths or experiences simultaneously. In intimacy, for example, once we get beyond the romantic ideal of $1 + 1 = 1$ (where differences are obliterated), we see a more mature version of $1 + 1 = 3$ (where the differences of "I" and "thou" held in a unified field of consciousness give birth to a third, shared "us"). Later in this chapter, I describe how shifts in identity engender the need to hold opposite or multiple frames simultaneously, and examine further how altered states of consciousness are inevitable at this time. I also describe how these altered states are symptomatic or therapeutic, depending on whether the opposites are regarded as complementary or as irreconcilable, and whether a common field is felt to underlie and imbue both simultaneously. For now, I would like to simply suggest that aesthetics is an approach to identity that seeks to see or feel through different images to what T. S. Eliot (1943/1952) has called "a further union, a deeper communion" (p. 129). In holding multiple images or descriptions simultaneously, one is freed from the tyranny of what Bateson (1970/1972) described as the pathology of operating from a single position.

THE PREMISES OF SELF-RELATIONS

With these general distinctions in mind, we are now ready to examine how self-relations theory approaches the question of identity. There are three basic premises.

1. Self as Consciousness: The Principle of Beingness

The first premise is meant as an alternative to the three major causal metaphors used in psychotherapy—namely, (1) you are your past (personal history); (2) you are your biology; or (3) you are your social context (ethnicity, gender, family, etc.). Self-relations acknowledges that these are immensely important factors in shaping your experience, and that you must come to terms with each of them. Like ignoring money in modern times, ignoring them is the kiss of death. But if you make any of them primary, you'll also go down. So, while respecting the importance of personal history, biology, and social place, self-relations says that you are something more: You are a one-of-a-kind being of consciousness.

This can be expressed as the principle of beingness:

1. The beingness of life is distinctively present in each person.

Its corollaries are:

2. When the direct experience of beingness is ignored, denied, or cursed in a person, symptoms are likely to develop.
3. To alleviate symptoms and relieve suffering, first connect with the basic goodness of beingness in a person.

The felt sense of distinct beingness is represented in Figure 10.1 by a simple circle, to indicate an existence ("ex" and "stand"—to stand out). The point is that you really do exist as a human being. Your beingness is blessed. To forget or to ignore this leads to great suffering.

This may sound a bit esoteric, so let me give a few simple examples. If you were to meet my young daughter, Zoe, I could say to you, "Behold Zoe consciousness!" and you would get it. You would understand that she's no story, she's no description—she's consciousness itself, she's the real thing! Or if you've ever had the privilege of sitting with a person dying, you probably felt a deep consciousness in his or her process of letting go. A client of mine recently spoke of her struggle to come to terms with her dying father. He had been a terribly abusive man all her life, violating her in many ways. She had had no contact with him for years, but visited him upon hearing that he was dying of cancer. When she saw him on his deathbed, she was shocked to see that his mask of hatred and violence had dissolved, and a gentle, lonely man was exposed. She described it like the scene at the end of *Return of the Jedi*, when Darth Vader ("Dark Father") is unmasked to reveal his atrophied human face. Her heart felt opened, but her behavior was still paralyzed by what had happened over the years. In the therapy session, she struggled to reconcile the lifelong image of her father and her last experiential sensing of the consciousness behind the image.

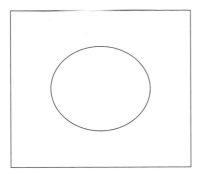

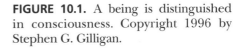

FIGURE 10.1. A being is distinguished in consciousness. Copyright 1996 by Stephen G. Gilligan.

In a similar way, we all become caught in fixed images or static stories that obscure and deny the dynamic life force pulsating through everything. It is easy to become seduced to fixating on the image, and more difficult to feel through it to the self as consciousness. But I believe that this is one of our challenges as therapists—to sense and reconnect consciousness to itself.

The experience of beingness is first known via *blessings* from influential others. Most people can remember someone in their lives—a family member, teacher, or friend—who really saw them as special and unique. This is not a cognitive event; it is about seeing and calling forth the spirit of life that infuses each person. Blessings are crucial acts in the emergence of each person into the world. Without them, love and other skillful human acts are not possible.

The opposite of a blessing is a *curse*. Curses are prominent in most traumatic events that are the forerunners of many symptoms. A trauma typically involves not only a physical violation, but also a curse: The perpetrator invades and imprints life-denying ideas such as "You exist only to serve me," "You are stupid," "You deserve to be punished," "You are unlovable,", and so forth. Self-relations refers to these events as "invasions by aliens," to emphasize that such ideas are not intrinsic to a person. They represent a sort of autoimmune disease in the "psychological immune system"—the part of a person that is needed to differentiate what's "me" from what's "alien to me." In other words, violence tears the "sheathing" that surrounds a being, and through the tear pour the aliens.[2] A person almost inevitably comes to misidentify these

---

[2]The sheathing that surrounds each being can be seen graphically in the response of young children to strangers or unfamiliar situations. A three-year-old may be exuberant and completely outgoing while playing at home with friends or family, but may show great changes when a stranger arrives. Everyone has seen how such a child may grow shy and hide behind a parent's protective body while sizing up the stranger. Because a child's sheathing is so delicate, a parent is responsible for shielding it from events that might tear it.It is in this way that the idea of a "tear in the sheathing" is meant.

alienating ideas as his or her own and to act accordingly. Self-relations looks to discriminate alienating ideas from self-affirming ideas, and suggests methods by which a person may "externalize" these aliens and reconnect with internally resonant descriptions (cf. White & Epston, 1990).

Children rely exclusively on blessings at first to experience their beingness. But as they mature, they develop the possibility for knowing their beingness via self-generated means. Self-relations terms such methods *centering practices,* and is interested in identifying which ones might work for a given person. Such practices—such as walking, meditating, talking to a friend, or creating art—bring a person to a calming, nonintellectual center of being. Through a combination of blessings and centering practices, a person may overcome the curses of alienation and recover the primacy of beingness.

2. Self as Relational Field:
The Principle of Belongingness

Self-relations suggests that the beingness of self is revealed in two complementary domains: (1) *a relational field* and (2) a *relational form.* The first is a felt sense of belonging to something bigger, to a field of consciousness; the second is a dynamic form of relationship playing through that field. To get a sense of the experience of self in a relational field, one might inquire along the following lines:

1. When do you feel most like yourself?
2. When you need to reconnect with yourself, what do you do?
3. When is life not a problem for you?

Typical responses might include playing or listening to music, going for a walk, being in nature, talking with good friends, reading, knitting, creating or performing art, dancing, and so forth. These activities constitute what I call "traditions of the aesthetic." They are traditions in that they are pulled from a large body of cultural practices that have been developed over many years, and aesthetic because of the nature of the experiences generated by such practices. If asked to describe what existential or phenomenological shifts occur during such events, most people will include responses such as decreased internal dialogue, timelessness, and an expansion of a felt sense of self. If you ask where the sense of self ends during such experiences, people will look at you quizzically, because no sharp boundary exists. *This expanded feeling of self beyond boundaries of skin and either–or ideology, while maintaining a center, is the experience of self as relational field.*

This relational field is described by the principle of belongingness:

1. The consciousness of self belongs to (or is part of) a larger relational field.

The corollaries are as follows:

2. When a person experiences a sustained "break in belonging" to a relational field, symptoms are likely to develop.
3. To relieve suffering and reconcile symptomatic conflict, reconnect consciousness to its relational fields.

This relationship may be represented in the traditional figure–ground or figure–field diagram (see Figure 10.2). The relational field may be spiritual ("I belong to a higher power, and he or she or it moves through me"); organismic ("I belong to nature, and it moves through me"); social ("I belong to my marriage/family/culture, and it permeates my consciousness"); or psychological (My experience/perspective is embedded within a larger field of experiences/memories/archetypes, and they guide/inform me").

Self-relations makes the observation that this experience of the field is present when life is working for a person—when life is not defined or perceived as a problem. At the same time, a person struggling with a symptom has experienced a "break in belonging" to the field; such a person does not feel a connection or sense of connection to a power or place greater than himself or herself. The experience of self is contracted and split, and a unified field supporting self and other is not felt. This cutoff from context leads to identification with the intellect and its fear-driven strategies of control and domination (and experiences of being out of control and reactive), rather than to curiosity and connectedness. Again, this is the basis for fundamentalism.

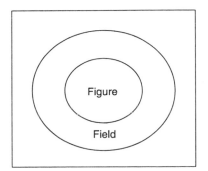

FIGURE 10.2. Each distinction of consciousness belongs to a larger field. Copyright 1996 by Stephen G. Gilligan.

The disconnection from field occurs in many ways, most of them involuntary. Some disconnections are the healthy first steps to individuation, as when an adolescent rebels against his or her family. Thus, breaks in belonging are not necessarily bad; they are inevitable steps of separation, and are ideally followed by a reunion with the field. But some experiences (such as traumas) don't allow such reconnection to occur. If the conditions or violence or trauma prevail, a sustained break occurs in which the person or experience is split off from its larger contexts of resources.

In this regard, symptoms are seen in part as unsuccessful attempts to reconnect with the field. For example, an addiction—whether to drugs or alcohol, food, sex, or cults—is initially an experience of losing one's self to a larger field. However, because the person attempts to get rid of part or all of his or her personal identity in this process, the results are emptiness and depression, followed by a downward spiral of further attempts to reconnect with the field by self-destructive activities. In this way, one part of the symptom is an attempt to return to the ground of being, while another is an reenactment of the violence that exiled one from the field in the first place.

Thus, a major focus of self-relations is on the nonviolent restoration of the felt sense of the field. It gently seeks to help a person unloose the grip of egoic control and rediscover the dynamic ground of natural being. In any performance art—dance, music, acting, aikido, sculpting, writing—one will hear from an artist the important of "relaxing" and feeling the rhythm. This is not the experience of a stuporous drool, but rather one of feeling centered and grounded in a way that allows the presence of the life force to move through one's being. In psychotherapy we help clients do this via many relational methods, including joining and validating experience, being in rhythm with the clients, encouraging centering and a felt sense of experience, and so forth. Disciplines such as prayer and meditation, service, and other mindfulness practices are explored and gently encouraged. In this regard, therapy is a process of reconnecting a person with his or her natural ground of being, so the sense of self as a relational field can be felt and used to gently ground and guide the person's activities.

3. Self as Relational Differences: The Principle of Relatedness

In time ("successive moments of now"), the relational self comes to know itself by proceeding through conversations between relational differences: different positions, different truths, different people, different times or places, different values, and so on. As Bateson (1979) repeatedly emphasized, *mind is relationship,* and *difference is the basic unit of mind.* Self-relations suggests the self as the experience of a dynamic relatedness between differences. This is described as the principle of relatedness:

1. To learn (or become) who you are, relatedness between differences is required.

Its corollaries are as follows:

2. When a "break in relatedness" persists, the experience of self disappears, the fundamentalist ego-mind reigns, and symptoms are likely to arise.
3. To reduce suffering and to reconcile symptoms, reestablish dynamic relatedness between positions of identity.

Self as the conversation of differences is represented in Figure 10.3 by the simple figure of two interconnected circles. In terms of psychological identity, this may be described in terms of a subject–object relationship, in which the person is identified with one position (the subject, or what we might call the "me" position), while directing his or her attention to another position (the object, or what we might call the "not-me" position). Thus, the relational self is a pattern of connections between "me" and "not me," experienced in a relational field.

Other pairs of relational differences relevant to psychotherapy include the following:

> self (me, us, I)–other (you, them, it)
> good–bad
> power–love
> inside–outside
> masculine–feminine
> healthy–sick
> problem–solution
> therapist–client
> thinking–feeling
> mind–body
> conscious–unconscious

In healthy situations, these relational differences operate in a conversational connectedness, the sort of "I–thou" relationship described by Martin Buber (1923/1958). In intimacy, there is an experience of a

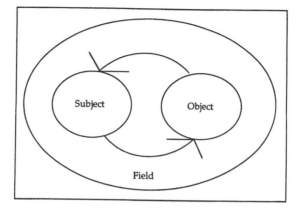

FIGURE 10.3. The relational self as the pattern that connects differences. Copyright 1996 by Stephen G. Gilligan.

"me," a "you," and the relational self of "us" that is felt when both the "I" and "thou" are validated. The experience of therapeutic trance (Gilligan, 1987) reflects a similar "self-(other) self" relatedness. The fictional terms of "conscious–unconscious" are provided, the suggestions to do something while just letting it happen ("Your hand can lift involuntarily") are given, and the resulting experience of "It's happening but I'm not making it happen" (e.g., "My hand is lifting, but it's old Mr. or Ms. Not Me that's lifting it!") is central to every hypnotic happening.

An exceptional example of how this happens in art has been given by the Chilean writer Isabel Allende. In an interview with Michael Toms (1994) appearing in the journal *Common Boundary*, she described how the characters in her novels first appear as "beings in her belly." She holds these beings in a sort of pregnancy. Her process of "giving birth" to them includes practices of falling in love with them on their own terms, accurately describing them, and listening to the story they have to tell. (How much this sounds like good parenting!) In the first stage of the process, these "beings in the belly" are guiding the story; in the second stage, her writer's ear and editor's craft are more active. *In both stages, the creative self is the experience of relatedness between these two orders of being.*

The examples above suggest that relatedness between differences is played out in different domains: Relational differences require a container, or a "temenos," as Jung (1916/1971) described it. The boundaries of "mind" may be intrapersonal or interpersonal; "mind" could be the individual, the couple, the family, the group, or the nation. For therapy purposes, self-relations generally emphasizes three types of relatedness required for conscious learning. The first is the *interpersonal,* involving the "I" and the "thou" described by Martin Buber. The second is the *embodied intrapersonal,* a felt sense of vertical relatedness between the cognitive/social self in the "head" and the emotional/archetypal consciousness in the "belly." The third is also intrapersonal—a horizontal *interhemispheric relatedness* required for experience to be processed and integrated (cf. Shapiro, 1995; Rossi, 1977). Self-relations posits that a sustained "break in relatedness" in any of these domains will result in an image of self that is "frozen in time," unable to learn, and thus likely to produce symptoms.

In problem situations, relatedness between different positions is denied or ignored. An interpersonal "thou" becomes an objectified "it," and the "beings in the belly" are reduced to an inhuman "other" to be removed by any means necessary. But as Jung (1957/1967) pointed out:

> We think we can congratulate ourselves on . . . having left the [archetypal] gods behind . . . but we are still as much possessed by autonomous psychic contents as if they were Olympians. Today they are called phobias, obsessions, and so forth; in a word, neurotic symptoms. The gods have become diseases; *Zeus no longer rules Olympus but rather the solar plexus.* (par. 54; emphasis added)

When life is working, life moves through us as we move through life, and is represented by the psyche in terms of different positions. The key is to find ways to respect and value each position as it moves through its ever-changing forms. This is a difficult process, as anyone involved in an intimate relationship soon realizes. It requires a centering within one's beingness, a grounding in one's field, and an openness to dialogue. Even under the best conditions, imperfection reigns. But as T. S. Eliot (1943/1952) encouraged, humility is endless. Or as Bill Wilson (1967), the founder of Alcoholics Anonymous, noted: "This is no success story in the ordinary sense of the word. It is a story of suffering transmuted, under grace, into gradual spiritual progress" (p. 35).

As we come back to relatedness, our experience of the relational self as dialogue develops. Holding the tension between differences nurtures a deeper harmony and capacity to act with love and integrity. At some point in the cycle, what Jung (1916/1971) termed the "transcendent function" occurs: The opposites integrate into a united form, where a difficult contradiction moves into a beautiful paradox—a movement Jung described as the central means of individuation of self. At that moment, we realize that the kingdom of God is within.

A SELF-RELATIONS MODEL OF HOW SYMPTOMS DEVELOP

The three principles of beingness, belongingness, and relatedness suggest questions to hold for sensing a person and not getting trapped in a problem-defined self:

1. Can you feel the beingness?
2. Can you sense the belongingness?
3. Can you hold the tension of the opposites?

Conversely, the principles suggest that symptoms reflect three types of sustained breaks: a "break in beingness" (and the awareness of goodness or blessedness), a "break in belonging" to something bigger (spiritual, organismic, social, psychological), and a "break in relatedness" between differences.

From these premises we can build a working model for self-relations. Figure 10.4a represents a healthy learning situation involving three aspects of a relational self: (1) the *normal self,* (2) the *experiential/archetypal self,* and (3) *influential others.* The *normal self* refers to the basic, everyday egoic sense of self that a person is aware of when life is not a problem. It is the cognitive/social self, based on the person's present age, and centered in the head. It includes competencies, resources, associations with present social others, skills, and multiple perspectives. It uses frames and models to plan, evaluate, and otherwise try to manage the world of experience. It is "normal" in the sense that it is what most people would

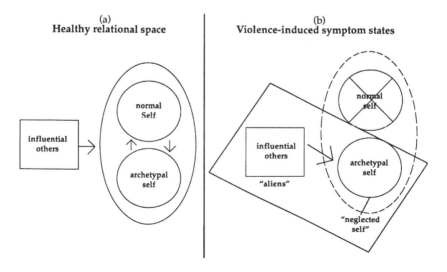

FIGURE 10.4. Relational space of the normal self, archetypal self, and influential others: (a) Healthy relational space and (b) violence-induced symptom states.

think of as their typical sense of self. In a symptom, this sense of self disappears, contracts, dissociates, or is otherwise nullified. Some clients will talk about just wanting to get back to their "normal self."

The *experiential/archetypal self* lives in the belly. It is experiential in that it is a directly felt sense of self, and archetypal in that it is connected to many generations of psychological experiences. Some traditions call it the *center;* others call it *soul.* Self-relations asserts that life moves through a person (except when it doesn't), radiating out from this center. It assumes that this order of mind is, at its roots, collective and transpersonal. In healthy situations, there is no fixed text or single image tied to this center. It is not an inner child, although the inner child may at times be one of the "beings in the belly," as Isabel Allende described them. Just as children have multiple forms of expression moving through them, so does the archetypal self in the belly. Whenever a particular form becomes fixated in a person's expression—as the Mental Research Institute folks say, whenever "the same damn thing happens over and over again" (see Watzlawick, Weakland, & Fisch, 1974)—it can be said that the archetypal self is disconnected from the cognitive self. This becomes the main objective of self-relations work: to restore the spirit of relatedness that joins the two selves into a relational self.

The normal self and the archetypal self constitute a dual-processing model of the relational self. As Epstein (1994) has effectively argued, there is tremendous support for this type of model of human processing. He summarizes the many descriptions of this dual processing, including "holistic–analytical," "affective–logical," "receptive–active," "nonverbal–verbal," "experiential–rational," and "narrative–analytical."

A third aspect of the relational field can be described as *influential others.* One's sense of identity is always a function of the intrapersonal relatedness between the normal self and archetypal self, as well as the interpersonal and transpersonal relatedness between oneself and influential others. These others may include social individuals, such as parents, friends, enemies, children, spouses, and so forth; they may also include spiritual beings, such as one's sense of a higher power. The point is that one is always being influenced and influencing identity via these interpersonal or transpersonal connections. Self-relations is especially interested in identifying which influential others are in a person's current circuitry, and what types of conversations are taking place.

Of special interest is whether these influential others offer blessings or curses of one's beingness. In healthy situations, a person is seen and blessed by influential others; in unhealthy situations, curses reign, and self-denigration and other alienating practices are the order of the day.

Thus, as Figure 10.4a illustrates, a healthy relational process involves life-affirming processes at both interpersonal and intrapersonal levels. At early developmental stages these two levels are barely distinguishable, since the normal cognitive/social self is very undeveloped, such that the interpersonal others (e.g., parents) must fill in for and model the normal self. Maturity involves gradually developing one's own unique cognitive/social self that can both be "a part of" and "apart from" influential others, such that a person's intrapersonal relatedness becomes an increasingly important factor. The earlier example of Isabel Allende illustrates one way in which this occurs.

As Figure 10.4b illustrates, a symptomatic self occurs when one or more influential others invade the boundaries of self, leading to a break in relatedness between the cognitive and archetypal selves, as well as a break in belonging of the self to its larger field. These breaks are what allow alienating ideas ("curses") to be internalized. If processing of the traumatic event is inhibited, the alienating ideas are mistaken for one's own voice, and the traumatic relationship is mistaken for one's identity.

An identity based on traumatic experience leads to three types of symptoms (cf. Herman, 1992). First, the person's normal sense of self is constricted, dissociated, fragmented, or otherwise inaccessible. Second, the archetypal self is gripped in a state of "neuromuscular lock," a frozen state distinguished by out-of-control emotions, hyperarousal, hypervigilance, somatization, and regression. Third, the person cannot shut out intrusive, negative images and voices that define the self as bad, unlovable, deserving of violence. and so forth. Thus, in the language of self-relations, the normal self becomes disconnected; the archetypal self becomes neglected, literalized, and frozen into a fixed form; and the influential others lock into alien(ating) presences.

A PROTOTYPE MODEL FOR SELF-RELATIONS WORK

Self-relations suggests some basic interventions that may be helpful in psychotherapy. The first is dissolving rigid attachment to a single text or description, so that other frames may be made equally available. The second is returning consciousness to a felt sense of the relational field, so that a person has a direct sense of belonging to the community, to the environment, and to an intelligence and power greater than the isolated ego. The third is reconciling or at least resolving the relational differences between the "me" and "not-me" positions in a person's identity.

In the development of practices along these lines, a simple seven-step prototype has emerged. This is not a fixed prescription for how to do therapy with every person, but rather a pattern that suggests coherent principles that can be applied in various ways. In applying this model, it is important to reiterate the aesthetic base of self-relations: *The goal is to find a middle way between the alienation of intellectual discourse and the inflation of catharsis or regression processes.* The client should be helped to stay in the present, while also feeling a variety of experiences via the "other self." To allow for the emergence of this processing of the relational self, the relational connectedness between therapist and client must be developed and maintained throughout the application of the technique. This is not a model to be explored without a felt sense of ongoing connectedness; to put it bluntly, if you can't get it, don't use the model. This is difficult to convey in writing, but crucial to understand in practice. Based in part on the earlier legacy of Milton Erickson, a main focus of the method is on gently opening mind–body circuits, to move language from an "in-the-head" intellectual analysis to an "in-the-body" felt sense that evokes multiple levels. It should be used with a soft rather than a hard intensity, with relational grounding and nonverbal pacing. Many of the ideas, especially those of "aliens" and "neglected selves," will be unhelpful if they are not apprehended in the more primary felt sense.

With these considerations in mind, let us consider each step in turn.

Step 1: Identify the Problem

In this first step, the therapist seeks to identify what the problem is, where and when it is occurring, and what specifically happens that moves an experience from mere unpleasantness (e.g., "I feel sad") to an identity-defining, self-disturbing symptom. The therapist's frame is something like this: "A funny thing happens on the way to this person's becoming more of his or her self. What is it?" Thus, after receiving the client's general description of the problem, the therapist may ask something like this: "If I were accompanying you on a day [or week, or month] in your life, where and when would I see this problem occur?" Clients often have difficulty getting specific, or may say something like "It happens all the time," so the therapist may need to be gently persistent—perhaps by asking, "When did it happen recently? Where was it really disturbing?" The movement into specific times and places helps to move the experience of the problem back into the body and other important realities, so this step is crucial.

As the person identifies a time when the problem occurred, the therapist slows down the processing to try to get a moment-by-moment, frame-by-frame description of the problem sequence. Clients will frequently rush through frames, so the therapist must try gently to get the details of both external behaviors ("And then he did that") and internal experiences ("And then I felt angry" or "Then I thought I was wrong"). The basic idea guiding the therapist is that circumstances at some point trigger the activation of the neglected self, which prompts the person to "leave time" (i.e., "successive moments of now"). This dissociation sticks the person in a loop; since he or she has left time, life moves from "one damn thing after the next" to "the same damn thing over and over." This is the "break in belongingness" as well as the "break in relatedness" that moves a difficult, unpleasant event to a symptom-producing clinical problem.

Here is an abbreviated example of this part of the interview:

CLIENT: Well, I guess the last time I got anxious was this morning when my friend came over.

THERAPIST: Your friend came over. . . . May I ask your friend's name?

CLIENT: Bill.

THERAPIST: Bill. And before Bill came over, how were you doing?

CLIENT: Okay. I was feeling okay that morning, just making some phone calls and stuff.

THERAPIST: You were feeling pretty good, and then this event with Bill started happening. When exactly—if you can just take a moment to relax and remember back—when exactly did you feel the first moment of disturbance? Was it before Bill came, or was it when he actually was there, that you began to feel the first suggestion that the problem of anxiety was going to happen? [The therapist softens the tone to allow experiential accessing.]

CLIENT: (*Pauses to think*) Well, I began to feel a little weird as soon as he walked in.

THERAPIST: As soon as he walked in. And where were you.?

CLIENT: I was sitting at my desk.

The therapist now asks a series of detail questions about the other furniture, what each person was wearing, what specifically was said, what was felt in the body at each point, and so forth. This procedure is an outgrowth of Ericksonian hypnotherapy procedures (see Gilligan, 1987), whereby associational questions are asked in a hypnotic-like focus to move attention to experiential revivification of the problem sequence, so that the emotional/imaginal/psychological components of the sequence can be heightened and utilized. (Remember, trance is the repoeticization of experience.)

Step 2: Identify and Somatically Locate the Neglected Self

At some point in the problem sequence, a felt sense of the problem will begin to develop in the client. This marks the appearance of the neglected self. An easy way to identify the neglected self is to ask the client to fill in the following statement: "If only I didn't experience/do [or could get rid of] X, then this really wouldn't be a problem." X marks the spot of the neglected self. For example:

If only I didn't feel so inhibited, I would be successful.

If only I didn't feel so angry, I could get on with my life.

If only she wasn't so cold (and I didn't feel rejected as a result), our marriage wouldn't be such a problem.

The idea is that when this unacceptable experience or behavior arises, the person has to "leave town" or dissociate, because he or she cannot hold the tension between the opposites—between this experience and his or her egoic normal self. In other words, this is where the break in relatedness occurs, and where symptomatic behavior is likely to arise. Thus, self-relations seeks to bring the neglected self back into the field of the relational self in three subsidiary steps.

Step A: Locate the Somatic Center

The therapist should ask the client: "When the problem is present, where in your body do you most feel its center of disturbance [or discomfort]?" Many people point immediately to their stomach, solar plexus, or heart area, even before conscious or verbal awareness has developed. If a person has difficulty understanding the question or feeling anything, a bit of relaxation helps to open awareness of somatic sensation. A major purpose of locating the neglected self is to form a relationship with it, so it may be both "apart from" the ego identity (to reduce what Jung (1928/1971, p. 88) called "psychic inflation") and "a part of" the relational self (to reduce "alienation" from the archetypal self). When the neglected self is brought into the body, experience is brought back into the reality of time ("successive moments"), where change is a constant process. Locating it in a specific center causes it to lose its amorphous quality and takes a specific "otherness" that allows related-ness.

Step B: Identify an Age

The archetypal/experiential self has many identities and many ages. In fact, through its center in the body flows a progression of different psychological forms. A symptom represents a point where that flow of the psyche through the belly has been arrested, and its form fixed and "frozen in time." Reintroduction of trauma cues can reactivate the symptom, and it may be experienced without conscious understanding or meaning as an out-of-control feeling in the body that must be ignored, denied, repressed, or otherwise disconnected. In order to allow it to enter the change process of life, the self-relations therapist not only identifies its location but asks the person, "If you were to let a number come to mind that represents an age for that experience in your [identified somatic location], what number do you become aware of?" The language here is somewhat hypnotic, as should be the therapist's soft but focused attention. If a person tries intellectually to guess a number or has difficulty letting one develop, more relaxation is in order, so that the age can flow freely from the neglected self into conscious awareness.

Again, the point is not that the neglected self is always that age. It may help to point out to the client that a person's center carries every age and every emotion and every psychological form, but a particular one (such as the one the client keeps coming back to in the symptom) stays until it is accepted and loved. Acceptance allows release, and release allows new psychological ages and identities to emerge.

Step C: Shift Pronoun from "It" to "He or She"

A crucial question in psychological relationship, either internal or external, is whether the other is regarded as an "it" or a "thou." Self-relations looks to move the neglected self from an "it" that needs to be controlled or otherwise disregarded to a "thou" that can be accepted. For example, say the client responds to the question regarding age with the number "Three." The therapist may continue: "So ['seeing' and sensing the person at three] . . . *she* is three." A number of clients will respond to such a comment, when it is delivered with appropriate empathic qualities and soft attentional focus, with gentle tears or other emotional softenings. Such a response will usually be experienced as coming from someplace other than one's intellectual, "in control," normal self.

Other clients may feel something stirring inside when the neglected self is directly named, but may cognitively be confused and ask, "What do you mean, *she?*" The therapist may respond:

> Well, I mean that there appears to be something or someone other than yourself that gets active when the problem kicks in. If I'm hearing you correctly, you're saying that when the problem develops, one of the things that happens is you get an intense unpleasant feeling centered in your body that doesn't feel that it's coming from you or even belongs to you. Is that right? [Client usually agrees.] And it seems one of the most disturbing things is that when that feeling develops, somehow you feel like *you* disappear or disconnect or feel out of control. Is that right? [Client usually agrees.] So I guess an important question is this: If that response isn't coming from your normal self, who is it and where is it coming from? [Brief pause to let this sink in.]

There's obviously a lot of ways of talking and thinking about it, and certainly the more traditional way is to think of that response as an "it" that has no meaning, that should be ignored or destroyed or gotten rid of. It seems, if I'm hearing you correctly, that you've tried that many times and have failed miserably. It keeps coming back over and over, more and more. . . . It may be helpful to consider that the feeling belongs to *her,* to another aspect of you that is listening even right now. . . . She has her own feelings, her own thoughts and images, her own way of listening. . . . She's been ignored for a long time, but it doesn't seem like she can be denied any further.

Other comments may elaborate this theme of thinking of the neglected self as a separate autonomous being. If this sounds too strange, it should be reminded that appreciation of and relationship of this "other self" is the basis for much of artistic expression. When the therapist delivers such comments in a relational, experiential, absorbing manner, the client has a hypnotic-like response of feeling that another part of his or her is activated and listening.

Step 3: Activate and Locate the Normal Self

One of the great dangers of attending to the neglected self is that one can become identified *as* it, rather than feeling a way to be *with* it. For example, a person may feel an emotion so strongly that his or her identity regresses to an earlier age. The goal in self-relations is to feel the presence of this neglected self in one's center, but to also stay present with one's normal cognitive/social self, thereby generating a felt field that holds and harmonizes both. Thus, it is important to activate and shift attention to the normal self periodically, especially when a client seems to be getting overwhelmed by and drawn into the neglected self. This method is akin to a form of systematic desensitization, in which the aversive stimulus (the neglected self) is progressively paired with a positive image.

The shift to addressing the normal self should generally be accompanied by a shift in nonverbal communication to a less hypnotic, more straightforward, but still engaging and gentle tone:

THERAPIST: So she's three . . . and, by the way, how old are *you,* in reality?

CLIENT: (*Makes a nonverbal shift, coming out of light trance*) I'm 43.

THERAPIST: Yes, I can see that you're 43. And can you tell me, what's the best thing about being this age compared to three?

A majority of people will say that the best thing about their present age is that they have more freedom, more ability to choose. Further questions to reconnect a person to his or her normal self includes associations to work, present family and friends, interests, and so forth. It is important for the therapist to be connecting with the client relatively nonhypnotically during this time, or the client may slip back into the neglected self.

Step 4: Identify and Externalize Aliens

A major obstacle to activating or maintaining the normal self is the presence of alienating ideas. This can be observed when clients appear unable to stay connected with themselves or the therapist; they withdraw, become critical, shut down, or the like. Such a "break in relatedness" signals that the alienating ideas have "taken over" the cognitive self.

I often approach the idea of "alien possession" with an "Irish twinkle" that conveys a gentle humor along with gentle, serious compassion. For example, with a person caught in negative internal dialogue, the therapist may say:

THERAPIST: As we're talking, I'm wondering if you're aware of *them*.

CLIENT: Them?

THERAPIST: Yes, it seems like you're coming under the influence of aliens.

CLIENT: Aliens? (*Looking at therapist, not sure if therapist is kidding or serious, but intrigued*)

THERAPIST: (*With mock somberness*) I'm afraid so . . . my professional opinion is that you're possessed by aliens. (*Pauses, then smiles gently*) I'm only half kidding, but it seemed like when we were just talking, all of a sudden you weren't quite present. It seemed like some other presence came in and you had to leave, to withdraw, to go away. Did you feel that?

CLIENT: Yes . . . I felt bad all of a sudden.

THERAPIST: Yes, I saw that. Are you aware of what those voices or ideas are saying about you then, or even right now?

CLIENT: They're saying it was my fault. [Other alienating ideas might be "You're unlovable," "You're stupid," "You're never going to be okay," etc.]

THERAPIST: That it's your fault. . . . Whose voices are those, anyway?

CLIENT: Well, mine, of course.

THERAPIST: (*Gently, with serious focus*) Where did you ever get the idea that those voices are yours?

CLIENT: Well, whose else could they be?

THERAPIST: I'm not sure, but they sure don't feel to me like *your* voices.
. . . Because I notice that when they show up, you have to leave. . . .
When they activate, you seem to feel smaller and less of a person. Is
that right? (*Client nods*) So whoever they are, they sure as hell don't
seem like they represent you. . . . I use the term "aliens" partly
humorously, because you can't survive in these situations without at
least a little bit of humor, but also with great seriousness, to suggest
that whatever happened to you, you got invaded by something that
led you to believe that the negative stuff that was conveyed to you
was your voice. (*With Irish twinkle*) But you may be possessed by aliens
. . . if so, there's a way out.

CLIENT: What's that?

THERAPIST: Reconnecting with that part of you that was wounded and
had to be abandoned. Because when the relationship between you
and her [the neglected self] is disconnected or abused, a break in
relationship occurs—the elevators stop going up and down—and the
aliens come. But there are other times when you feel that good
connection between the cognitive stuff in the head and the feeling
stuff in your belly—the elevators are going up and down. [The
therapist might ask about times when the client doesn't feel alien-
ated—i.e., the traditions of the aesthetic practices described above—
to point out that sometimes the aliens aren't around. The suggestion
can then be made that such experiences reflect times when there is
a connection between the egoic center and the archetypal self.]

Many clients find the idea of "aliens" exceptionally helpful. Like a
meditation technique that teaches a person to detach from the thoughts
in his or her mind, it helps to free a person from identifying with negative
influences, thereby allowing reconnection to a calm "thinking center" in
the belly. Again, the term is meant poetically and is designed to generate
both lightness and seriousness, so the therapist needs to present it in such
a context. The intent of naming aliens is not to give primary focus to
them, but to differentiate them from a person's own voice and externalize them. The more primary relationship is the reconnection of the
normal self and the archetypal self.

Step 5: Connect Normal Self and Archetypal Self

When a person's consciousness is not subjugated by alienating influences, it is free to reestablish the circuitry of the relational self. The
present model uses a scaling technique to identify the intensity levels of
the normal self, the neglected self, and the spirit of connection between
them. The therapist asks the client:

1. On a scale of 1 to 10, where 1 is the low end and 10 the high end, how much do you feel the presence of your neglected self in your solar plexus right now? Just let a number come to your mind.
2. On a scale of 1 to 10, where 1 is the low end and 10 the high end, how much do you feel the presence of your normal, everyday self in your head (looking out from behind your eyes) right now? Just let a number come to your mind.
3. On a scale of 1 to 10, where 1 is the low end and 10 the high end, how much do you feel a sense of connection between the normal self in the head and the neglected self in the belly? Just let a number come to mind.

Again, the goal here is to foster a felt sense of each relational component. Once this has developed, the therapist can ask whether the client would like to experiment with lowering or raising an intensity value 1 or 2 points to see what happens. For example, if the normal self is at 5 and the neglected self is at 8, the client will often feel out of control. If the therapist helps the client to go inside and gently "shift knobs on the intensity controls," the normal self may be moved to 7 and the neglected self to 6. This small difference in relative values can often make a significant difference in the person's overall quality of experience.

When the therapist asks about the level of connectedness between the two selves, some clients will look blank, as if the idea of such a connection is entirely new. This is often the case; the normal self and the neglected self frequently have little or no history of coexistence. When a person feels normal, the archetypal self is ignored and forgotten; when the archetypal self is activated (i.e., whenever identity is at issue, via symptoms), the normal self disconnects (and is hence replaced by alienating influences). Thus, the goal of self-relations therapy is to examine what happens when a person feels a connectedness between the two selves. This is a structural description of wholeness, intimacy, love, and cooperation.

When the felt or "telepathic" sense of connection is made, the person will usually look different; a sense of beauty will often imbue his or her being. The person will feel aware but not identified with each self. It is important to note that the connection is not the ego speaking (down) to the "inner child," but to a felt spirit that runs in full orbit.

Step 6: Return to Original Problem Sequence

Since a problem degrades into a symptom when a sustained break in relatedness occurs, a reparation of the break will allow a person to move though a problem sequence without becoming symptomatic. The therapist may suggest that the client take a few minutes to close his or her eyes, feel the connection between the selves, and then imaginally go back through the problem sequence (as defined in the first step), this time keeping the telepathic inner connection.

Step 7: Identify Further Tasks

An old saying laments, "We abandon our souls a hundred times, no, a thousand times each day." Thus, self-relations therapy is not a cure-all procedure, but the beginning of a tradition of being in relation with one's center regardless of circumstances. Much practice is needed, and the therapist should always be exploring with the client workable practices for continuing to nurture this tradition. We cannot hope never to disconnect, but we can grow stronger and more gentle in our commitment to keep coming to the relational self.

CONCLUSION

This chapter began with a question of identity: "Who the hell do you think you are, anyway?" Now we can see that self-relations suggests that the answer to this perennial question is always dynamic and always relational. When the beingness of belonging, separateness, and relatedness is broken, bad things happen. Psychotherapy can be seen as a devotional practice of restoring the sense of beingness of the relational self, in its field and dynamic form.

Walking this path, we are reminded of T. S. Eliot (1943/1962, p. 144):

> Who then devised the torment? Love.
> Love is the unfamiliar Name
> Behind the hands that wove
> The intolerable shirt of flame
> Which human power cannot remove.
> We only live, only suspire
> Consumed by either fire or fire.

As we learn to hold the fire in the belly, we are guided further by Kahlil Gibran (1923, p. 51) in *The Prophet*:

> Among the hills, when you sit in the cool shade of the white poplars, sharing the peace and serenity of distant fields and meadows—then let your heart say in silence, "God rests in reason."

And when the storm comes, and the mighty wind shakes the forest, and thunder and lightning proclaim the majesty of the sky—then let your heart say in awe, "God moves in passion."

And since you are a breath in God's sphere, and a leaf in God's forest, you too should rest in reason and move in passion.

May the force be with you.

REFERENCES

Bateson, G. (1955). A theory of play and fantasy: A report on theoretical aspects of the project for study of the role of paradoxes of abstraction in communication. In G. Bateson, *Steps to an Ecology of Mind.* New York: Ballantine Books. (Original work published 1955)

Bateson, G. (1972). Form, substance and difference. In G. Bateson, *Steps to an Ecology of Mind.* New York: Ballantine Books. (Original work published 1970)

Bateson, G. (1979). *Mind and Nature: A Necessary Unity.* New York: Dutton.

Buber, M. (1958). *I and Thou* (R. G. Smith, Trans.). New York: Scribner & Sons. (Original work published 1923)

Eliot, T. S. (1952). Four quartets. In T. S. Eliot, *The Complete Poems and Plays, 1909–1950.* New York: Harcourt, Brace & World. (Original work published 1943)

Epstein, S. (1994). Integration of the cognitive and the psychodynamic unconscious. *American Psychologist, 49*(8), 709–724.

Gibran, K. (1923). *The Prophet.* New York: Knopf.

Gilligan, S. G. (1987). *Therapeutic Trances: The Cooperation Principle in Ericksonian Hypnotherapy.* New York: Brunner Mazel.

Herman, J. (1992). *Trauma and Recovery: The Aftermath of Violence from Domestic Abuse to Political Terror.* New York: Basic Books.

Jung, C. (1971). The structure and dynamics of the psyche (Section on the transcendent function). In J. Campbell (Ed.), *The Portable Jung.* New York: Penguin Books. (Original work published 1916)

Jung, C. G. (1957). Commentary on "The secret of the golden flower." In H. Read, M. Fordham, & G. Adler (Eds.) and R. F. C. Hull (Trans.), *The Collected Works of C. G. Jung* (Vol. 13). Princeton, NJ: Princeton University Press. (Original work published 1957)

Jung, C. G. (1970). Mysterious conjunctions. In G. Adler & R. F. C. Hull (Eds. & Trans.), *The Collected Works of C. G. Jung* (Vol. 14). Princeton, NJ: Princeton University Press. (Original work published 1957)

Jung, C. G. (1971). Relations between the ego and the unconscious. In J. Campbell (Ed.), *The Portable Jung.* New York: Penguin. (Original work published 1928)

Keen, S. (1986). *Faces of the Enemy: Reflections of the Hostile Imagination.* San Francisco: Harper & Row.

Koestler, A. (1964). *The Act of Creation: A Study of the Conscious and Unconscious in Science and Art.* New York: Dell.

Rossi, E. (1977). The cerebral hemispheres in analytical psychology. *Journal of Analytical Psychology*, *22*, 32–51.

Shapiro, F. (1995). *Eye Movement Desensitization and Reprocessing: Basic Principles, Protocols, and Procedures.* New York: Guilford Press.

Toms, M. (1994). Writing from the belly.: An interview with Isabel Allende. *Common Boundary*, *12*(3), 16–23.

Watzlawick, P., Weakland, J., & Fisch, R. (1974). *Change: Principles of Problem Formation and Problem Resolution.* New York: Norton.

White, M., & Epston, D. (1990). *Narrative Means to Therapeutic Ends.* New York: Norton.

Wilson, B. (1967). *As Bill Sees It: The AA Way of Life.* New York: Alcoholics Anonymous World Services.

Yeats, W. B. (Ed.). (1979). *The Poems of William Blake.* London: Routledge & Kegan Paul. (Original work published 1905)

CHAPTER 11

No Self? No Problem!
Actualizing Empty Self in Psychotherapy

ROBERT ROSENBAUM
JOHN DYCKMAN

> Whether you are pulling a tooth, lancing a carbuncle, or
> whatever it happens to be—no matter how simple or how
> complicated—you ought to keep the following in mind. Your
> patient is one person today, quite another person tomorrow,
> and still another person next week, next month, next year. Five
> years from now, ten and twenty years from now, he is yet
> another person. We all have a certain general background, that
> is true, but we are different persons each day that we live.
> —MILTON H. ERICKSON (1985, p. 3)

SELF IS NO THING

You tend to assume you exist, separate from me, separate from the chair in which you are sitting, separate from the book that you are reading. You assume things are either outside you or inside you. Material objects, business associates, friends, therapy clients, lovers, parents are outside you; perceptions, thoughts, intentions, consciousness, feelings of love and anger are inside you. You apply these internal experiences to the external world.

Or do you? Where are you and this book right now? At this moment, are these words "inside" or "outside" you? When a client speaks and you feel moved, and the client feels moved by your feeling moved, are you really so separate? We all tend to assume without question that we exist separately from other people. This, though, is a fundamental error—perhaps *the* fundamental error, leading to a great deal of suffering. It helps greatly if we can approach therapy without this burden.

Each of us lives our epistemology of what our self is. The quality of our feelings, our relationships, and our sense of identity depends on our understanding of how our self-nature is constituted. There is a deep tendency to assume that we each have some core identity that underlies our existence and defines each of us. Our usual epistemology sees the self as the repository and integrator of personal experience as represented in thinking, feeling, and actions. Unfortunately, the underlying (usually unstated) implication is that the self is ultimately a thing, an object with some "essence." Living out this implication, we get confused, so when we think we are asking "Who am I, really?" we are often asking "*What* am I, really?"—as if self could be characterized with fixed qualities and measurable quantities. This is looking at the world through the lens of philosophical realism, where real objects actually exist that can be discovered or interacted with by a separate, real observer. A constructivist position, in contrast, argues that neither reality nor observer can be determined independently of each other; knowledge is not of objects, but a creation of the act of knowing (Watzlawick, 1976, 1984; Neimeyer & Feixas, 1990; Omer & Strenger, 1992; White & Epston, 1990). In this view, there are no "things" existing "out there," but rather a continual mutual co-arising of creator and created.

Most individualist personality theories assume that we all exist as atomistic, quantifiable entities walking around within bags of skin; then, however, they get into difficulties accounting for how we exist in interaction with each other, such as in our families. If therapists adopt a view of the self as an object, a residue that contains states and experiences, they then may think that relationships "contain" a certain "amount" of a certain type of feeling. Then there is also a danger that a therapist will share a client's delusion that the client's problems come from having either "bad stuff" or "insufficient good stuff" "inside" him or her. A more sophisticated view within this paradigm holds that there is "not enough harmony" in either the internal states of a client, or the interpersonal goals and desires of family members.

In any case, one cannot quantify harmony or touch a bad introject. In adopting a theoretical perspective that treats the self as existing with real characteristics (or deficits) "in" it, therapists join their clients in implicitly treating the client's self as a thing. In a thing-self, feelings and relationships are treated as quantities. In fact, though, the felt sense of experience cannot be predicted from its physical magnitude. A firm but gentle touch that is reassuring doesn't become more reassuring with "more" touch (which may be experienced as pain or intrusion), and may not become less reassuring with "less" touch (which may be experienced as a caress or a playful tickle). Feelings and relationships are not quantities, but qualities. Emotional distress generally cannot be alleviated by providing a certain amount of a missing emotion; a client who feels unloved does not need a certain number of hugs and nods of approval, but rather a certain quality of experience within a relationship.

A patient in the hospital asked to see a therapist. The patient had been widowed two years previously, when his wife died of cancer. On her deathbed, his wife asked him to take care of their three children, ages 8 to 12. It became important to him to be an especially devoted father.

Two weeks before seeing the therapist, he had taken his children to a family reunion. On his way back, on a narrow stretch of desert road, strong winds began buffeting his rented van. He lost control of the van and struck a telephone pole. The patient was thrown clear; the van burst into flame. The patient went back into the van and rescued one son. The patient then went back again into the van and rescued his daughter, though she was burned badly, and the patient also sustained severe burns. He turned back once more to go rescue his third child—his favorite son—and the van exploded into a bonfire, immolating his son.

The patient was in the hospital after recovering from burn surgery. His daughter was in another hospital, with third-degree burns over most of her body. The patient was an insightful man who had been in therapy before, when his wife died. He was consciously processing the thoughts and feelings of this traumatic incident, and he realized that it would take time to recover psychologically, as well as physically.

The therapist, (R.R.), a father himself, was profoundly moved by the patient, as indeed virtually any human being would be upon hearing this story. The very intensity of the tragic accident, with its invocation of mortality and loss, inspired an "existential meeting" in the moment. The client, though, was asking for something more specific. He complained that although he could deal with the psychological pain during the day, at night he would experience hypnogogic "flashbacks" of the burning car, as he tried to fall asleep. Was there anything that could help him with these?

The therapist knew a hypnotic technique involving invoking and viewing of the traumatic scene as if on a video screen, while intentionally altering some minor detail. He helped the patient to enter a trance and perform the technique, and the patient experienced some relief. After rousing from trance, the patient offered his (burned) hand to the therapist, to thank him. As their hands met, there was a special, nonverbal "meeting" of client and therapist.

Is it more useful here to think of the *quantity* of comfort or the *qualitative* "feel" of the encounter? It may sometimes be appropriate to take into account the number of times a client needs to tell and retell his or her story, but we believe that this may obscure the defining features of an encounter and its meaning to both the client and the therapist. We believe that we come to know ourselves in the process of experiencing others knowing us.[1] Client and therapist were able to meet here in a meaningful mutual horizoning, which was independent of the quantity of time they had known each other.

Self is not a quantity, yet many family systems theories rest on erroneous assumptions that quantify the experience of self. Some family systems theories often begin with a version of this statement: "Everybody has a certain amount of self, and nobody has enough" (R. Ayllmer, personal communication, 1978). Fogarty (1978) went on to develop this concept explicitly, ascribing the lack of "enough" self to the quest for emotional closeness, fusion, and distancing. Certainly, when people pursue or distance themselves from other people, they act as if they had a certain amount of self that could be gained or lost.

But what is it that the self can gain or lose? Experience. Memories. Feelings. Habits. Thoughts. Sensations. Awareness. There are volumes about the development of the sense of self in children (Stern, 1985), but essentially all of them adopt the idea of "self by accretion." In this view, we do something or have something done to us; we then encode it in some form of representation, to be remembered later. Our selves become an accumulation of all that we have thought, felt, and done; these residues lie "within" us and determine how we will react to new experiences.

Most people feel that they may change certain aspects of themselves, but not others. When experience is discordant with our concepts of what the self "ought" to be or is, our attempts to sustain self-image may result in psychological symptoms. In such situations, our clients don't "have" a self; they are "had" by their self. This is, after all, what therapy is about: A person or family comes to therapy when some "core essence" of his or her self or of the family identity is perceived to be threatened or challenged. Usually as therapists we attempt to increase the flexibility or broaden the scope of the definition of identity. We rarely challenge the concept of "identity" itself, because we tend to share the naive view of self—that there is some essence underlying the changeable parts. Our unexamined acceptance of this concept of self can constrain our therapies unnecessarily. When self has no fixed qualities or characteristics, change can happen quite rapidly, as the following case shows.

A 56-year-old woman, Mrs. A., was referred by her neurologist for "relaxation training" because of a seizure disorder. Mrs. A. had a history of meningitis in adolescence and had been involved in a motor vehicle accident several years later, at which time she struck her head against the windshield with a possible brief loss of consciousness. Her seizures began approximately six months after this. She had had seizure episodes on a regular basis since then, with an average incidence of once a week.

---

[1]D. W. Winnicott (1964) eloquently illustrated this process in the infant, whose self develops in the process of being "heartwarmed" by seeing his/her own pleasure (at nursing) reflected in the true pleasure of the mother witnessing this pleasure. He went further, saying, "There is no such thing as a baby . . . a baby cannot exist alone, but is essentially part of a relationship" (1964, p. 88). What Winnicott described for an infant is true for people at all ages.

Some of these were generalized grand mal seizures, but the majority were complex partial seizures involving automatisms, confusion, absences, and loss of muscle tonus. In the 12 months prior to her referral to the psychiatry department, she had been seen 13 times in the emergency room, and hospitalized once for seizure activity.

Mrs. A.'s seizure disorder had proved refractory to all medical treatment, despite therapeutic blood levels of anticonvulsant medications. She was treated over the years with all of the major anticonvulsants; she was also evaluated for surgical intervention, but was not found to be a good candidate for this. Her neurologist suspected that the patient's seizures were connected to significant life stress.

When first seen, Mrs. A. appeared worn, haggard, and worried. She said that she would "do anything" to rid herself of seizures. She knew little about hypnosis, but was willing to learn. A relaxation induction was attempted, but it soon became apparent that she had a great deal to say about her life and was interested in using her time to discuss this. One of her concerns was the fact that others in her family had moved the furniture to suit themselves, without regard to her wishes. The therapist (J.D.) employed a naturalistic hypnotic technique (Erickson, 1985), which involved listening to the patient's language, joining it, pacing, and finally leading by interspersing suggestions framed in the patient's words or metaphors. Many of these suggestions were conveyed via the theme of furniture arranging.

Mrs. A. came from a very conventional background in which women were expected to defer to their husbands and families, and not directly express their own needs. It soon became apparent that she maintained this deference only at great personal cost. A folk expression for this kind of suppression of one's own desires is to "Bite your tongue!" Perhaps it was not accidental that in her "fits" she would on occasion bite her lip or tongue.

Mrs. A. was extremely concerned about her husband. For many years she had "never crossed him" openly, her only harsh words to him coming during some of her "spells" when she would, as she put it, "get meaner than blue blazes." Whether these particular episodes were temporal lobe seizures or pseudoseizures seemed less significant than the way in which her seizures were embedded in her social context.

Mr. A. refused to travel with his wife, for fear that she would have a seizure while they were away from home or far from medical attention. At the same time, he feared leaving her alone. Mrs. A. wanted to travel, but felt compelled to honor her husband's wishes. The compromise solution she arrived at was to plan small trips with friends. Mr. A. also suffered from a chronic and painful physical condition. In some ways, Mrs. A.'s seizure disorder thus afforded the family system a way to avoid the potential discomfort of travel without having to directly acknowledge limitations arising from Mr. A.'s health; this preserved his status as provider and protector.

Their biggest difference was in regard to their adult "kids," who took shameless advantage of the couple, financially and emotionally. Mr. A. was so attached to the idea of family that he was unwilling to question the children's behavior, no matter how exploitative it might be. Mrs. A. was resentful but silent, and the burden of the caretaking fell to her. She spontaneously began to question this in the first session. Interestingly, when the patient was seen for the last time (the sixth session, 20 months after her first visit), she was able, with trepidation, to broach this with her husband, who to her surprise agreed that the "kids" should not be allowed to move back into their house.

After three sessions, the therapist sent Mrs. A. a letter, in the style of the narrative therapists Michael White and David Epston (1990). All of the "reframes" embedded in this letter had been introduced (although not spelled out completely) in the three sessions that preceded it.

Dear Mrs. A.:

I enjoyed talking with you on Monday and thought to write to you to summarize my understanding of the changes you have made as you have "cleaned house" and reclaimed your own interests.

You said that even though you used to have a seizure at least every Monday, you had not had any blackouts since we talked, and you decided to speak up for what you wanted and needed. You decided that you really wanted to change your wardrobe, and to get rid of old outfits that no longer fit or suited you. [Mrs. A. referred to her seizures as "spells" or "fits."]

You arranged your furniture to suit yourself and not to please others. You are in charge of deciding to "fix up" your house, and of arranging for necessary repairs.

You asked your "kids" to help pull their own weight, rather than dragging you down, and are beginning to teach them what they need to know: how to cook, clean, and fend for themselves. Even though they are not really children any more, you are teaching an important lesson that you have learned for yourself—namely, that it is okay to take responsibility for yourself, and that it is even necessary to do so to be really grown up.

You are feeling much better about pleasing yourself; cooking food that you like, wearing clothes that you fancy, and exploring some places that you would like to visit with friends, like [here followed a list of specific sites she had mentioned].

But perhaps the biggest thing that you have told me is that you have overcome your fear to do things that you have "always been scared to death to do." This includes not being so afraid of blackouts—and you said that when you felt a blackout trying to come on, you just went and lay down, did your deep breathing, and told everyone to "just leave me alone." When you did this, you felt much better. It sounds like you are feeling that you are more in control of your life, and the blackouts are less in control of your life. I wonder how long it will be until you feel in complete control?

You have said that you feel that there is "less of a pressure on me since I stopped worrying what anybody's going to say." Now that you are listening to what you are saying, do you think it will be sooner rather than later that other people will listen too?

You have said that you now "feel human, and not a servant of a sort."

I am impressed that you can now consider being your own helper, as well as the helper of others, and it seems like you are finding a new and more comfortable balance. This process can move forward and backward, but as it is going, your direction is clear. Good luck with your "housecleaning!"

I am pleased that you have shared your story so far with me, and hope that I have got it right. If you want to add another chapter or let me know how it is going, please feel free to contact me.

Overall, Mrs. A. was seen six times: three visits about a week apart on first referral, then 12 months later for two more sessions, and finally for a single session 20 months after her initial visit. By most measures her improvement was dramatic. Following her first three sessions, she had a period of almost seven months of markedly reduced seizure activity. In the 12 months prior to therapy, she was seen in the emergency room 13 times for seizures, as noted earlier; in the next 12 months, she was seen there once. During this period she required hospitalization once, for a grand mal seizure and medication adjustment, and that episode led to referral back to the psychiatry department. In the 12-month period following this, she again had only one emergency room visit for seizures. At the time of this writing, Mrs. A. had reported to her neurologist that her "spells" were light and infrequent.

A perspective that views people as having a stable, underlying self-structure has difficulty explaining such improvement from what seems like a minor, "surface" rearrangement of the house furniture. "Filled-self" theory would say that if this woman were "an epileptic," then she could not have stopped her seizures so quickly; it might conclude that if her seizures did stop, then she probably wasn't "a *real* epileptic" to begin with. Filled-self theory would probably argue that the therapy of this woman was incomplete, that numerous underlying aspects of her self-structure were not addressed, and that both psychological and physical vulnerabilities would remain. In filled-self theory, we are all in the position of the university professor in the following story:

Nan-in, a Japanese master, received a university professor who came to inquire about Zen.

Nan-in served tea. He poured his visitor's cup full, and then kept on pouring.

The professor watched the overflow until he no longer could restrain himself. "It is overfull. No more will go in!"

"Like this cup," Nan-in said, "you are full of your own opinions and speculations. How can I show you Zen unless you first empty your cup?" (Reps, no date, p. 5)

THE FLUIDITY OF THE SELF

When self "empties out its cup" so that it is not full of defining opinions and speculations about itself, self gains considerable freedom. When self is "empty"—that is, contains no fixed defining characteristics—then no one is "an epileptic," though some people may sometimes experience seizures. When there is no "core" self that must be addressed, there can be rapid and dramatic shifts in experience; we can focus on selective attributes of our clients, and especially on clients' strengths. In the case of Mrs. A., she felt that her seizures were "part" of her, but was able to find a different way to express herself that did not involve seizure activity. When this client told a therapist of her dissatisfactions, it was already a change from her passive, "victim" stance in the world, and precipitated an avalanche of positive change. The avalanche metaphor is chosen deliberately. It is a powerful reminder that although we often think that change in the natural world occurs continuously in small increments through gradual evolution, recent geological evidence suggests that the world can also change abruptly through "punctuated evolution," in which sudden, discrete events such as meteorite strikes cause profound, long-term "structural" changes (Gould, 1980).

> When one of us (R. R.) was initially enlisted by colleagues to work on a project investigating single-session therapy (Rosenbaum, Hoyt, & Talmon, 1990), he had serious doubts about the enterprise. Shortly after beginning the project, he was taking a hike in the mountains. As he walked along, inspired by the stability of the huge mountains that loomed on either side of the valley he was traversing, he mused about the futility of single session therapies.
>
> "Perhaps some change can occur in a single session," he thought, "but surely not *significant* change. Lasting change requires the gradual processes that mold mountains. Time, slow erosion, wind, and rain sculpting the face of the stone over and over again are required."
>
> At that point, the trail turned around a bend, and he came face to face with a huge avalanche chute. Half of a mountain, seemingly, had slid down into the valley the previous winter, changing both mountain and valley forever—all in the course of less than 30 seconds.
>
> He decided to respect the possibility of sudden, rapid change.

Cybernetic epistemology maintains that all change is maintained through stability, and all stability through change (Keeney, 1983). The fluid dialectic between change and stability in an ecosystemic view helps provide a basis for rapid, long-lasting changes based on relatively small perturbations of a system; it provides a basis for brief therapy. Consider the simple experience of standing completely still with your eyes closed. It is very hard to do this without swaying slightly. You keep your balance through movement; you must rely on activity to support your stillness. You also know what it is like to try to step forward on slippery ice. To go forward, you must first find someplace that doesn't slide beneath you. You must support your movement on something that doesn't move.

Now most of us usually think that what doesn't move is *us;* we try to plant our feet in a stable self-identity, to anchor us in a changing world. Careful observation, though, reveals self-identity to be fluid and constantly evolving; the stories we tell ourselves about ourselves vary according to the contexts and relationships involved. At work, we may be decisive and authoritative; when out to dinner with our spouses, we may be hesitant and deferent about what to order for dinner. Yet we believe ourselves to be the "same" person, even in the face of events that radically alter our perceptions of ourselves. If we lose a limb, we think of ourselves as basically still our same (albeit altered) selves. We may think ourselves to be dutiful sons or daughters, but when our parents die, we are still our (altered) selves.

We all would agree that we can put on different pairs of shoes and not change our essential selves. If a client comes to us after the amputation of an arm and insists, "I don't feel like my old self any more," we may try to bolster a widened view of a self that is not dependent on having two good arms. But how far can we take this? Isn't there some point at which, if too much is taken away, the self disintegrates? Most of us would sooner or later answer this question in the affirmative. Within the field of therapy, there is an often-held assumption that certain subordinate parts are expendable or changeable, but that there is a "core essence"—a "superordinate self-concept" (Horowitz, 1988) or core set of relationships, homeostasis, or coherence that, if upset or destroyed, means the destruction of the self as well.

This is ultimately the fear that fuels symptoms: that the self is threatened, will be overwhelmed, or will disintegrate. This is why clients say things like "I can't do that; it's not me." The problem is that, to the extent therapists believe that any client has a core "me," any intervention they engage in will not address the fundamental point. When therapists reassure clients by saying, "You can just try it out [i.e., your self will still be there]," they still do not address the core incorrect belief: that the self is a thing. If the self is a thing, it may be lost, damaged, or hurt.[2]

Self is not a thing, but a process. This process is constantly shifting. Even as an individual breathes in and breathes out, the atoms that make up his or her body are being exchanged. Although most of us consider ourselves "the same self" from day to day, this is probably closer to a wish than to a reality. Though our lives consist of discrete actions, the choices we make mistakenly become seen as relatively stable preferences, or even as enduring attributes (e.g., "I am a Democrat," instead of "I voted Democratic at the last election").

Of course, there is nothing wrong with saying "I am a Democrat" (or "I am an artist," "I am a man," "I am a psychotherapist," etc.) as a convenient shorthand expression. It is important, however, not to reify these shorthand expressions into fixed traits and become attached to them, in an effort to maintain a "stable" self. When we are comfortable with the idea of a fluid self and can see change as the only constant, it becomes somewhat easier to imagine transforming problem behaviors. This leads naturally to the examination of "exceptions" or "unique outcomes" that contravene the problem (de Shazer, 1985; White, 1986). When clients' curiosity about the exceptions to the problem is aroused, they begin to let go of overgeneralizations and other behaviors that may support the problem, and to experience themselves as already "different" than when they came in. The Mental Research Institute group similarly works to undermine the erstwhile "problem-solving" behaviors of a client or family that in fact maintain the unsatisfactory status quo, by redefining ("reframing") the presenting problem (Fisch, Weakland, & Segal, 1982). Narrative and constructivist approaches inherently imply a notion of self as constantly changing—a work in progress rather than a set piece. When we identify a problem in the language of "qualities" we tend to believe that change will be slow. When we locate this problem in our "self," we may believe that we cannot "be" ourself without having the problem.

> Ted, a young man, came to therapy complaining that he was depressed, suicidal, and couldn't control his temper. He had been severely physically abused as a child, and felt that this had scarred him forever. He had lost his job about a year before during a layoff in the aircraft industry. Because of money problems, Ted, his wife, and their young infant were forced to live with his mother-in-law. He felt worthless; he felt he "never did anything and never will do anything." He didn't even

---

[2]A therapist may collude with a client in the illusion that the client is missing something. Such collusion can be very tempting for the therapist, who can then pretend he/she "has" something that the client needs. Then the therapist may feel very helpful, and may have a very grateful client, but both run the risk of spending therapy looking elsewhere for solutions when the solution is right at (the client's) hand. Therapists often ally themselves with clients' wishes for security and stability, but this alliance may be founded in a chimera that reflects the therapists' own existential insecurity. Therapists, like clients, prefer to imagine themselves "the same self" from day to day, but sometimes holding on to the safety of consistency comes at the expense of openness to new experience.

help out around the house. Even in high school, when he'd been on the football team, he'd been injured and hadn't been able to fulfill his potential. Ted had a fixed idea that he had been and would always be a "loser."

After spending some time empathizing with Ted's situation, the therapist (R. R.) attempted to discover some exceptions to the client's overgeneralizations about himself. It turned out that when Ted had been laid off, he had not only contacted each of the airlines in the area looking for employment; he had done so every week for six months. The therapist questioned whether this was a profile of somebody who "never did anything"—it sounded more like the actions of someone who didn't quit easily. Ted did recall then that in high school nobody had ever thought he'd ever make the football team to begin with; he persisted, though, and became a starter. The therapist said he found it hard to believe that someone who could be so persistent, even if he would occasionally get discouraged, never did anything now. Ted did admit that he occasionally helped out around the house—it just seemed he never could do anything to his mother-in-law's satisfaction. The therapist and Ted discussed the family situation in more detail. It also turned out that Ted had found part-time work, though the changing shifts he worked made him tired. The work also made it hard for him to exercise as much as he wanted. Ted lifted weights. The therapist asked whether Ted ever felt, after lifting weights for a while, that the weights felt heavier than at the start of the session. Sure, Ted said; that was when he just would reach inside himself and make an extra effort. That was how he got stronger. The therapist suggested that Ted pay attention, next time he was exercising, to how he "reached inside" himself to lift those weights just when they felt heaviest.

By the end of the first visit, Ted remarked on how he'd been treating himself like a "piece of garbage," but now realized he was a person who had his ups and downs. On his next visit several weeks later, he reported that his depression had remitted almost completely. He was doing more around the house, felt more optimistic, and generally felt better about himself. He resumed looking for work, and soon found a job in an entirely new field he was excited about. He promptly moved his family out of his mother-in-law's house. On follow-up two years later, he was enjoying his job, buying his own house, and looking forward to the birth of his second child.

Self is not unitary, but the product of multiple drafts. The view that the self is not one but many has been ably presented in social psychology by Mischel and Peake (1982). Self is a composite experience. We are not only different in different social contexts, but at any given instant we are engaged in a process of "summation" of different selves-in-action that produce the working "draft" of our consciousness (Minsky, 1986). If we adopt this view, it immediately recontextualizes our view of "split," "multiple," or, as recently renamed, "dissociative" identity disorders (see American Psychiatric Association, 1994). If we speak in terms of multiple contextual selves for us all, the focus becomes not on how the personality is "split," but on how the dialogue/summation of the "selves" is interrupted. Holding this view produces the salutary effect on the therapist of normalizing these somewhat dramatic clients and increasing empathic connection, for in this view they are not so "different" from the rest of us. It also allows for more rapidly establishing reintegrating conversations between the "selves," once the trauma-induced emotional barriers to this exchange are explored and reduced.[*]

Often clients complain, "I'm not myself." Who, then, are they? The therapist who relies on a real "inner" self may be tempted to help such a client find a "better" self or return the client to some comfortable image of himself or herself. The therapist who is not attached to such a view, however, is free to eschew any images or ideas about what self the client "should" be or "have," and recognizes that none of us can escape being ourselves each and every moment for all time. In order for therapists to adopt this useful stance, it is helpful to view self as empty—not a thing; not created, not destroyable. *The self is not an accrual of experience but an ongoing, ever-changing manifestation of potentiality.*

> A 29-year-old woman came to a therapist (R. R.) asking for hypnosis to lose weight. She mentioned that she had recently moved back in with her parents, and felt her mother was scrutinizing her weight "for her own good." The client also said that she had one brother, a drug addict. Sighing, she remarked that she had "always had the weight of being the ideal child" in the family.
>
> The client felt she needed to lose weight for herself, not for anybody else. Since it wouldn't be possible for the client to hide the fact from her mother that she was going on a diet, the therapist suggested she tell her mother she was going on a diet, and post a chart on the refrigerator of her daily caloric intake; however, to ensure that the client was doing this on her own, the therapist further advised that the client should, without her mother's knowledge, put *inaccurate* figures on the calorie chart. The client was greatly amused at the idea of misleading her mother and taking charge of her diet.
>
> During the formal hypnosis, the therapist helped her imagine she was shopping with her mother for clothes and going into a "changing room" by herself. Within the changing room, the client took off layers of clothes and put them on, repeatedly, until she reached a point where

---

[*]*Editor's note:* See O'Hanlon's discussion of treating a person who was functioning as a "multiple personality" in Chapter 4, and Gergen's related discussion in Chapter 16.

"having found what's comfortable to take off, from now on you can keep it off."

The therapist was attempting to emphasize autonomy while giving indirect suggestions for weight loss. For this to be successful, the client needed to realize she did not have to be bound by a particular "filled" vision of herself she needed to present to her mother; she could shed and "try on" multiple versions by and for herself.

On follow-up a year later, the client had moved out of her mother's house, had gone back to school to get a graduate degree, had lost weight, and had kept the weight off. Posing alternative possibilities to this client was important; it was also important, though, to contextualize the client's identity within the framework of an important relationship in her life.[3]

SELF AND RELATIONSHIP

As soon as one assumes that a substantive identity exists which has an intrinsic essence separate from its interactions with the world, then a gap arises between "I" and "it," "me" and "you." Treating self as nonempty, containing "things" "inside" an "ego," leads inevitably to a wildly solipsistic viewpoint. If "I" am what is "inside" a "me"—if I have an internal reality separate from my ongoing being-in-the-world—ultimately my "I" can exist in isolation, eternally separate both from what I do and who I'm with. The self becomes an observer, separate from what it participates in. It then becomes difficult to account for human relatedness. I can never know your experience, since we are each ultimately separate, each holding some private, core existence. If we each have a core existence, we must be "true to ourselves" to live a good life; then there are conflicts between selfishness and altruism.

The most common way out of this dilemma is to assume an "interpersonal" perspective, which sees the self as having a fundamental essence, but acknowledges that much of the enduring sense of self derives from the interpersonal matrix. This perspective follows Sullivan (1953) by stating that self consists of the reflected appraisals of others. If we are consistent in this position, though, we must then consider that the other's self is also a reflected appraisal, and that our selves are reflections of reflections.

This kind of circular causality—mirrors within mirrors, in which my perception of you is affected by your perception of me, which is affected by my perception of you— is no surprise to family therapists, who daily encounter its clinical manifestations (Tomm, 1987; White, 1986). Con-

[3]A nearly complete transcript of this case appears in Rosenbaum (1993b) and is also cited in Rosenbaum (1994).

ceptually, however, this presents challenges to the naive view of self. If "self" and "other" are treated as real, rather than as analytic fictions, then introducing the idea of a self with its own coherent identity "inside" it produces an inevitable chasm between self and other, which cannot be fully traversed through interpersonal bridges. Stating that the self "interacts" with others is not sufficient to explain how the self crosses the chasm to be related to the other.

The way out of this dilemma is to acknowledge that it is an analytic fiction to see an object as existing independently of its context. In a lived world, objects exist *only in relationship*—a crucial point made by postmodernist and feminist writers (e.g., Jordan, Kaplan, Miller, Stiver, & Surrey, 1991), who stress the inherent relational and contextual nature of self. Although this emphasis is helpful, it often stops short of fully developing the ramifications of this view: that identity is always fluid, lacking any core essence. There is no such "thing" as self and no such "thing" as other. This realization, of course, appeared long ago in Buddhism, which teaches that self and other are empty. This does not mean that they are void, but that they have no independent, permanent existence other than their appearance in relationships, which are constantly arising in immediate experience in the present moment.

As contexts change, self changes—or, more precisely, self-in-context is a constantly changing process. It is not as Zucker (1967) pointed out, that persons *have* problems, but that they *are* their problems; that is, their lived experience is problematic to them or to others. The notion of a "full" self promotes an illusion that people are somehow separate from what they do. Experience, however, need not be represented "in" an actor who is separate from his or her action. Just as "self" and "other" are not things, neither is the experience of relationship. Indeed, it would be more accurate to talk of experience not as an ordinary noun, but as a gerund: experienc*ing*. Experiencing does not involve discrete stages of function, perception, and cognitive representation, but rather a total immersion in the actions of being alive (Bohart, 1993). Varela, Thompson, and Rosch (1991), attempting to reconcile modern cognitive psychology with a Buddhist epistemology, conclude that cognition is embodied *enaction*, and, like the philosopher David Hume, posit that the self does not exist apart from these enactions. In baseball, the pitcher pitching, the batter batting, and the catcher catching all meet in a common activity, just as do therapist and client, parent and child, lover and beloved. When one is immersed in the immediacy of the moment, the separateness of "self" and "other" drops away; there is neither "knower" nor "known," but only knowing.* In other words, *self is undivided activity.*

Editor's note: See Gergen's discussion in Chapter 16 of this relational field.

SELF AND ACTION

Self is self-in-action, and as such is always contextual. Views of self-identity
that treat it as internalized representations or schemes tend to ignore the
action component. As Piaget (1952/1963) pointed out, intelligence is at
base a sensorimotor process. That is, actions always take place in a
context, a lived-world. Internal symbolic structures, archetypes, can be
seen as generalized representations of interpersonal *acts,* to borrow and
extend Stern's (1985) terminology.

Moreover, self is *embodied* action. Self appears in mind-and-body as
a necessary unity (Bateson, 1979). From the time Freud (1923/1961)
argued that the ego is first and foremost a projection of bodily experience, psychologists have long recognized that the way the body and mind
present themselves to each other constitutes a critical area for defining
self-identity. This of course is consonant with the reemergence in psychotherapy of body-oriented techniques (cf. Kellerman, 1979, Juhan, 1987)
and the work of family therapy researchers such as Minuchin, Rosman,
and Baker (1978), whose studies of free fatty acid levels (serum markers
of physiological pathology) in juvenile diabetics and their families suggest that there is a physiological as well as psychological homeostasis in
these families. That is, there is a "family body" as well as a "family psyche."
This further stretches our common-language notions of a skin-encapsu-
lated "self."

When we consider self as embodied action, new avenues for the
treatment of problems in living open up. The treatment of panic disorder
is a useful case in point, since 10 of the 13 DSM-IV diagnostic criteria for
panic attacks are bodily sensations or experiences (American Psychiatric
Association, 1994). Barlow (1988) describes the utility of body-focused
techniques such as diaphragmatic breathing and relaxation training in
the treatment of panic disorder. We have found that awareness "with"
(not "apart from") the body helps create the confidence and reinterpre-
tation of bodily sensation needed to proceed with exposure exercises.

> Ms. B. was a 32-year-old nurse who had come to the emergency room
> five times in the previous six months complaining of chest pain and
> shortness of breath. She was worked up medically, and no organic
> illness was found. She accepted the referral to the psychiatry depart-
> ment with some reluctance, since one of her physicians had told her
> that her problem was "all in your head." She participated in a structured
> group therapy for "panickers," which uses a number of different
> interventions: cognitive restructuring, interoceptive exposure, training
> in relaxation, diaphragmatic breathing, and bodily awareness
> (Dyckman, 1994). After an exercise designed to increase awareness by

dividing attention—simultaneously noticing the sensations in all 10 toes, both heels, and both ischeal tuberosities—she spontaneously remarked that "I lost track of myself," and that instead of this being another occasion of anxiety, she felt calm, secure, and capable. She reported a subsequent marked decrease in the incidence and severity of her anxiety episodes, and her improvement continued, so that at a three-month follow-up she was symptom-free despite some significant intervening life stressors.

As clients become curious about the perceptual qualities of a sensation, they almost always notice that sensations are constantly changing, and are doing so much faster than their ideas about their sensations. Jon Kabat-Zinn (1990) has shown the utility of this in his work with patients suffering from chronic pain. When these patients attend to the quality of sensation, they open up the "story" that they have made up about the sensation, and create space for a new view.

When clients focus "with" immediate body experience in this way, they often spontaneously comment, "I lost track of myself," and are surprised to find themselves doing things that had previously been terrifying or even unthinkable. When a client says, "I lost track of myself," we are faced with the question of who is "the" self here: the person losing track, or the person being lost track of? A therapist subscribing to full-self theory might attribute the client's experience to dissociation, but a therapist comfortable with empty self may note the similarity of this type of un-self-conscious action to the experience of "no-mind" that is described frequently in religious contexts, though only rarely in psychotherapy (Greenleaf, 1971). In this experience there is no separate "doer" and "deed," just "doing."

We are used to thinking of ourselves as "doers" who perform "deeds." This view is fine for describing a world where separate subjects act unilaterally on isolated objects; however, as soon as we enter into relationships where there is *mutual* influence, the nature of identity becomes fuzzy. In a healthy ecology, each person and his or her environment coevolve with each other through making choices. But the question remains: "Who" makes these choices? This question is based on a misconception: that we exist fundamentally apart from our actions and separate from each other. There is choosing, but without a *separate* chooser or chosen. As Yeats (1928/1989, p. 217) put it:

> O chestnut-tree, great-rooted blossomer,
> Are you the leaf, the blossom or the bole?
> O body swayed to music, O brightening glance,
> How can we know the dancer from the dance?

The issue is not one of how the body is represented "in" the mind. This view perpetuates a mind–body dualism that is particularly pernicious, and leads to fruitless debates regarding whether the locus of the "self" resides in body, mind, or somewhere "in between." Varela et al. (1991) point out that the essential problem here is the idea that experience needs to be *represented* by a self separate from that experience. When self and experience are united in embodied action, there is no need to "re-present" experience "out there" to a self "in here." Varela et al. offer the image of "laying down a path in walking" as appropriate for activity by an empty self.*

One consequence of this view is a greater emphasis on the manner in which we create and walk this path, and less on the exploration of our motives for walking, or even on the explanation of how we walk. Experience becomes more important than explanation. When we tell a story with a client, we are inviting actions on a different path. In the following case, a client's self-criticism served to maintain a very restricted sense of herself. The therapist attempted to help the client by altering the role of her internal critic, and by telling a story he invited her, quite literally, to lay down a path while walking.

> A 40-year-old woman with a long history of depression (which included two hospitalizations) came for therapy with the presenting issue of wanting to have a relationship with a man. Her father had died when she was quite young, and she had suffered a number of career losses before plunging into depression. Since its onset she had gained a significant amount of weight and felt unattractive. She was highly critical of herself, and (somewhat less visibly) of others. Her violent self-criticism was not easily dislodged. She had a list of complaints, and added new ones faster than she could remove the old. The therapist (J.D.) finally suggested that her judge would make an excellent "*consiglioro*" (an ethnic reference not lost on this Italian-American client), but that as with any *consiglioro*, the actual decisions would rest with the "prince" (or in this case the "princess"). This move to externalize the critic (White, 1988) eased her paralyzing self-criticism. It also opened the door to more direct criticism of the therapist by the *consiglioro*, who would judge each therapy session as "productive" or "unproductive." When the therapist inquired as to the criteria, she responded that sessions that led to physical activity were more likely to be judged productive.
>
> The therapist asked the client whether she knew the story of Hansel and Gretel. The client laughed, flushed, and became attentive. The

---

Editor's note: See the discussion by White in Chapter 2 of the spirit with which we choose to construct our path.

therapist noted that there were different versions of the story. In one version, the children first dropped shiny pebbles in the forest to find their way home after being abandoned by their woodsman father; the next time they left a trail of breadcrumbs, which the birds ate, leaving them to wander in the forest to confront the witch, and finally to return home triumphant and changed. The therapist then proposed that the client take a daily walk carrying a bag of sunflower seeds. As she walked, she was to select a seed and to assign it a specific complaint that she was ready to leave behind, drop it, and leave it for the birds and the squirrels to devour. She was to take a different route home each time, so that the complaints couldn't find their way back to her. She appeared puzzled and bemused, but agreed. She came back the next week reporting that her walks made a kind of "one-way bridge" to her self-criticism. She was more realistic and planful, and was beginning to exercise regularly. She also began to make tentative plans to attend a "singles" dance at her church.

SELF AND CONSCIOUSNESS

When we no longer re-present experience "out there" to a self "in here," the varieties of self-experience widen. The actual experience of living is broader than the way we represent our experience to ourselves in language. Language is a useful means for communication, but an inevitable consequence of language is that whenever we label an experience, we always limit it.

Self knows itself through consciousness, but consciousness need not be restricted to language and labeling. Varela et al. (1991) point out that consciousness always arises through *activity*. Much of self exists outside the realm of verbal experience. Is a preverbal child without self? How about a monk sitting in silent, wordless meditation? What about two lovers touching each other? How about the skier, zooming downhill with the wind on his or her face and no words for the flashing images that streak by? If self is language-bound, where does self "go" during sleep?

One can distinguish at least three types of consciousness: (1) consciousness *of* an object separate from the observer (e.g., looking at a rock); (2) consciousness *by* an experience, in which awareness is subsumed by the action, such that there is an intentional act without self-consciousness (e.g., tying one's shoelaces without "thinking" about it); and (3) consciousness *with* a process. The third type of consciousness straddles the previous two: Awareness coexists with a changing stimulus in such a way that it simultaneously is determining and being determined by the shifting quality of awareness (e.g., sitting on a rock and experiencing it as variously rough or smooth, depending on one's position; meditating on a candle flame; listening to a piece of music; working with a client/family).

It is possible to locate self not just in language, but in the inherent activity and experience of *autopoesis*—the self constituting itself through a bootstrap operation (Maturana & Varela, 1992). "I" arises not just in observing myself observing, but also in touching myself touching (Merleau-Ponty, 1964). Self exists immanently in the context of a boundary that creates an interface of experiences. I may touch myself touching others or touch myself touching myself; "where" I touch is not so important as the act of touching itself.

Touching constitutes a self, but it is a self without a locus. Since touching operates *at* a boundary (not *within* one), a touching self is immanent in the act of relationship, throughout a boundary. Touching yourself touching yourself, the precise locus of the self becomes confused; where is "you" in this experience? You are neither "within" your body nor "absorbed" by the object, nor are you somewhere "in between." Think of this the next time you touch yourself touching a client. Doing therapy, being a person, involves touching.

Touching is quintessentially a present-time experience. It occurs only in the now, at the immediate present of the current interface. It has no history and no future, and provides the model for therapy that the psychoanalyst Bion (1967) advocated: entering a session "without memory and without desire." A touching self is an experiencing, self-reflecting self, but not necessarily an observing self, in that the kind of consciousness involved in touching is not consciousness *of* an object, but rather consciousness *with* a coparticipant. Touching is a horizoning of each with the other; it generates self and other, not as entities separate from each other, but as coparticipants in the creation of the boundary.

———

Roth and Chasin (1994) have developed a wonderful method of working with couples that takes advantage of the transformative aspects of touching with a coparticipant. Each partner illustrates his or her goals for the relationship. Then the following is done for each partner in turn: The client describes or reenacts a painful childhood experience with a parent or caretaker when similar goals might have been desired but were blocked, with the therapist taking the role of the client's frustrating parent/caretaker. The client then creates a scene of what the parent/caretaker's life "should have been" like when this person was growing up, so that he or she could have acted differently toward the client when the time came. This usually involves enacting a scene in which the partner plays the part of a (benevolent) parent/caretaker to his or her own parent/caretaker (whose part is played by the client's partner). Finally, a revised version of the client's painful past is enacted, with the client playing the young version of himself or herself, while the client's partner enacts the client's "re-formed" parent/caretaker in a way that enables the client to achieve the desired goal.

This complex and powerful technique often loosens the attachment that each member of the couple feels to his or her current, problematic story. Imaging the re-formed past for the deficient caretaker and for himself or herself with the current partners, each partner touches himself or herself touching multiple others across changing relational boundaries. The past, "frozen" relationship, with its echoes of disappointment in the present, is reexperienced through several modalities of consciousness, with a deliberate mixing of "identities" or roles within the system. A new relationship arises, with fresh possibilities for the definition of the "other."

SELF AND HISTORY

Touching, which occurs in the present moment, is not by itself sufficient to account for our lived sense of self; in addition to the current boundaries where an organism and its coparticipants actualize themselves, there are also historical dimensions involved in transformation. The subjective sense of individual history, past and future, also plays a role for empty self.

Whereas touching is centered in the immediate moment, defined by discontinuity and by intersections at boundaries, history is defined by a seamless *absence* of boundaries over an extended period of transformations. If you examine a growing child, you can say that the child was 53 inches tall last month, and is now 54 inches tall. You can never say, though, at what precise moment the child passed from being 53 to 54 inches tall because it did not occur as a discrete quantum jump, but rather in infinitesimally small bits. However fine your measuring stick and your stopwatch, you will never be able to find a precise moment for the phase transition. At ever-decreasing intervals of time, you will need to measure ever-decreasing intervals of space until, finally, you will have to make an arbitrary decision as to where to mark the point of transition.

We call this historical aspect of growth in the individual "proceeding-from becoming," to capture the past-future-in-the-present aspect of individual (and human) existence, as opposed to the immediacy of present-time touching. In this view, though, individuals are not accruals of experience, but constrained sets of potentialities.

Modern historians acknowledge that there is no single "reality" in the past that can be captured and codified. Rather, each history text constitutes a particular present-time reconstructing—another version of the story. *We make our pasts in the present.* The history of humankind is not the mere collation of more or less accurate recollections of "real" past events; nor is the history of an individual self made up simply of memories of things that happened to the self.

Modern theories of memory reject the idea of an encoded engram that is recovered from an attic or storeroom in the brain, in favor of a processive view of memory. Memory is always a present-time construction, although the act of constructing it may be facilitated by previous, similar acts (Friedman, 1993). Memories are created moment by moment, through successive associative processes that pick up on current partial information received from the activity of the subject in relation to his or her total environment; from a categorically organized information pool, bits and pieces are assembled until they form a familiar "fit" with experience. Memory does not necessarily involve a process of going to a storeroom, retrieving a videotape of a past event, inserting it in a VCR, and replaying it. Rather, memory can be more like being an actor in a scene in a live production of a play; even though the same scene from the same script may be repeated night after night, each time it must be reenacted with a slightly different rhythm between the players, a slightly different interpretation, a varied expression (Edelman, quoted by Levy, 1994).

The history of individuals and of species is not what they have done or what has happened to them; this would consist of crystallized "engrams." Rather, the history of individuals and species consists of what they have *excluded* from their set of possible actions. Our genes do not carry instructions about standing on two feet; rather, they carry a set of potentialities that includes walking, crawling, somersaulting, and so forth. There are individuals who are human but who don't walk, because of either socialization (e.g., the case of a child who was raised by wolves [Rymer, 1992]) or accident (e.g., quadriplegics). What our genes do is eliminate certain possibilities: They don't make us walk, but they ensure that we can't physically fly. Our genes eliminate certain sets of possibilities; they are restrictive, but not prescriptive.

This is how the individual self develops—not by accruing experience, but by eliminating certain possibilities. I may be used to saying of myself, "I am a psychologist," but this is shorthand for saying "I am not a carpenter [candlemaker, etc.]." It's easier to state my identity as a positive, but it creates, through language, a dangerous illusion: that there is a "thing" called "being a psychologist," which is "in" me. Instead, I can recognize that my "identity" is not a characteristic "in" me, but merely a convenient label that marks the excluding of certain pathways. Eliminating pathways is convenient and efficient; I don't have to spend time considering all possibilities for every decision. From this point of view, I need not consider my self as "filled" with certain "attributes"; rather, I can recognize my self consisting of a wide range of potentialities, many of which I have excluded, but which are still potentially available to me.

Clients are often disinclined to look at potentialities they define as outside of their immediate vision of self, when it is precisely this restriction of vision that traps them. If you carry a long board of lumber on your shoulder, it will be hard to look to one side or to turn easily. Therapy is about dropping the board and looking around. This can happen in a moment, as long as you're not holding on to the board too tightly. Psychotherapy consists in part of the unlocking of the roads less traveled, but if we are attached to our current road, saying, "This is my self," we will be less likely to look at alternative pathways. If we conceive of the self as the set of the pathways taken—past experiences—it is hard to jettison these or find new paths. However, if we conceive of the self as the entire nexus of potentialities, with certain ones being manifested at this particular time, then changing the self requires no act of subtracting to the self, adding to the self, or "rewiring of the pathways." Self-changes require a turning, a rediscovery of potentialities that have always been there but have been temporarily excluded. The self as an accumulation of experience is a prison; the self as empty, as shimmering potentiality, is a prism that, depending on its turning, gives forth many different colors.

Angela had been having panic attacks for 20 years, since she was 18 years old. She was frequently worried about the safety of her children, husband, and other relatives, having a vague dread that "something bad" would happen to them. She was frequently tearful and depressed. She had been through several courses of psychotherapy and had been tried on several varieties of psychotropic medications, all to no avail.

The therapist (R. R.) saw her during a particularly bad time for her: Over the past year her beloved stepmother, her grandmother, her aunt, an uncle, a cousin, and a close friend had all died. It turned out that each of these deaths reminded Angela of her father's death 20 years ago—about the time the panic attacks started. Angela had been very close to her father and had depended on him greatly. In particular, Angela had a memory from about six months prior to her father's death. At a family Christmas gathering, her father had saved the biggest and most enticingly wrapped gift for last, to give to Angela. He told Angela he knew she had always wanted this gift, then started crying. When Angela happily opened the gift, she saw it was a picture of her biological mother, who had died when Angela was a toddler. Angela gazed at the picture in horror; her father had told her years earlier that she would get the picture when he died. She felt the gift presaged that her father was ill, although he denied it. A few months later, he was indeed dead.

Since her father's death, Angela had experienced visual memories of the Christmas gathering almost daily, replaying it in almost exactly the same form each time. She felt bereft, and believed that she would never get over the death of her father. However, after several sessions in which she and the therapist developed a strong relationship, Angela agreed it might be time to do something about her grief, and consented to a session of eye movement desensitization and reprocessing (EMDR; Shapiro, 1995).

During EMDR, Angela's memories alternated between repeated images of the Christmas scene and of her father's deathbed. She sobbed almost nonstop. Eventually she had an image of her sister, and was able to express a previously unvoiced thought: that her sister had "pulled the plug" on her father's respirator. She voiced considerable anger, but then resumed crying. With continued EMDR, she had more images of the Christmas gathering, but then had an image of being a little girl on the beach with her father. In response to a question from the therapist, she mentioned that her father was "overprotective" at the beach, and laughed. She then had a series of other images and, distressed, asked whether something were wrong with her mind. Shouldn't she just have the same image over and over? She had trouble believing the therapist's reassurance that new images and associations were normal, but she eventually derived comfort and some relief from the session. Over the next several weeks, her symptoms gradually became less severe.

This client felt compelled to remain faithful to a memorial image from many years ago, which she had been continually rehearsing on a daily basis in her current life. But a snapshot of an experience is different from the experience itself; photographs always lie. A similar thing holds true for emotional pathways: We always relive them in the present, rather than recall them from the dead past. We cannot be frozen in the past unless we keep refreezing, working to keep the temperature cold. Life is always moving. However, time is not linear, but lived. In life, each moment expresses the entire person.

BEING TIME

A "full" self is generally felt to be a participant in linear time. Here, we become our memories of the consequences of our desires. We think we keep telling ourselves who we are, but in fact are telling ourselves who we've been. It is hard, in such a view, to account for how we can ever do anything discontinuous or qualitatively new, since even our futures—our hopes and wishes—are basically projections from past residues.

Something very different transpires when self is empty and time is experienced not as clock time, but as the articulation, in this physical locale, of our self-expression. In the words of a 13th-century Zen teacher, Eihei Dogen (Dogen, c. 1246/1985a, pp. 76–77):

> Even though you do not measure the hours of the day as long or short, far or near, you still call it 12 hours. Because the signs of time's coming and going are obvious, people do not doubt it. Although they do not doubt it, they do not understand it. . . .
>
> The way the self arrays itself is the form of the entire world. See each thing in this entire world as a moment of time. Things do not hinder one another, just as moments do not hinder one another. The . . . mind arises in this moment; a . . . moment arises in this mind.
>
> Thus the self setting itself out in array sees itself. This is the understanding that the self is time.

We have trouble believing this, since we have very naive views of time. One way we cling to the idea that our lives are reasonably stable is to try to hold onto a frozen self-image that is timeless; we then view time as something outside our selves, separate from our selves. We see our selves as traveling "through" time but not being "of" time. One form this takes is to think to ourselves, "It takes time for a person to change."

It is true that if we think of time as some *thing* that exists "out there" and is measured by clocks, then "it takes time for a person to change." It is true that if we think of a person as some real entity that exists with a core identity separate from immediate experience, then "it takes time for a person to change." It is true that if we think of change not as a constant flow, but as something that has a beginning and end, then "it takes time for a person to change." It is also true, though, that these ways of approaching time are some of the primary ideas that bind us in the prison of our imaginings. These thoughts are conceptualizations about experience, rather than experience itself.

Psychotherapy is about helping people let go of outmoded ideas they have about themselves, which get in the way of their current experience. Once we let go of the ideas we carry about ourselves, once we let go of the ideas we carry about what an experience should be, self becomes each moment. Then, once we let go of the ideas we carry about what a "moment" is and what an "experience" is, we become our experience, and manifest ourselves through being time. Being one's self does not "take" time, since it is not being in time: rather, it is time being.

If we think of time in the conventional way, and break time down into a linear "before and after," then each second the clock ticks, time is lost. In this view, time is outside of us: we pass through it, we live in it. Time elapses; things take time. We think "I was this; I want to become that later."

But something different occurs when you find this moment completely. The paradox is that to open up fully to the moment, you must let go both of yourself and of the moment. Bringing your entire self to bear on one moment, where will you find it? What does it consist of? How do you hold it? The more you try to catch hold of time, the more it slips away. As you reach out to it, it is already gone. Yet even as you try to catch it, and think it slips away, you are embodying it. This *is* time.

Self functions the same way. Your existence here, in this space, reading, on this chair, is an expression of time. Or, to put it another way, you *are* time. Change does not *take* time. Change *is* time, and time *is* change. Time and self become both infinite and infinitesimal in the moment, so long as you stop looking ahead or gazing behind you. At this moment, you and all your clients are completely free.

This doesn't mean that we live from moment to moment in stepwise fashion. Just as there is no ether-like medium through which waves of light travel, so there is no moment "within" which the self exists. The self is not this, then that, then this. Since the self and the moment are not separate—there is no moment outside of the self, and no self outside of the moment—we could also say that the moment arises and passes away in the self. Both moment and self are constantly changing, ultimately empty.

If the bottom-line question in therapy is "Who am I?", ultimately the answer has to be "Here I am." If this leads us to ask, "What or where is 'here'?", we must answer, "Now." We *are* the expression of here and now.

Psychotherapy does not occur *in spite of* time that is measured as short or long; psychotherapy *depends on* the time being. Therapy can only take place a session at a time; each session can only take place a moment at a time; and when we are in that moment, we don't measure the time, but simply experience it. In therapy, we need to pay attention to what our clients and ourselves are *being* at this very moment. Instead of asking clients, "What have you been doing? What do you want to be doing?" perhaps we should be asking, "What is your being, now?" We don't ask this explicitly, since clients probably would not know how to answer in words. But we ask it implicitly with our gaze, our listening, our every interaction with every client. In this way we join with the client, practicing mutually with each other, and each becomes the session's time being. The time being is each of us and each client's whole life, here, right now. As Eihei Dogen noted:

> Since there is nothing but just this moment, the time-being is all the time there is. . . . Each moment is all being, is the entire world. Reflect now whether any being or any world is left out of the present moment. (c. 1246/1985a, p. 77)

> [When] the moon [is] reflected on the water . . . although its light is wide and great, the moon is reflected even in a puddle an inch wide. The whole

moon and the entire sky are reflected in dewdrops on the grass, or even in one drop of water. . . .

The depth of the drop is the height of the moon. Each reflection, however long or short its duration, manifests the vastness of the dewdrop, and realizes the limitlessness of the moonlight in the sky. (c. 1246/1985b, p. 71)

Most of the people consulting us are in pain and turmoil about their lives. They want to be different from the way they are now. To say, "This [painful] moment is your whole life, right here, now," may seem cruel and counterproductive. Certainly if we do this in a way that makes clients feel stuck and attached to this transitory experience, implying that this is what they "really" *are*, it could increase their pain and intensify their anxiety. However, if we join with them compassionately in being time, in a way that helps them appreciate rather than fear the fluidity of self-identity, we have found that the resulting disidentification with a fixed self paradoxically often brings a client a sense of relief and increased freedom. It does not generally help to talk philosophy with clients. The task, instead, is to enable a client to have an immediate experience of self-emptiness. This often brings an acceptance of the ubiquitousness of change that leads to an increase in compassion and a befriending of one's own experience (Nishitani, 1982).

During the course of a couple's therapy,[4] as her husband's obsessive self-recriminations lessened, Mary began to feel flooded with painful childhood memories of sexual abuse and humiliation. She asked to be seen individually. She then told the therapist (R.R.) how when she was growing up her parents, both nudists, would embarrass her if she brought friends home; they also forced her to pose for "cheesecake" photos, and conspired to give her sexually to their friends. Her primary feeling was one of self-disgust; she felt as though she had an indelible "stain on her soul." She felt that she had been treated like shit, and that this made her like a piece of shit on the inside, no matter how competent she appeared on the surface.

After several sessions, she remained mired in self-disgust. The therapist looked for some way both to acknowledge her terrible experiences and to free her from them, and said, "You know, when you take a mirror, and hold it up to a piece of shit, it looks like the shit is in the mirror. It's easy to believe this illusion. Imagine what it would be like being a mirror, if you believed you were everything you reflected. But you are making this mistake here. You look at yourself, and see the shit in the mirror, but fail to see that *you are the mirror*, and the mirror isn't sullied."

[4]More details of this case appear in Rosenbaum and Dyckman (1995).

Mary stopped. She looked transformed, as if a great weight had fallen off her shoulders. "I'm me," she stated, in some wonder. "I'm not what *happened* to me." Mary had begun to realize that her self transcended her historical experiences: her self being empty, it was and always would be free.

TECHNIQUE

Approaching self as empty does not result in a particular technique that a therapist should administer to specified patients, like an internist prescribing antibiotics. Neither of us (R. R. or J. D.) has said to another client, as was said to Mary, "You are the mirror." Just as self is always changing, so the manner in which we work with clients is always moving. The view of self as "having" an "identity" is fine for the simple step of observing, recording, and recalling experiences in linguistic self-statements. We do not wish to suggest that people lack any coherence to their experience and actions. At the next level of recursiveness, however—that of observing the observing observer—an infinite regress occurs where naive notions of identity fail to apply, as language tends to fall silent.

Approaching self as empty does not generate a list of things to do, but rather encourages a certain attitude toward the encounter between therapist and client. Knowing that sound arises from silence, that motion arises from stillness, the therapist cultivates the empty field of potentiality that actualizes itself in specific interactions between client and therapist.

Therapists may rightfully ask "Okay, this theory is nice, but will it have any effect on my therapeutic technique?" This kind of question, though, implies a kind of separation between what therapists think and what they do—between their "inner" life and their "outer" actions in the world. Experiencing self as empty helps obviate such a split, so that therapeutic technique and the existential encounter with the client depend on each other. A case example may be helpful.

The therapist (R. R.) was seeing a client who was incessantly self-derogatory. Five years ago she had reluctantly gotten divorced, when her husband was unfaithful. Previously, she had been very dependent on her husband; since the divorce, she had not even attempted to balance her own checkbook. However, she had managed to raise two children as a single mother. The older son was involved with drugs and had become abusive toward her. In order to safeguard her younger teenage daughter, and to get away from this son, the client had recently moved out of her apartment. She was financially strapped, trying to save money for her daughter's college education, so she moved in with her mother. Her mother, unfortunately, was very critical and controlling; she objected if the client even went out to church socials, and would call her a "tramp." Many relationships had been cutoff in the mother's family of origin, generating a great deal of isolation and bitterness.

The client spoke in a whining voice, complaining about how awful her life was. The immediate precipitant for coming to therapy was that her car had been stolen; she couldn't afford both to get another car and to move out of her mother's house. She couldn't decide which to do. She was scared to buy a car, and scared to continue living with her mother. She took this as evidence that she had ruined her life—that she was fatally flawed or incompetent. She explicitly stated that she just wanted to give up and have somebody take care of her, but nobody was available. She would plead for help from the therapist, but anything the therapist offered was rejected. If the therapist tried empathizing, the client switched to talking about the concrete aspects of the car problem. If the therapist attempted to emphasize the client's strengths and past successes, the client disqualified them. If the therapist tried problem solving about the car and living situation, the client would find one objection after another, insist that she was incompetent, and retreat to whines and tears about her inevitable misery.

Frustrated, the therapist noticed that he was starting to mentally label the client a "help-seeking, help-rejecting, dependent personality." He realized that his frustration was leading him to categorize and pathologize the client, distancing from her rather than meeting her. He also realized that he needed to open up to the situation more, but had no good ideas about what to do. So he took several deep breaths and attempted to let go of his expectations, feelings, and frustrations. He tried to cultivate feelings of compassion for the client's suffering, impartial acceptance, loving kindness, and sympathetic joy. Utilizing this "technique" helped the therapist feel somewhat calmer.

The therapist then confessed apologetically to the client that he found it hard to know how to help her. He acknowledged that the choices she faced were difficult, and none of them were ideal, but suggested that some might be better than others. He then offered a long "laundry list" of all the options for the future he could think of.

Among the options the therapist suggested was that the client could enlist an ally. What about her siblings? At this point the client started talking, with some emotion, about how her older sister was also "on the outs" with their mother, whereas her younger sister, from the day she was born, could do no wrong. The client had tried and tried to be the "good daughter," but had never gotten any approval. The therapist attempted to empathize with her feelings about this, but this still led only to yet another rehearsal of her car difficulties rather than to any emotional contact.

The therapist then suggested a paradoxical intervention involving exaggerated advice seeking from the mother on virtually all decisions. The client began to smile. When the therapist mentioned that the idea of this "reverse psychology" was for the mother to eventually encourage the daughter to live her own life, the client then said, "But I'm not sure I want that. I have to admit I still want her approval."

At this point, the client began to respond to empathic exploration. She related childhood experiences, expressed her pain, and talked about how she still tried hard to be the "good girl" to win her mother's approval. The therapist and the client were able to work together through some metaphors, and the client was able to externalize her problem by naming it and mapping its influence on her life.

As she concluded the session, the client commented on how much better she felt. She thanked the therapist, who told her (genuinely) that it had been a pleasure working with her. The two shook hands, and felt they had made contact with each other.

The session had required numerous technical interventions, but none of these would have been effective without a willingness to let go of expectations arising from belief in a fixed, core self. When the therapist was able to stop objectifying the client into a static, pathology-laden identity, he was able to stop worrying about being a "helpful therapist," and the client was able to stop holding on to being a "pitiful waif." They managed to avoid becoming overly bound up in their narrow definitions of their roles, and avoided mistaking their roles for their selves. Groping toward and finally finding an empty field of potentiality, both were able to meet new self and new other for a moment.

With self empty, we bring ourselves to that horizon where other people and the world at large arise to greet us. Realizing self as empty, we are able to experience ourselves and others without making ourselves or others into objects; psychotherapy is ultimately about meeting clients in a way that doesn't turn them (or us) into objects. The dreariness of publicly always proclaiming oneself a "full self," and the pleasure of meeting in emptiness, have been nicely expressed by Emily Dickinson (c. 1861/1960, p. 133):

> I'm Nobody! Who are you?
> Are you—Nobody—too?
> Then there's a pair of us! Don't tell! they'd advertise—you know!
>
> How dreary—to be—Somebody!
> How public—like a Frog—
> To tell one's name—the livelong June—
> To an admiring Bog!

Although the meeting of empty selves is fundamentally natural, it is easy to lose our way in admiring (or pathologizing) bogs. When we are stuck in a bog, it is helpful to have the firm ground of some technique to fall back on. Technique, from this standpoint, is not some *thing* we as therapists perform "on" clients with the expectation of making some *thing* happen (Rosenbaum, 1982; Rosenbaum & Bohart, 1994). Rather, technique is a vehicle for expression, a particular framework to facilitate an encounter. Language is a technique; it is separate from the experience it attempts to capture. Direct experience cannot be captured, though; we need some vehicle—language, art, movement—as a medium for the expression of experience (Rosenbaum, 1988, 1993a)

There is no contradiction between the "naturalness" of empty self and the inescapable need for technique. All therapists must use technique; technique is necessary for communication. In addition, by giving therapists something to "do," technique can help bind therapist anxiety and create more space for a genuine encounter to take place. Therapists must neither avoid technique nor get trapped in it. Rather, technique must arise to meet the needs of the particular client and the particular moment: then it becomes an existential meeting. Ericksonian, narrative, and constructive therapies are not techniques, but ways of *collaborating* with clients; to do this, a therapist must rely on some technique. Seeing self as empty, the therapist is able to engage in technique freely, playfully, without getting caught in either its mechanics or in expectations of what the technique will "produce." Paradoxically, when the therapist can give up producing a particular result, both the therapist's and the client's actions become congruent expressions of their (empty) selves, and integral change emerges naturally. Technique is a way of "calling" the client and "clearing" one's self to create an unforced openness to change.

> Recently, one of us (R. R.) was attempting to pull weeds, in order to make his yard presentable before having a group of friends over. Despite his attempts to cultivate nonjudgmental acceptance, he was feeling annoyed both with himself and with Nature for letting the weeds grow so high (three feet tall!). They had already gone to seed, so that they'd be back again next year; the weeding felt futile. The sun was hot, and the ground was rocky and hard. The weeds' roots went down deep. He would attempt to dig down as far as he could, but couldn't get very far; he would grasp the weed's root and pull, and the root would break off in his hand.
>
> After an hour or so of fighting the weeds, making little progress, it came to him that he could help himself relax by using a "technique." He got off his hands and knees, and planted both feet firmly on the ground. Reaching down as far as he could, he took hold of one weed's root. He then closed his eyes and stopped opposing himself to the weed.

Instead, he let himself "feel" the weed's root all the way down to its deepest tip, appreciating it fully. He let himself feel the earth surrounding it, and the whole earth under foot. The activity shifted from extirpating something bad to first encountering the root in its present place, acknowledging, meeting, and cherishing it; then helping it move to another place where, as mulch, it would have an opportunity to join with the garden in a different way.

He let his whole body join with the root, the earth, and the sky. With all involved fully engaged, pulling in one direction, the root came up effortlessly. The remainder of the weeding became a joy, and passed swiftly.[5]

When a client joins a therapist in the "garden," if someone is carrying chemical weedkillers, both therapist and client should wear protective masks and gloves. Working to eradicate "bad stuff" "in" or "around" the client's land will result in seeing only the weeds, not the flowers or the healthy deep roots. It may not be necessary to move from a "bad" piece of land to a "good" piece of land if one can realize that the field in which client and therapist meet currently includes not only what is visibly growing, but also the past growths whose death and decay now give their nutrients to the soil; the seeds and bulbs that, presently quiescent, hold future blooms; the worms to turn the soil; animals to dig it; and birds and insects to carry the seeds to new places. This vast field also includes the earth, the sun, the rain, and the sky. Knowing this, a therapist can meet a client humbly, with tremendous respect for the client, in a way that says, "Our whole self, our whole life, is here in this moment."

The "technique" of empty self being time actualizes itself when you, the therapist, meet a client in the waiting room and shake hands. Don't shake hands as a "preliminary" before starting work. The meeting can occur, right there, as you shake hands, and make eye contact, in a way that is different from usual social behavior. You communicate to the client that you are working to be totally present with the client. So when you sit down with the client, you must bring your whole self to the encounter, body and mind. Take a few extra seconds to sit down, and align yourself with the moment; sit up straight, let the breath go deep, place full attention on the client, and empty yourself of any preoccupations, expectations, hopes, or fears you have for yourself in this encounter. Realize that you and the client are not ultimately filled "things," separate atomistic islands, but rather are intimately interlinking, arising, and

---

[5]"We say, 'Pulling out the weeds we give nourishment to the plant.' We pull the weeds and bury them near the plant to give it nourishment . . . you should rather be grateful for the weeds, because eventually they will enrich your practice." (Suzuki, 1970, p. 36).

creating yourselves in the interaction. Realizing this, fully treasure your-self and your client meeting.[6]

With the pressures of a busy day; with our insecurities, hopes, and fears; and with the ways the client may press us to respond in habitual ways that may not prove helpful, it is not always easy to maintain the attitude of openness that facilitates the meeting of empty selves. A useful "technique" can involve consciously cultivating what Buddhists call the "four heavenly abodes": feelings of compassion for others' suffering, impartial acceptance, loving kindness, and sympathetic joy. Of course, we realize we are always falling short of fully realizing these abodes. The illusions of our "filled self" get in the way, so we need to use all the interventions we know (hypnotic, interpretive, strategic, narrative, medi-tative, etc.) in the service of our work. When we attempt to meet our clients by simultaneously opening up and letting go, we can also take joy in the fullness of their (and our) experience. Even when this experience brings pain, and we let ourselves open to experience the pain in sympa-thetic resonance with the clients, there is joy in the process of growth and transformation that is constantly occurring—a whole life in each moment.

CONCLUSION

Experience is always richer than the stories that we make up about it. Because there are more "degrees of freedom" in an experience than in any one story, we can make up alternate stories that are also consistent with experience. No one tale captures "the" person, since "the" person doesn't exist except as an ever-changing flow of experience. This is the essence of constructivist and narrative approaches to psychotherapy (Shafer, 1976; Spence, 1982; White & Epston, 1990). We can go further and say that attempts to tell the story of the "self" will *always* fall short, because the tale has no separate teller, only the tellings.

In our tellings, we must give self-identity boundaries. It is important, though, that these not be the rigid boundaries of penned-in lines on a political map; wars are fought over such boundaries, despite the fact that on the land itself these map lines cannot be seen, smelled, heard, tasted, or touched. Our boundaries must rather reflect living shores, where sea and winds constantly change the form of cliffs and cove, inlets and jutting rocks. Boundaries are always expressed in action. Humans' boundaries

---

[6]One of us (R. R.) has made it his practice to have the client enter his office first, and bow to the client. He does this out of sight of the client (so as not to make the client uncomfortable with unusual social behavior), but finds it useful as a way of orienting himself to the upcoming encounter.

are not abstract conceptual schemas, but always embodied; being embodied, they are not stationary things, but are in constant interaction with a world from which they are not separate. World and self mutually influence and create each other; self and other arise to meet each other in each moment. An empty self does not mean an egolessness of diffuse boundaries and confused pseudofreedom that seeks to abandon all constraints (Epstein, 1992). Rather, seeing self-identity through the lens of emptiness can help draw a map for a self whose territories are continually arising in the meeting of touching and proceeding-from. On the shorelines of such lands, the sun becomes the ocean disappearing into sand.[7]

It is important to understand that both Buddhist and radical systemic epistemological approaches say that not only self, but *all* "things" are empty, including emptiness. To say that self or experience is empty is not to say it is void; this would imply that self is marked by a particular quality of nothingness. Rather, saying that self is empty is simply a shorthand for saying self has no permanently fixed, defining, "thing-like" characteristics. The individual self and the family system manifest their selves in this emptiness, where there is no dichotomy between self and other. Self does not subsume other or other subsume self; nor does self exclude other or other exclude self. Self-identity not only tolerates, but actually embraces the apparent contradiction of being both self and other simultaneously (Rosenbaum, 1982, 1990). Separateness and oneness are not mutually exclusive: Buddhists say that the vast sky does not hinder the white cloud (Dogen & Uchiyama, 1983).

When both self and world are empty, they embrace each other fully. That point where history and immediacy meet, where boundary and infinity intersect, where touching and proceeding-from dance, is existence its-self. From this standpoint, each person constantly expresses his or her original self, and this original self has no unchanging characteristic that brands it permanently. That being so, original empty self has no surfeit or lack; to call it perfect is not right, but it cannot be blemished. It is like when the wind strikes the water: Water and wind meet for a moment in a wave, which crashes on a shore that is then wiped clean by the wind. Therapist meeting client is like this.

Fundamentally, *empty self is connected self.* When we see selves as full, there are vast chasms that separate people. When selves are empty,

---

[7]A self with boundaries of infinite length but finite area is a self where "inner" development and "outer" contact with the world are two faces of the same coin. We can view such a self as consisting of the intersection of immediate relationship in the present with historical growth—the intersection of touching and proceeding-from/becoming. Self arises at an intersection of multiple planes, but this intersection is expressed at a single point (which, like all single points, is dimensionless and empty).

arising in response to immediate experience, we are all intimately connected to that well from which all experience comes—the "singularity" that cosmologists tell us created (and is perhaps constantly creating) a universe from nothing. Looking deeply into emptiness reveals that "each can only inter-be with all the others" (Nhat Hanh, p. 27, 1992). Families actualize themselves through individuals; individuals actualize themselves through families. The therapist meets the family, but is created by the family; the family meets the therapist, but is created by the therapist. The therapist creates himself or herself creating the client, and the client creates himself or herself creating the therapist.

When identity is empty, there is room for wood and woodcarver, individual and family, self and society. People encountering each other have a direct experience, in which each realizes his or her self in the other, the other in his or her self, the other in the other, and the self in the self. When therapist and client meet; when individual and family meet; even when a reader picks up a book chapter, and eye and word meet, there is no need to worry about "self" and "other." Once freed from clinging to an illusory fixed identity, self and world arise to meet and actualize each other, and therapy—like drinking tea or baking bread—becomes spontaneous activity. In such spontaneous activity, we rediscover the wonderful joy of a natural interconnectedness; there, love and compassion arise.

Dear reader, you are a particular person, holding a particular book, at a particular time. Still, as you hold this page, you are connected to the tree that gave itself up to become paper; to the sun and rain that helped the tree grow; to the people who worked the wood, printed the print, and made the book; to the earth whose mass keeps us all from spinning out into space. Your family, your clients, your students, and your teachers are all here now in your thoughts and your feelings, just as our families, our clients, our students, and our teachers are all here in these words we write and you read. As you experience this, we are all meeting one another. We thank you for touching us and for allowing us to touch you.

REFERENCES

American Psychiatric Association. (1994). *Diagnostic and Statistical Manual of Mental Disorders* (4th ed.). Washington, DC: Author.

Barlow, D. (1988). *Anxiety and Its Disorders: The Nature and Treatment of Anxiety and Panic.* New York: Guilford Press.

Bateson, G. (1979). *Mind and Nature: A Necessary Unity.* New York: Bantam.

Bion, W. R. (1967). Notes on memory and desire. *Psychoanalytic Forum, 2,* 271–280.

Bohart, A. (1993). Experiencing: The basis of psychotherapy. *Journal of Psychotherapy Integration, 3*(1), 51–68.

de Shazer, S. (1985). *Keys to Solution in Brief Therapy*. New York: Norton.

Dickinson, E. (1960). *The Complete Poems of Emily Dickinson*. (T. Johnson, Ed.) (p. 133). Boston: Little, Brown. (Original work written c. 1861)

Dogen, E. (1985a). The time-being. (D. Welch & K. Tanahashi, Trans.). In K. Tanahashi (Ed.), *Moon in a Dewdrop: Writings of Zen Master Dogen* (pp. 76–83). Berkeley, CA: North Point Press. (Original work written c. 1246)

Dogen, E. (1985b). Actualizing the fundamental point (R. Aitken and K. Tanahashi, Trans.). In K. Tanahashi (Ed.), *Moon in a Dewdrop: Writings of Zen Master Dogen* (pp. 69–73). Berkeley, CA: North Point Press. (Original work written c. 1246)

Dogen, E., & Uchiyama, K. (1983). *Refining Your Life* (T. Wright, Trans.). New York: Weatherhill.

Dyckman, J. (1994). A communications model of panic disorder. *Anxiety Disorders Practice Journal, 1*(2), 77–82.

Epstein, M. (1992, Spring). Freud and Dr. Buddha: The search for selflessness. *Tricycle: The Buddhist Review*, pp. 51–53.

Erickson, M. H. (1985). *Life Reframing in Hypnosis*. New York: Irvington.

Fisch, R. Weakland, J. H., & Segal, L. (1982). *The Tactics of Change: Doing Therapy Briefly*. San Francisco: Jossey-Bass.

Fogarty, T. (1978). On emptiness and closeness. In E. Pendagast (Eds.), *The Best of the Family* (pp. 70–90). New Rochelle, NY: Center for Family Learning.

Freud, S. (1961). The ego and the id. In J. Strachey, Ed. and Trans.), *The Standard Edition of the Complete Psychological Works of Sigmund Freud* (Vol. 19, pp. 3–66). London: Hogarth Press. (Original work published 1923)

Friedman, W. (1993). Memory for the time of past events. *Psychological Bulletin, 113*(1), 44–66.

Greenleaf, E. (1971) *A Spontaneous Experience of "No-Mind" During Hypnotherapy*. Unpublished manuscript.

Horowitz, M. J. (1988). *Introduction to Psychodynamics*. New York: Basic Books.

Jordan, J., Kaplan, A. G., Miller, J. B., Stiver, I. P., & Surrey, J. L. (1991). *Women's Growth in Connection: Writings from the Stone Center*. New York: Guilford Press.

Juhan, D. (1987). *Job's Body: A Handbook for Bodywork*. Barrytown, NY: Station Hill Press.

Kabat-Zinn, J. (1990). *Full Catastrophe Living*. New York: Delta.

Keeney, B. P. (1983). *Aesthetics of Change*. New York: Guilford Press.

Kellerman, S. (1979). *Somatic Reality*. Berkeley, CA: Center Press.

Levy, S. (1994, May 2). Dr. Edelman's brain. *The New Yorker*, pp. 70–71.

Maturana, H., & Varela, F. (1992). *The Tree of Knowledge: The Biological Roots of Human Understanding* (rev. ed., R. Paolucci, Trans.). Boston: Shambala.

Merleau-Ponty, M. (1964). *Signs* (R. McCleary, Trans.). Evanston, IL: Northwestern University Press.

Minsky, M. (1986). *The Society of Mind*. New York: Simon & Schuster.

Minuchin, S., Rosman, B. L., & Baker, L. (1978). *Psychosomatic Families: Anorexia Nervosa in Context*. Cambridge, MA: Harvard University Press.

Mischel, W., & Peake, P. K. (1982). Analyzing the construction of consistency in personality. *In Nebraska Symposium on Motivation* (233–262). Lincoln: University of Nebraska Press.

Neimeyer, R., & Feixas, G. (1990). Constructivist contributions to psychotherapy integration. *Journal of Integrative and Eclectic Psychotherapy, 9*, 4–20.

Nhat Hanh. (1992, Spring). Commentary on the heart sutra. *Tricycle: The Buddhist Review*, pp. 26–27.

Nishitani, K. (1982) *Religion and Nothingness*. Berkeley: University of California Press.

Omer, H., & Strenger, P. (1992). The pluralist revolution: From the one true meaning to an infinity of constructed ones. *Psychotherapy, 29*(2), 253–261.

Piaget, J. (1963). *The Origins of Intelligence in Children* (M. Cook, Trans.). New York: Norton. (Original work published 1952)

Reps, P. (Compiler). (no date). *Zen Flesh, Zen Bones: A Collection of Zen and Pre-Zen writings*. Garden City, New York: Doubleday Anchor Books.

Rosenbaum, R. (1982). Paradox as epistemological jump. *Family Process, 21*(1), 85–90.

Rosenbaum, R. (1988). Feelings toward integration. *International Journal of Eclectic Psychotherapy, 7*(1), 52–60.

Rosenbaum, R. (1990). Strategic psychotherapy. In R. Wells & V. Gianetti (Eds.), *Handbook of the Brief Psychotherapies* (pp. 351–404). New York: Plenum.

Rosenbaum, R. (1993a). Comment: Integration and translation. *Journal of Psychotherapy Integration, 3*(1), 73–78.

Rosenbaum, R. (1993b). Heavy Ideals: A strategic single-session therapy. In R. Wells & V. Gianetti (Eds.), *Casebook of the Brief Psychotherapies* (pp. 109–128). New York: Plenum Press.

Rosenbaum, R. (1994). Single-session therapy: Intrinsic Integration? *Journal of Psychotherapy Integration, 4*(3), 229–252.

Rosenbaum, R., & Bohart, A. (1994). *Psychotherapy: The Art of Experience*. Unpublished manuscript.

Rosenbaum, R., & Dyckman, J. (1995). Integrating self and system: An empty intersection? *Family Process, 34*, 21–44.

Rosenbaum, R., Hoyt, M., & Talmon, M. (1990). The challenge of single-session psychotherapies: Creating pivotal moments. In R. Wells & V. Gianetti (Eds.), *Handbook of the Brief Psychotherapies* (pp. 165–192). New York: Plenum Press.

Roth, S., & Chasin, R. (1994). Entering one another's worlds of meaning and imagination: Dramatic enactment and narrative couple therapy. In M. F. Hoyt (Ed.), *Constructive Therapies* (pp. 189–216). New York: Guilford Press.

Rymer, R. (1992, April 13). A silent childhood. *The New Yorker*.

Shafer, R. (1976). *A New Language for Psychoanalysis*. New Haven, CT: Yale University Press.

Shapiro, F. (1995). *Eye Movement Desensitization and Reprocessing: Basic Principles, Protocols, and Procedures*. New York: Guilford Press.

Spence, D. (1982). *Narrative Truth and Historical Truth: Meaning and Interpretation in Psychoanalysis*. New York: Norton.

Stern, D. N. (1985). *The Interpersonal World of the Infant*. New York: Basic Books.

Sullivan, H. S. (1953). *The Interpersonal Theory of Psychiatry*. New York: Norton.

Suzuki, S. (1970). *Zen Mind, Beginner's Mind* (T. Dixon, Ed.). New York: Weatherhill.

Tomm, K. (1987). Interventive interviewing: Part 1. Strategizing as a fourth guide-line for the therapist. *Family Process, 26*, 3–13.

Varela, F., Thompson, E., & Rosch, E. (1991). *The Embodied Mind*. Cambridge, MA: MIT Press.

Watzlawick, P. (1976). *How Real Is Real?* New York: Random House.

Watzlawick, P. (1984). *The Invented Reality*. New York: Norton.

White, M. (1986). Negative explanation, restraint, and double description: A template for family therapy. *Family Process, 25*(2), 169–184.

White, M. (1988). The externalizing of the problem. *Dulwich Centre Newsletter, No. 2,* 3–20.

White, M., &. Epston, D. (1990). *Narrative Means to Therapeutic Ends*. New York: Norton.

Winnicott, D. W. (1964). *The Child, the Family, and the Outside World*. Harmondsworth, England: Penguin.

Yeats, W. B. (1989). Among school children. (1928/1989). In R. Finneran (Ed.), *The Collected Poems of W. B. Yeats* (p. 217). New York: Collier Books. (Original work published 1928)

Zucker, H. (1967). *Problems of Psychotherapy*. New York: Free Press.

CHAPTER 12

Core Transformation
A Brief Therapy Approach to Emotional and Spiritual Healing

CONNIRAE ANDREAS
TAMARA ANDREAS

Core Transformation® is a process through which our limitations become the doorway to greater wholeness and well-being.[1] A great many limitations melt away naturally as we get in touch with our own inner nature, our core essence. The following characteristics make the Core Transformation process unique:

1. *It is remarkably effective in changing "symptoms" or complaints.* Unuseful behaviors and feelings melt away. Instead of a person's having to use willpower and struggle to change something, the new, more resourceful responses and behaviors become as automatic as the old, unresourceful ones were.

2. *It addresses a very broad range of limitations,* including virtually any unwanted emotions, behaviors, or thoughts. These include the effects of past trauma and abuse, poor self-image, negative habits and addictions, eating disorders, self-criticism, shyness, and emotions that we feel are out of balance (such as rage, persistent grief, jealousy, or fearfulness). We have reports from therapists who have successfully used this process with limitations such as learning disorders in children, and schizophrenia.

3. *The process itself is intrinsically kind and compassionate.* People describe the process as "a kindness toward myself that I didn't think

---

[1]In this chapter we use the words *therapist* and *client* only when someone is taking one role or the other. When we are discussing human characteristics, using *we* and *us* makes it clear that we are talking about all of us. Also, please note that Core Transformation is a registered trademark to maintain quality standards. For training information, contact NLP Comprehensive, 4895 Riverbend Road, Boulder, Colorado 80301.

possible." Particularly when dealing with serious issues such as rage, depression, grief, and abuse, many people have expectations such as these: "If I really deal with the issues, I will have to go through a lot of pain," or "If I really go within myself and discover what's there, I'm sure to find something awful." With this process, people are usually surprised to discover an undreamed-of kindness and re-sourcefulness within.

4. *The process itself can be used to deal with resistance to change*. Many processes do not get results with "resistant" clients. Frequently clients have reservations about change, or their personal thought/feeling styles seem to interfere with their progress. With Core Transformation, any resistance or interference to the process can be easily included in the process, and actually becomes an asset.

5. *The process tends to bring about "deep-level" change*, whether we are working with our life's most trivial issue, or our life's toughest issue. There is a shift in our awareness of our deepest sense of self. Inherent in the simple procedure is a path that leads to a profound experience that many call spiritual, yet no spiritual beliefs are required. Clients often say, "This experience cannot be described by language." Some of the words that people often use that come the closest to the experience are "oneness with all," "inner peace," "universal love," and "wholeness."

In this chapter, we briefly describe the development of the Core Transformation process, provide some concepts underlying it, and out-line the first five steps of this 10-step process. We provide a transcript of using these five steps with a woman who felt stifled by self-criticism, and close with more conceptual understanding, enriched by examples of results of this process in dealing with depression, abuse, and resistance.

We feature the first five steps of the 10-step process because this will provide the key exercise in the process, which can be used independently. A more in-depth discussion of these five steps, and a presentation of the remaining five steps, are available in the book *Core Transformation: Reaching the Wellspring Within* (C. Andreas & T. Andreas, 1994).

THE DEVELOPMENT OF THIS PROCESS

During my (C. A.'s) graduate studies in clinical psychology in 1977, I encountered the new field of neurolinguistic programming (NLP; Bandler, 1985; Bandler & Grinder, 1975, 1979, 1982; Grinder & Bandler, 1976). Finding the field a significant paradigm shift from traditional therapy, I appreciated its ability to go directly to results that were observable in a wide range of situations. After years of work as a trainer, writer, and developer in the field of NLP, I gave myself a personal challenge: I decided to work with people who had tried "everything" with their life's biggest issue, and nothing had worked. My task was to sit down with them and talk until they had what they wanted, without my using any of the approaches I already knew how to use. I had found that the field of NLP had provided me with many ways to assist others in making significant changes in their lives, often quickly (see S. Andreas & Andreas, 1987, 1992; C. Andreas & Andreas, 1989). Yet I was seeking a way to go deeper somehow—to bring about transformation more completely or more effectively than we in the field already knew how to do.

A strong part of my motivation came from the fact that I found myself to be much more effective with others than with myself. I was sometimes envious of the changes that clients and workshop participants reported, and found that these same processes rarely made a significant difference for me.

As I worked with these clients, committed to enabling this deeper level change to occur, the process that we now call Core Transformation began to emerge. Many got results from one session that they described as "profound," or even called "a miracle." These were clearly stronger results than I was accustomed to getting, particularly given the kind of limitations I was working with. I carefully reviewed these sessions to distill the 10 Core Transformation steps, creating a process for anyone to use.

Since that time, as the two of us and our colleagues and clients have gained more experience with the process, we have enriched our conceptual understanding of how the process works. However, it is significant that this process originated from intuitive work with clients, to which a conceptual framework was added afterward, in contrast to a process that is developed through applying a theory. We regard the experience of doing the Core Transformation process to be more important than the theory.

CONCEPTUAL BACKGROUND

Parts

When doing the Core Transformation process, we think of whatever we don't like in ourselves as a *part*. For example, we might say, "I lost my temper when I would rather have remained calm and collected. It was as if a part of me got angry anyway, even though I didn't want to." When we use the phrase "a part of me," we do not usually mean a body part, such as a kidney or an arm. We do not usually mean a "little me" inside, either. We mean one aspect of our experience.

We can think of any limitation as "a part of me" that does something

"I" am not so happy about: "A part of me generates experience X, even though I don't consciously want this experience."

One woman was conflicted about her career. She said, "A part of me wants to leave my job, but a part of me wants to stay." Any inner conflict can be described in terms of two or more parts. Many psychological complaints involve two or more discrete behaviors or feelings. For example, a bulimic person will sequentially binge, then purge. One would expect to work with at least two parts to resolve bulimia.

Resistance to change can also be described in terms of parts: "A part of me wants to change, but another part is reluctant."

The Unconscious

Most complaints that we have about ourselves are patterns of emotion, behavior, or thought that happen automatically—or "unconsciously." This is the sense in which this process works with our unconscious. In the first step, we get in contact with the unconscious part that produces the unwanted experience.

Although this process involves communication with the unconscious, it is not necessary to go into a formal hypnotic state. The state useful for doing this process is simply inner-focused and attending to inner experience, in contrast to intellectualizing.

Positive Purpose

In this process, we assume that every behavior, thought, or emotion has a positive purpose. Even if the behavior or emotion is experienced as negative, it arises out of a positive motivation. So the part of us that gets angry wants something that is positive; perhaps it wants to get our needs met, or to set boundaries. When we experience fear, the part that's afraid typically wants protection or safety. When we're overly critical of ourselves, the part may want to improve our behavior, or to protect us from being criticized by someone else.

The concept of positive purposes is foundational to a number of effective therapy interventions. Virginia Satir often relabeled people's behavior in a positive light. For example, she might redescribe clients' "wimpiness" as their "flexibility," or their "stubbornness" as their "ability to stand firm" (see S. Andreas, 1991; Satir, 1989). The NLP process of six-step reframing is based on discovering a positive purpose (C. Andreas & Andreas, 1989). The following transcript and explanatory outline show how Core Transformation takes the concept of positive purposes to a new depth. Rather than stopping when a positive purpose is discovered, the process leads us to an experience of a profound sense of wholeness or oneness that can have powerful healing qualities.

TRANSCRIPT AND CASE EXAMPLE: INNER CRITICAL VOICE

This session is drawn from a Core Transformation seminar,[2] in which Connirae demonstrated this process with Alicia, a 47-year-old woman. The transcript is edited for brevity.

Step 1: Selecting a Limitation to Work With, and Finding a Part

CONNIRAE: Alicia, what do you want to work with?

ALICIA: I want to overcome the fundamentalist "shoulds" and "shouldn'ts" I feel constantly constraining me, to release the free spirit within.

CONNIRAE: And how do you experience the "shoulds" and "shouldn'ts"?

ALICIA: I hear a voice saying, "You should . . . this," and "You shouldn't . . . that." (*Alicia's voice sounds loud and domineering as she quotes her inner voice*)

CONNIRAE: That sounds like something good to work with. Alicia, when you hear this voice speaking to you, where is it talking from?

ALICIA: It's in a box, over here. (*Alicia gestures to the left side of her head, where her inner "box" is*)

CONNIRAE: Wonderful. So now we're going to be talking about this voice as a "part" of you. And the first step is to welcome this part of you. Probably you have been pushing this part away, and trying to get rid of it, right? Most of us do this with parts of ourselves we don't like. We try to push them away.

ALICIA: Definitely!

CONNIRAE: And now we're going to do the opposite. Instead of trying to get rid of it, you can take a moment to welcome it, because this part of you actually has something wonderful to offer that we're going to be discovering. . . . (*Pauses as Alicia turns inward to welcome the part*) And what happens as you welcome the part?

ALICIA: It seems like it relaxes a little bit.

---

[2]A number of the cases reported herein are drawn from two- or three-day seminars. These followed a semistructured format: A trainer provided didactic background and demonstrated each of a series of experiential exercises which participants then did in pairs. All exercises were supervised by the trainer and a team of small-group leaders. Seminars usually involved 30–80 participants.

Step 2: Discovering the Positive Purpose of the Limitation

CONNIRAE: (*Nods*) And now, as you sense this part of you, the next step is to ask a simple question inwardly. (*Connirae's voice softens*) Ask this part, "What do you want?" and notice what answer you get. You may hear, feel, or see something as an answer.[3]

ALICIA: The answer came right away. "To prevent me from being rejected . . . and criticized."

CONNIRAE: Okay, wonderful. And thank this part for giving you an answer.

ALICIA: It says the "shoulds" and "shouldn'ts" are to keep me from being rejected or criticized by God, mother, and other people.

Step 3: Discovering Deeper Levels of Positive Purpose—The Outcome Chain

CONNIRAE: So now, Alicia, the next step is to invite this part to step in and experience what it would be like to completely *have what it wants*. So this part is going to step into what it is like if it succeeded at keeping you from being rejected or criticized, *completely*.

ALICIA: But that's not possible, to never be rejected or criticized.

CONNIRAE: That's right. Often what our parts want is not possible in the real world. Yet we're honoring what this part of you *wants* right now. And it can be important to be clear we realize that this imagining is not something that could be real in this world. So knowing that, you can invite this part to step into what it *would be like*, to completely have it, anyway. . . .

ALICIA: Okay. (*Closes her eyes, turns inward, and begins to look more relaxed*)

CONNIRAE: And when your part has stepped into that, you can ask your part, "What do you want, through keeping me from being rejected or criticized, that is even more important?"

ALICIA: "Peace and serenity." The answer came right away.

CONNIRAE: Okay. Great. So now, invite this part to step in and experience *having peace and serenity*—fully, the way that this part wants it. . . . You can nod to let me know when your part has done that. (*Alicia nods*) And ask, "Having this, what do you want through peace and serenity that is even more important?"

ALICIA: "Bliss."

---

[3]See the book *Core Transformation* (C. Andreas & Andreas, 1994) for more information about how to make it easy to receive an answer.

CONNIRAE: Okay, so thank this part for wanting bliss. And now invite this part to step into bliss—whatever bliss is, for this part. (*Alicia's breathing deepens, and more color comes into her face; she nods*) And you can ask, "Having bliss, fully and completely, what do you want through bliss that is even more important?"

ALICIA: I'm getting a visualization instead of words. When I was experiencing the bliss, it was like going back to a community drum circle I was in, where I closed my eyes— it was almost like we all became one spirit. Then the answer I get to your question, it's "To take that spirit and to widen (*she gestures with both hands*), encompass."

CONNIRAE: To take that spirit and widen and encompass? (*Connirae repeats Alicia's hand gestures*)

ALICIA: Yes.

CONNIRAE: Good; wonderful. So is there any one word or phrase that we can use to name this experience?

ALICIA: "Freedom."

Step 4: Reaching the Core State

CONNIRAE: And you can invite this part to step into having freedom, fully and completely. . . . (*Alicia nods*) And ask, "What do you want, through having freedom, fully and completely, that is even more important?"

ALICIA: . . . It's "Oneness with the earth and everyone." (*Alicia looks relaxed in a way that goes through her whole body; even more color has come into her face, and her breathing has become increasingly full*)

CONNIRAE: And so invite this part to step in and fully experience the oneness now. And ask this part, "Experiencing the oneness, is there anything that you want through oneness that is even *more* important?"

ALICIA: I don't think it's more important, but there's this sense of energy and love that goes with it. And there's something coming up about restoring my body. I think this part's been shutting down parts of the body, so that I can't get out and get myself in trouble.

CONNIRAE: That may be. And now this sounds like a shift. Instead of getting a deeper level of outcome, what we're getting is most likely the consequences of having the core state. When we get to the core state, the part will either let us know, "There is nothing more," or the part will start telling us how our life would be different if we lived out of the core state. This sounds like what your part has done.

Alicia's Outcome Chain and Core State

See the outline below ("Overview of the Steps . . .") for an explanation of outcome chains and core states.

> *Limitation to work with*: Voice that says "You should . . . this," and "You shouldn't . . . that."
> *Outcome Chain*: Prevent me from being rejected and criticized → Peace and serenity → Bliss → Freedom.
> *Core state*: Oneness.

Step 5: Reversing the Outcome Chain

CONNIRAE: Now your part, it turns out, thought that the best way to get oneness for you is to start off by speaking critically to you: "You should do that," and "You should do this." Right?

ALICIA: By making everybody happy and being a good girl, and being perfect. . . .

CONNIRAE: Yes, and avoiding criticism.

ALICIA: Uh-huh!

CONNIRAE: So it's almost as if this part thought, "Okay, if you want oneness, first you talk to yourself and tell yourself all kinds of things you should do and shouldn't do." Right? Good first step. "Then what you do is you make sure nobody rejects you. For anything." Right? "And once you've succeeded at that, then you can feel peace and serenity and bliss and so on down the line." And each of us will find that we have parts like this. We have sequences mapped out where we need to do certain things to get access to core states of being like oneness.

  Now, the only problem with these nice little scenarios that we work out is that they don't succeed. This is because states of being, like oneness, cannot be earned through our actions. They are not given or received. When it comes down to it, the only way I know to really experience profound oneness is to *step in and have it*.

  I think there are ample examples in our world showing that even when we succeed at meeting our goals in the world, it doesn't necessarily lead to the deep sense of well-being that we are seeking. The most obvious examples are the movie stars and famous people who are often not very satisfied inwardly, despite their outer success. Or the business executive who has made millions but feels hollow. These people have what a lot of people want, and yet they still haven't gotten what they are most deeply seeking. So even if Alicia could succeed at having no one criticize her, would she have what she wanted? Not really. It's not likely to lead her to the oneness that this part of her is really seeking.

So that's the deal. Somehow, unconsciously, we get these little scenarios mapped out for ourselves that basically can't work. It's a fortunate thing, though, because what does work is so much easier. You know, if she had to succeed at getting no one to reject her, this would be impossible. But to step in and feel oneness—that she can do. That's an easy thing. Does this make sense to you, Alicia?[4]

ALICIA: Yes. (*Nodding*) I think the method this part of me was using was that if it didn't get to me mentally, it started getting to me physically. And it would have progressed to the point of being bedridden and not doing anything, and who can criticize someone who can't do anything? (*Laughs*)

CONNIRAE: So it's a good thing you chose that to work with, because now you have the opportunity to reorient your whole future. So, are you ready for another approach?

ALICIA: Sure.

CONNIRAE: All right. So, turning inward, thank this part of you for wanting oneness, and ask this part of you if what I've been saying makes sense, and ask if it wants to have oneness by stepping into it and experiencing it.

ALICIA: . . . What's interesting is this part is totally crying and exhausted. It's been trying so hard.

CONNIRAE: And you may have a sense of comforting this part now. Because it's crying and it's exhausted. Because this part has been willing to go to great lengths to try to succeed at getting something so important as oneness. And that's the aspect that always touches me the most—how dedicated these parts of us are.

ALICIA: They work so hard.

CONNIRAE: Yes. *So* hard. Fortunately, this part can now experience a whole new direction with this, because you can invite this part of you now to just experience what it's like to step in and have oneness as a way of being in the world. Just because this part likes it. . . . So is this part experiencing the oneness already?

ALICIA: Right this second, I think it's experiencing grief.

CONNIRAE: Grief usually comes out of knowing that there's something you want, but not having it yet. Or not having it any more. We know

---

[4]When doing the process, people are often surprised to discover that stepping into even a profound state they have never known before is quite easy, because the unconscious inner part that wants the core state has the knowledge of it. If we had to step into these states consciously, it would usually be impossible.

what we could have; in a sense it's right close to us; but we're not fully stepping into it yet. So that's why this part is feeling grief. So as soon as this part steps in and has the oneness, the grief will flow out. Does that make sense? (*Alicia nods*) So you can let this part do that now. That's right. . . . Really letting that flow out as the oneness flows in. And this oneness, in a sense, will be emerging from deep within this very part that had been grieving. That's where the knowledge of it is. That's where the experience itself is. So in a sense we're just releasing that now.

ALICIA: (*Her eyes are tearing–she is obviously feeling strong emotion*) My tears are like the tears of a new birth. . . .

CONNIRAE: And that's fine, that's wonderful. You can let them come, because these are the tears of reconnection. It's like reawakening something that's always been there.

ALICIA: And acceptance.

CONNIRAE: Yes. And really letting this oneness spread even more, within this part of you. You can ask inwardly of this part, "Having oneness already there as a way of being in the world, how does this make things different?" And you don't have to put the answer into words. You can just let this part sense the answer and experience it and enjoy it.

ALICIA: There's total acceptance—a sense of unconditional love . . . and joy.

CONNIRAE: Yes. And now we get to take this oneness through all the other outcomes this part has had for you. So invite this part to experience how already having oneness as a way of being, radiates through freedom . . . transforming and enriching. Now that this part is already fully into oneness, and this oneness radiates through this part, the oneness can spread. And, whoosh,[5] it literally spreads through the next domain of what the part wanted, freedom. And it just does whatever it does—perhaps it melts, softens, changes the freedom. There's no need for you to figure it out, or understand it, or even to know what's happening; yet you can sense it spreading, deeper and deeper. . . .

ALICIA: The craziest words are coming out: "I can be a dope; I can be a fool; I can be . . . "

CONNIRAE: All right! (*Both laugh; applause from the audience*)

ALICIA: I never *dreamt* those words!

CONNIRAE: You probably never would have guessed that you would be

[5]Connirae makes this sound to amplify the unconscious processing.

thinking this, and it would be progress! Isn't there a Tarot card where the fool is the wise one?

ALICIA: Yeah, I learned to be a fool here at the seminar. That's progress! (*Laughter; Alicia takes a deep breath, and looks even more relaxed and vibrant*)

CONNIRAE: And we're hearing now the integration of something that had been put aside as "not me." And that's what we're all doing when we do this process. In taking *anything* from human experience and deciding "It's not me," we limit ourselves. So by including the things that we think are not so great, and not so wonderful, we actually enrich ourselves. So now it's like, "I can be that, too. I'm so much more now."[6] So now you can experience how already *having the oneness as a way of being* transforms, radiates through bliss. Whoosh . . . letting that be even more.

ALICIA: Yeah. Because if I go out into the mountains and do that and people go "God, she's crazy, stay away from her!", I'll laugh. (*Laughter*)

CONNIRAE: And this part can notice how already having this oneness—how this radiates through the peace and serenity. And now that's going to be enriched and transformed with the oneness, whoosh, spreading through that. Whatever was before, now is—

ALICIA: . . . Now I have an image of a sun. All those things like "stupid" and "fool" are all part of what I can be now. It's all together, with rays coming out.

CONNIRAE: Wonderful. The glory of it all together. And now, one more thing, to have even more fun. . . . Invite this part of you to experience how already having the oneness, whoosh, radiates through those experiences in which *before* that voice would have said the "shoulds" and "shouldn'ts." And you can sense how having this oneness already fully there—how this radiates through those experiences, and what they're like now. . . . And to some extent, you'll experience *now* what they'll be like, and to some extent you'll be surprised in the future as it unfolds, with the oneness already there fully, now, as a way of being.

ALICIA: I can't wait to watch that.

CONNIRAE: Yes. And feel—

---

[6]As we integrate parts of ourselves that we have been pushing away, there is a sense of coming into balance. For instance, if we have been overly rigid in following rules, we may need to reclaim the aspect of ourselves that can "act like a fool" to have the most complete resolution. If we feel that we have gone too far toward the other extreme, rather than toward balance, this is a sign that there are *two* parts, one overly constrained and one rigidly foolish. Working with the second part can then bring about a complete balance.

ALICIA: I can feel it throughout my body. And while we were working, the box with the voice kind of just dissolved out. (*Her eyes are still closed, allowing the inner processing to continue*) All that criticism—now I think of it and it's like, "Oh, well."

CONNIRAE: Yes. We see a different expression and demeanor now, as she thinks of all those things that used to be buttons. But now it's a button for oneness. It's just another opportunity to experience more of that. Great.

ALICIA: Yeah. If someone says, "You're stupid," I might go, "Thank you." (*Laughter*) That means I get to have room to learn.

CONNIRAE: Wonderful. Yeah. So, Alicia, you can thank your wisdom within, and especially thank this aspect of yourself that's now integrated within you in a new way, and the gift of oneness that's there for you. Within and throughout. Thank you very much, Alicia.[7]

Follow-Up Information from Alicia

Eight months after doing the process, we called Alicia, who told us that there were many changes in her life after doing the process. She reported that before the process, she was so afraid of making a mistake it was "almost paralyzing." She was afraid of being called "foolish" or "stupid" and of being rejected.

After the process, she said that she became more apt to take a risk. She described telling people what she thought, saying "I disagree," saying "no," and setting a boundary with someone and going by it. She said, "I had a roommate who was becoming undesirable, so I gave her a time limit and I ended up kicking her out."

Alicia talked of having had this fear of making mistakes and appearing foolish as long as she could remember. She thought it started when she grew up around people she "couldn't please," and was reinforced in her marriage. She remembered her mother saying, "If you do that, nobody's going to like you," and "If you don't behave, you're going to kill

---

[7]For an extended, step-by-step script of how to guide someone through the process, see the book *Core Transformation* (C. Andreas & T. Andreas, 1994). Training is strongly recommended to learn (1) nonverbal cues that can indicate what is happening, and suggest what to do; (2) increased skill with the language—how to vary it and optimize impact (the wording for this process is very carefully selected. Often even highly trained people change the words and inadvertently dilute the impact); (3) how to identify the underlying structure of a difficulty, and how to translate this into parts to work with; (4) how to utilize this process with groups of parts; and (5) how and when to utilize this process at an entirely unconscious level. Certain background steps lead to greater effectiveness and protect the client from abreaction.

me and I'll drop dead and you'll be alone." Alicia commented on similarities between her mother and her ex-husband: "My husband was always there with toxic words and putdowns."

One change resulting from the work surprised Alicia. For at least 10 years, she had been afraid to drive a small car, and wouldn't go on freeways at all: "I often left several hours earlier and took back roads to avoid the freeways." She hadn't realized that her fear of driving was connected to her fear of making a mistake, but in retrospect it made sense to her. She realized she was afraid of making a mistake and being blamed for it, after being in a car accident several years earlier and being blamed for it by her husband. Right after doing the work with Connirae, Alicia drove through a major city in a small rental car, on a freeway, up and down hills. She subsequently purchased a small car and drove it comfortably on the freeways. "I drove to a town about 30 miles away from home, and I wouldn't have driven that distance before. I would have gotten someone else to drive me, or I wouldn't have gone at all."

This was Alicia's overall comment about the experience: "I feel like the process is still going on, and healing is still taking place. For me, it's really about freedom. I'm free, and if I make a mistake, so what?"

OVERVIEW OF THE STEPS TO CORE TRANSFORMATION

Use this outline along with the transcript above to understand how the process typically unfolds.

Step 1: Selecting a Limitation to Work With, and Finding a Part

In the first step, we ask, *"What do you want to change or work with?"*

This can be any feeling, behavior, or pattern of thinking that isn't wanted. In this step, we notice the inner *sensory experience* that goes with the limitation. The experience may be an annoying inner voice, a troublesome or off-balance feeling, or a compulsive or bothersome image. We treat this inner experience as an "inner part" that we welcome and work with throughout the process.

Alicia experienced "constraint" because of what she described as "fundamentalist 'shoulds' and 'shouldn'ts.' " Instead of dealing with this on an abstract or theoretical level, Connirae's first step was to help Alicia notice her experience of this. Alicia had an inner "box" from which a voice spoke to her.

Questions to help someone notice his or her inner experience of a limitation include the following:

1. "When do you [procrastinate, feel you are holding yourself back, feel shy, overeat, etc.]? . . . Put yourself back into a time when you were doing this. How do you know you are doing it?"
2. "Do you feel something, hear something, or see something?"
3. "Where is this [feeling, sound, image] located?"

Step 2: Discovering the Positive Purpose of the Limitation

In the second step, we say, *"Turn inward and ask this part of you, 'What do you want?' Then wait to receive the answer."*

Each limitation is only a way to accomplish some positive purpose. Alicia's part wanted to prevent her from being rejected and criticized.

Helpful comments to receive the answer include the following:

1. "You may sense the answer emerging from the location of the part."
2. "You don't need to figure out the answer. Just allow it to emerge. It may be something that surprises you."
3. "The answer may come in a feeling, words, or an image."
4. "Give the part time to sense for itself what it is wanting. This is a new question, and our parts often need some time to recall what they really want."

Step 3: Discovering Deeper Levels of Positive Purpose—The Outcome Chain

It turns out that our part's positive purpose is only the first in a series of increasingly meaningful and desirable outcomes or goals.

In the third step, we say, *"Invite the part to step into having [the outcome from Step 2], fully and completely. . . . Ask your part, 'What do you want, through [this outcome], that is even more important?' "*

We then thank the part for answering, and continue this question, filling in the last outcome each time, until the core state is reached. This series of outcomes is the *outcome chain.*

As noted earlier, Alicia's outcome chain was as follows: Prevent me from being rejected and criticized → Peace and serenity → Bliss → Freedom.

Step 4: Reaching the Core State

Through Step 3, we soon arrive at a profound state of being called the core state. This is the deepest purpose that the inner part is seeking. This state is often described as "being," "wholeness," "oneness with God," or "universal love."

When we follow this question, "What do you want?" in this specific, experiential way, our parts universally go to a level of being that many describe as a profound spiritual experience. It is as if our limitations are misguided attempts toward an experience of God, oneness, or wholeness. Discovering this is not a mental or intellectual activity; through the process, it is a *felt experience.*

We know we have reached the core state primarily when the part has reached a "being" level where what is wanted is no longer in relationship to something else. (The nonverbal state is more indicative than the word label for the state.) In addition, the part has nothing deeper that it wants, or the part begins to describe consequences—how life will be different if it had the core state.

As noted earlier, Alicia's core state was "oneness." Note that several of Alicia's intermediate outcomes were also on a being level; however, her part kept on going.

Step 5: Reversing the Outcome Chain

In the fifth step, we literally turn around our inner orientation to living. The inner part thought it needed to go through a series of purposes to get to some essential experience of being; it thought it needed to "do" or "get" things in relationship with others in order to have the core state. Often some of the purposes sought are unattainable. (For example, Alicia's part wanted to completely avoid making mistakes.) Even when the outcomes are attainable (such as "success"), achieving the outcome in the world does not usually lead to the profound inner state of being that our part is seeking. Achievement in the world does not lead directly to an experience of wholeness or oneness.

In Step 5, the core state that was released in Step 4 now becomes our beginning point. It becomes what we live out of rather than what we strive for.

We say, *"Invite this part to step in to having [core state] as a way of being in the world. How does already having [core state] make things different?"* . . .

"Now invite this part to experience how already having [core state] as a beginning, a way of being in the world, transforms, enriches, radiates through [previous outcome]." We do this for each outcome in the outcome chain.

We then say, *"Invite this part to experience how already having [core state] as a way of being, transforms the situation where you used to [have the limitation you began with]."*

Note that Alicia's part, when invited to step into the core state, did not immediately do this; it was "crying and exhausted." Although this is not a standard step, Connirae invited Alicia to comfort this part a moment before going on. The second time Connirae invited Alicia's part to step into oneness, Alicia's part experienced grief. This is also not a typical client response, but occasionally happens when the part stops just short of stepping into the positive state of oneness. Alicia's part was then ready to experience Step 5.

DISCUSSION

Reintegrating the Shadow

Our normal tendency is to fight with whatever we don't like in ourselves. If we overeat, we fight with our urge to eat more, and try not to. If we tend to blow our stack, to feel shy and insecure, or to be overcompetitive, again our normal human tendency is to try not to be that way. What we sometimes call "defense mechanisms" (e.g., denial, projection, and repression) are labels for some of the ways we do this—ways to say, "This is not me. I am not like this."

It is especially important and significant that with Core Transformation, whatever we don't like about ourselves becomes a source of tremendous, profound sense of wholeness and well-being. This fits with Jung's (1954/1966) idea of the "shadow" as something that needs to be reintegrated. However, the idea alone is not enough to do it. This process gives us a very complete and natural way to reintegrate the shadow, because once our "shadow" parts have transformed into their core states, they are in complete alignment with us as complete beings. There is nothing within us that any longer wants to fight them. At this point we can recognize the "gift" or "treasure" that is within each of these parts of ourselves.

How Are Parts Constructed?

Our "normal" range of thinking and experiencing as human beings is quite broad. When we take any human quality and try to make it "not me," it becomes a problem or limitation in our psyche. A simple example is a young boy who stumbles and skins his knee. Experiencing pain, the boy cries. If an adult emphatically tells him, "Don't cry! Big boys don't cry!", he is likely to push aside the pain and make it a "not-me" experience: "I don't hurt, and I don't show pain." For the child at the time, it is a good solution to a difficult situation. He wants to maintain love and approval from adults more than he wants to express his feelings, so he does his best to stiffen up and not show feeling. Unconsciously the boy may conclude that all feelings are bad. If this pattern continues, as a man this boy may have a wife or partner who complains that he is "too cold and unfeeling."

When something in our experience is judged as wrong or as "not us," and we do our best to push it away, it actually tends to become more extreme, as well as more stable and fixed. As children, when we are simply allowed to cry with a loving adult close by, soon the pain is over and our attention naturally goes to something else. However, when our natural response is stifled or judged, in a sense it is never allowed to complete itself naturally. It is as if some inner part of us still wants to cry, while another part of ourselves wants to "be a big boy/girl so nothing bothers us." An inner split has been formed.

How Does the Reintegration Happen?

When we become parents, and a small child tugs at our leg and yells for attention, the tugging and yelling get more dramatic if we ignore the child. If we pay attention and ask, "What do you want?" the small child may say, "I want a glass of milk." The child can then be satisfied and become quite happy and cooperative. So it is with parts of ourselves. When we judge an aspect of our experience as wrong or bad, we try to separate ourselves from it and dismiss it. This aspect then grows stronger. It "complains louder," as does the small child who is ignored. When we welcome this part and ask, "What do you really want?" in a very open, deep way, we discover the kernel of aliveness and wholeness ready to sprout within what we thought was a "negative" quality in ourselves.

Our Layers of Striving:
The Typical Progression of Our Outcome Chains

Through our work with many hundreds of people with this process, it has become clear that inner parts' outcome chains have a similar progression.

The first stage of an outcome chain is the *surface-level experience.* This is the *experience* (not mental analysis) that we sense limits us in some way. It may be a behavior, a feeling, an inner voice, and/or internal images that come up in a limiting way. Examples include a behavior of yelling at our children, a feeling of persistent sadness, an inner critical voice, or an inner image of a black cloud.

If someone has a mental analysis of himself or herself such as "I'm too codependent" or "I have an addictive personality," we try to find an example of being that way, and then to discover what internal *experience* is there, to use to begin this process. For example, someone who complains of codependence may notice that when they are with someone he or she cares about, he or she feels drawn to please the other person. More specifically, this person may experience a pulling sensation in his or her heart that feels as if it is drawing him or her toward the other person. This pulling sensation is a specific *experience.* We then work with this experience as a part by asking, "What do you want?" Since it is the *experience* that we want to have transformed, this is only possible if the process begins with the experience itself, rather than with mental concepts about the experience.

Next we discover what is wanted *through* the limitation. Typically, the first few positive purposes have to do with getting something from others, or in relationship to others. Acceptance or love from others, approval, protection, safety, control, success, and effectiveness are common examples. These are, of course, common "issues" that are dealt with by many kinds of psychotherapy. However, at this level resolution is very difficult because (1) the deeper motives cannot be known and addressed; and (2) the outcomes are, at least to some extent, dependent on other people and circumstances.

As we move to deeper and deeper levels of intended outcomes, they become less about the outer world and more about inner processes: fulfillment, satisfaction, "believing in myself," worthiness, "being connected with my mission," and so forth.

The final stage of the outcome chain is the core state. The core state no longer has anything to do with doing or getting something in relationship to something else. There is no longer a "do-er" or "do-ee," subject or object. It is beyond action, beyond separation and dichotomy, beyond conflict. At this level, we just *are*. The core state is a profound experience that is often difficult to put into words. When people are asked to describe it, they often use words like "beingness," "oneness," "wholeness," and "inner peace." We can describe it as either an awareness of our wholeness as individuals, or an awareness of the underlying fabric of experience where all is one.

Many people perceive their core states to be spiritual, yet no spiritual beliefs are required. Each of us is free to describe the experience in whatever terms seem most accurate to us at the time. However, for the process to be most effective, it is important to respect the experience that emerges, rather than to impose our beliefs on it. Those with strong spiritual beliefs sometimes discover more "mundane"-sounding core states, such as "okayness"; atheists sometimes find spiritual core states, such as "oneness with God."

Identifying the Part to Work With

Sorting out where to begin can make a big difference in how successful this process is. Clients often come in with a mental analysis of their limitation, and need a little bit of help to get back to their experience. Here is an example: Joe complains that "I overcompensate for low self-esteem," and that this interferes in his relationships. To assist Joe, we ask, "How do you know you are doing this?" Joe answers, "I try to be in charge a lot. I get kind of pushy." This is closer, but still not at the level of *experience.*

US: Put yourself back into a time when you were being pushy. What gets you to be pushy?

JOE: I think to myself, "You've just got to put yourself forward. Don't act like a wimp!"

US: How do you think this? Is it an inner voice, or a feeling or image?

JOE: I guess it is a voice. I hear it.

US: Okay, where is that inner voice located?

JOE: I hear it coming from right above me.

Now we have identified one part. However, Joe's initial statement is "I overcompensate for low self-esteem," so we know there is one part that experiences low self-esteem, and a second part that "overcompensates." For the most complete results in Joe's life, both parts can be worked with. Here is a way we can find the second part:

US: How do you know you have low self-esteem?

JOE: I just don't feel very good about myself.

US: Think of a time when you didn't feel very good about yourself. . . . When you put yourself back into that situation, what is your experience?

JOE: I feel like pulling away from other people and sort of disappearing.

US: Where do you experience this pulling away in your body?

JOE: It's almost like caving in, in my chest.

Now we have the second part to work with, in experience. As in this example of Joe, *any* limitation can be experienced in terms of the inner parts involved, and worked with in this manner.

Finding the Shadow Side

Knowing how to find all aspects of our "shadow side" makes a tremendous difference in how complete our results are when using the Core Transformation process. Basically, anything we don't like in ourselves *and* anything we consider "not me" become useful "shadow parts" to reintegrate.

Most of us have certain inner parts that tend to escape our notice. These parts are especially valuable to work with. If we are shy, afraid of being judged or rejected by *others,* we will easily notice the part of us that feels shy. However, we will benefit greatly from also reintegrating the part of *us* that judges and rejects. Similarly, if we experience ourselves as victims, we can reintegrate both the part of us that feels like a victim, *and* the blamer or persecutor within.

Usually one or the other side of an inner split is active and the other more passive. Usually we like one side better; the other one is disowned and projected, perhaps denied entirely. However, when we feel like a victim, we can be tremendously empowered when the part that is "hurt" or "wounded" is healed, *plus* when we acknowledge the "blaming/persecuting" parts within ourselves and heal them also.

In any situation where we blame others, it is obvious to work with our "inner blamer." In addition, we are empowered when we can notice and heal any parts of ourselves that feel hurt or victimized in some way. One aspect of blaming is blaming ourselves. When we work with both sides of this experience, old judgments against the self dissolve. Through all of this, we come to a loving and empowering sense of ourselves as "co-creators" of the situation.

DEEPENING OUR UNDERSTANDING:
EXAMPLES WITH DEPRESSION AND ABUSE

To assist in understanding how Core Transformation works, the range of applications, and the range of results to expect, we have selected examples of work with types of clients who are usually considered "difficult." Often therapists seek special procedures to use with each diagnostic category or complaint. Our experience in working with many individuals is that Core Transformation is effective with complaints as diverse as learning disabilities, mood disorders, shyness, nailbiting, smoking, and even schizophrenia.[8] This is because we are dealing with the underlying *structure,* rather than the "symptom." Our guess is that Core Transformation is effective with such a wide range of complaints because it works at a level of structure that is deep enough to address something universal that exists within all or most limitations. The structure of *any* limitation can be thought of as one or more parts of ourselves that are out of alignment with what we want.

Overcoming Depression

Nancy experienced a shift in depression after working with Core Transformation trainer Marilyn Veditz at a seminar. Nancy said at the seminar

---

[8]See *Core Transformation* (C. Andreas & Andreas, 1994) for case examples of most of these categories.

that she'd been depressed to varying degrees for five years, and seriously depressed for the last eight months. She had tried antidepressants, positive affirmations, support groups, and therapy, without noticing results.

Nancy was exhausted, yet pushed herself to stay busy to avoid being "overtaken by depression." When she was alone, she often started crying for no reason. Her description of her work was "I couldn't think straight, couldn't remember, was not organized at all, always was late, took long lunches, didn't care." Her boss threatened to fire her. She said that each thing she needed to take care of was "too much to handle." For example, she had gotten an insurance settlement for flood damage, and the money sat in the bank for six months because she "had no energy to fix the place up."

She believed that her depression started when she got in touch with some feelings from early childhood that overwhelmed her, and that the depression was her way of covering this up. Nancy felt unwanted by her parents, and felt like the family scapegoat.

> *Limitation Nancy worked with*: Needing to stay busy.
> *Outcome chain*: Needing to stay busy → Get things done and be in control → Sense of accomplishment → Security → Someone to take care of me → Safety.
> *Core state*: Peace.

After the seminar, Nancy said, "I woke up feeling like myself, excited about getting up in the morning." Her regular therapist corroborated her experience. Nancy said, "In my first therapy session after the workshop, my therapist couldn't believe the difference that she saw. In the next session, she was even more surprised that the change had lasted. She told me she had expected it to be a 'quick fix' that wasn't permanent."

Nancy has continued using the process on her own. She began repairing the flood damage to her home. In her job, work that would have taken her a week now took several hours, and she paraphrased her boss as saying that he'd never been so organized in his life as she'd helped him to be. She now felt she had outgrown her job, and she gave notice.

In summary, Nancy said, "I'm a whole different person! When I was depressed I couldn't picture tomorrow. Now I know where I want to go, I picture myself going, and I have faith that I can get there."

Working with Abuse

We present two examples of clients dealing with childhood abuse, Louise and Gail. These examples illustrate the usual range of response to Core Transformation work. Louise's experience was immediately dramatic, with a very strong sense of resolution after doing the process with only two parts. Gail used the process intensively for several weeks, and experienced ongoing healing. Our experience is that this process invariably produces some positive shift. Some people, like Louise, experience a dramatic positive change the first time they do the process. Others, like Gail, experience this shift gradually, working with parts over time.

Regaining Memories

Louise, in the first example to follow, reported having a spontaneous memory of early sexual abuse. Although early memories do not *usually* emerge, it happens often enough to warrant a few comments. Nowadays there is a lot of debate about whether memories gained as an adult in therapy are accurate, or have been induced by the therapist in a "false memory syndrome." When a memory emerges, one important distinction is whether the therapist did anything to "suggest" it, or whether the memory came up on its own.

In the Core Transformation process, we do not ask people to remember something from their past, or even suggest that they might. However, people spontaneously tell us of the emergence of early memories often enough that it is interesting.

Our best guess is that these memories emerge for different reasons on different occasions. One possibility is that people feel a kind of "safety" and trust in the Core Transformation process, and that these feelings make it less risky to become aware of incidents that might otherwise be overwhelmingly painful. They know from experience that they will not be "stuck" in whatever emerges. Instead, any part that experiences pain will be asked, "What do you want?" and invited to step into that. Already, at this point, an individual is out of the pain experience, and into another experience. This realization, that any pain will be the doorway to something very positive, makes dealing with unpleasantness completely different. Pain becomes profound experience remarkably quickly, and the person is then nourished by what had been painful.

Practically speaking, we assume that any painful images, sounds, or feelings that emerge do so because they are ready to be healed. We caution against trying to convince a client that a spontaneous memory is true *or* false, because as therapists we really have no way of knowing. Whether a particular image is literally true or whether it is metaphoric, our response is the same: to heal that part.

Sometimes the memories emerge after the healing is complete. A memory of abuse, or a terrifying incident that seems related to an adulthood "irrational fear," may emerge only *after* the adulthood complaint is completely healed and the troublesome behavior has changed.

It is as if the unconscious has realized, "This won't overwhelm or bother you now, so it's okay for you to become aware of it."

Louise

After attending a Core Transformation seminar with Tamara Andreas, Louise experienced a sense of resolution about childhood sexual abuse. Prior to the seminar, Louise had suspected that she had been sexually abused, because she drew many parallels between her own life and the people described in books about abuse. She had no memories from ages three to seven. When she was seven, she compulsively picked at sores on her legs and kept them from healing.

As an adult, Louise reported difficulties with shame, abandonment, and the need to be in control. After being abandoned by a "great love," she became sexually promiscuous. She described herself as "the office toy," leaving work at noon for sex, and meeting other men at night in their cars for sex. She fell in love with a series of married men. She said later, "Love was taken from me, but little if any was ever given to me, except in the form of the physical act." As she began to realize how unfulfilling these relationships were, and stopped them, she gained weight. "As I started to realize that the pseudolove I was getting was not enough, I used food to fill the emptiness."

She said that she had a need to plan things carefully, in order to be in control and avoid embarrassment. She often cried "for no reason." When something went wrong, she blamed herself, saying, "I should have known better."

During the seminar, Louise worked with a partner on her response when "I'm following the rules and someone comes along and wrongs me." When this sort of thing happened, she became enraged and vengeful to the point that she felt her behavior was sometimes dangerous. An example was when she was tailgated on the highway.

Louise's part discovered the core state of "sense of self." At a later point of the process, she said, "Wait, I can't go on right now. There is something in my mouth." She described an image of childhood sexual abuse that was "just there," and surprised both her and her partner. Louise reported that when she took the image of the man's penis out of her mouth, she could breathe more easily and had a sense of "everything opening up." However, she was left with feelings of regret, sadness, and anger about the memory and about how, in her perception, it had affected her whole life.

In the event that Core Transformation work seems to "bring an awareness of other parts that are suffering," as with Louise, we recommend doing the process directly with those parts as soon as possible. It is an indication that several parts together are involved in whatever present-day difficulty the client is working with. For Louise, working with a second part brought about resolution.

The next day, she did Core Transformation with the sadness, which she experienced as a "heavy, heavy weight on my chest." The core state was "oneness with God." She described the process as a rebirth: "I could feel everything slap together and align. I could feel the energy coming from my head into my arms and hands. I was stepping back into the self that I had lost so many years ago." After this, she couldn't find any other issues to work with about the memory of abuse.

Louise said it was important for her to realize that she did those self-destructive things for a reason. She said, "It's kind of like waking up from a deep sleep. I've always blamed myself, and thought, 'There's something wrong with me.' " After the workshop, her eating habits became healthier. She said that she made herself fried rice, rather than "popping anything into the microwave and then having a candy bar and potato chips."

Louise said, "The experience I had of regaining myself and connecting with something much greater than myself goes beyond words. When I do put it into words, the words don't have the power of the experience!"

Gail

This example illustrates the "safety" concerns that typically emerge in working with those who report a history of abuse. Safety concerns, like most other concerns, can be dealt with through the process in a very respectful and straightforward way that facilitates the effectiveness.

Gail burst into tears on the first day of a Core Transformation seminar, when she had simply contacted a part of herself. Since this is an unusual response, Tamara asked her what was happening. She said that she was an incest survivor, and had tapped into some feelings related to her childhood experiences. Tamara offered to assist Gail personally, as part of a demonstration for the group, and the next day she accepted the offer.

As the process began, Gail described a sense of being stuck that came up often, in doing personal change work as well as at other times. She used this as the part to work with. She felt this stuckness in the middle of her chest. When she asked this part what it wanted, it said, "To feel safe."

Tamara asked Gail to invite her part to step into feeling safe, and she said, "I can't. I don't know what safety is like." This is a fairly common obstacle, especially with people who report a history of abuse.

Tamara asked Gail to invite this part of herself to *pretend* as if it could feel safe. When she did that, she broke into a big smile. A frame of "pretending" or "acting as if" often allows people to step into experiences they don't believe they can have. As the process continued, Gail's outcome chain emerged as follows: Feeling stuck → Feeling safe → To be loved → Being me.

When they began reversing the outcome chain, Tamara asked Gail to ask that inner part of her, "When you have this sense of 'being me,' fully and completely, how does this transform your experience of being loved?" She processed silently for a moment, then responded, "I can see the love that's inside of people." Tamara asked, "How does having that sense of 'being me,' already there within you, also transform your experience when around someone who isn't expressing love toward you?" She responded, "I can still see the love inside them."

The reason Tamara asked Gail about having her core state while being loved *and* while not being loved was that she wanted Gail's experience of her core state to be independent of responses from other people. It's nice to get favorable responses from others, but it's not useful for our basic sense of well-being to be at stake.

Next, Tamara asked Gail to ask her part, "How does having the sense of 'being me' in an ongoing way transform or enrich your experience of feeling safe?" She responded, "I *am* safe." Tamara said, "Ask this part of you, 'Having the sense of "being me" and the basic sense of safety, how does this also help you notice if you're in a situation in which you'd want to do something to protect your safety?' Because when safety is an issue, it's like living in a house in which the fire alarm is constantly going off. It's impossible to know if there's really a fire. People generally find that when they have a basic sense of safety, this allows them to have more accurate inner signals, to know if they need to do something to keep themselves safe." After processing this, Gail nodded.

Next, Tamara said, "Ask this part, 'How does having that sense of "being me" in an ongoing way transform your experience in those situations in which you used to feel stuck?'" After a few moments, Gail said, "I feel free."

Tamara and Gail also did the next phase of the process, called "growing up the part," which primarily involves inviting the part to evolve to current age *with* the core state present (see C. Andreas & T. Andreas, 1994, pp. 62–81, for a detailed description of how to do this phase).

Three Weeks Later. In addition to the work described here, Gail used the Core Transformation process with other issues in exercises during the three-day seminar, and following the seminar. Three weeks later, Gail reported that the process had helped her get in touch with many issues related to her incest experiences, and to begin healing them. She attributed her gains to using Core Transformation in an ongoing way: "Any time I notice myself getting stuck, I'm able to ask myself, 'What do

I want?', and I imagine myself having it. . . . I use this process to get through it."

She described having had a "dysfunctional relationship" that she had continued obsessing about, even though she was now married to another man. The past relationship she considered a repeat of her dysfunctional past, where what had happened was denied, and she was blamed. "If I said something happened, my mother said, 'It's just a dream,' . . . " Gail recalled.

Gail described the Core Transformation process as having brought about a level of healing where she felt permission to "really feel my emotions and get in touch with my own knowledge about what had happened." As a result, she felt better able to let go of the past. She no longer found herself obsessing about her previous relationship, and "Now I feel like I've got energy for my husband."

Gail noticed that her changes also extended into her work relationships. She described going into a performance review with her boss, and asking for a promotion. "I felt flexible, whole—I had a nice sense of being, and did not get hooked by his behavior." Gail said that before, if she wanted to ask for something someone else did not want to give her, she got defensive and shut down.

Although Gail wisely felt that she had more to do, she reported now being on a trajectory of progress. She described coming to many new understandings about herself and others she had been in relationships with: "The technique has been very powerful for me. Before, I knew I had a lot of dysfunctional patterns because of my abuse, and I didn't feel I was making progress. Now I am definitely making progress and I feel myself becoming healthier."

Discussion. As often happens, Gail came to understand her past better through doing the Core Transformation process. However, it was significant that the understanding came *after* the transformation, in a natural way. The core state itself seems to bring about a new consciousness and new attitudes, for which the client then finds words. This is quite different from an approach in which the client is offered new insights in a more intellectual way.

As we have begun to discuss earlier, many people have found that this process makes it "safe enough" to address feelings and issues they have been avoiding. Having their sense of core well-being, wholeness, and inner essence intact can make painful feelings less threatening. The point here isn't that we always have to dredge up the past and deal with pain. It's that if we've been clouding over emotions or pushing them aside, this takes energy away from living our lives in the present. Transforming these emotions will free up our energy and enable us to be more fully present.

Core Transformation provides a safe way to work with abuse, because clients do not need to be overwhelmed with the negative feelings. We ask, "What do you want?" and the clients are immediately on a path that becomes increasingly positive and healing.

Action Steps. When we have our core states, we are empowered to act out of those states in whatever ways we choose. For example, Gail decided to go back to her home town and tell someone her memories of what had happened to her. This was her own decision. Someone else may choose different action steps. We assume that there is no right answer to the question of what to do to resolve past trauma, and that people can be empowered to decide for themselves what is most congruent with their inner nature and their life experiences. People often are surprised just to find themselves acting in new ways, as was Alicia (in the case presented earlier) when she found herself comfortably driving a small car on a freeway in the mountains. The more complete our healing has been, the more our action steps tend to arise out of a sense of clarity, compassion, and empowerment, without blaming either self or other.

TECHNICAL ASPECTS

Dealing with the Present (or Recent Past)

Like other brief therapy methods, the Core Transformation approach primarily addresses the present, rather than routinely dredging up the distant past or intellectually interpreting the meaning of experiences (Budman, Hoyt, & Friedman, 1992; Hoyt, 1994). We can think of a limitation as a configuration of emotion, thinking style, and set of behavioral choices in the present. For example, Alicia's limitation included *feeling* afraid of making a mistake, *thinking* critically of herself, and *behaving* so as to avoid the risk of appearing foolish (e.g., avoiding driving on freeways). Transforming this type of present configuration is our goal.

Addressing the Past, Present, and Future

Whatever our limitation, we can think of it as being a configuration with threads that run into the past and into the future. A limitation tends to be the best solution we could unconsciously generate in a time of difficulty. For example, a client was working with a present experience of pushing himself to write and publish. He suddenly got an image of being five years old, sitting at the dinner table as one of a large family; he wanted to express himself, but nobody paid any attention. It was as if an unconscious part of him thought he needed to continue to "push himself" to be heard. Through Core Transformation, we work with and heal the entire configuration that extends into the past, along with healing the present-day incidents that let us know "something is there."

Although this chapter has focused on the first five steps of this process, the last five steps include all time frames explicitly: past, present, and future. This gives a greater thoroughness of transformation, while remaining a "brief" process. These steps do not analyze the past, yet do extend the healing to include all past examples of the limitation on an experiential level. In addition, extending the healing into *future* experiences makes the transformation naturally available when future experiences arise.

Dealing with Resistance

We have found the Core Transformation Process to be ideally suited for respectfully acknowledging and transforming what is usually called "resistance." With the Core Transformation process, "resistance" is simply regarded as another part that also wants something positive. Several kinds of resistance or interference may emerge while doing Core Transformation. The client can be ambivalent about making a change; this just means we work with the part that does not want to change, as well as the one that is eager to change. Or the client's style may in some way interfere. For example, one client may intellectualize all answers, instead of waiting to receive an answer from the inner part. Another client may have a "style" of being pushy with inner parts, trying to force them to have the answers they "should" have. A third client may be impatient, irritable, or judgmental toward inner parts. All of these "styles" may interfere with Core Transformation's progressing easily. However, all we need to do is notice what is interfering, treat this as a part to be worked with, and do the Core Transformation process with this part. Accessing the core state of these parts and melting the interference not only make it possible to complete the Core Transformation work, but tend to transform the clients' ongoing style of moving through the world. The "style" that interferes with the Core Transformation process is likely to be the same "style" that is used to deal with life in general.

When there is interference, often it's obvious. A client can feel overwhelmed by a different feeling; an inner wall can emerge; or an inner voice can protest that the process should stop. For example, one client, Brian, was working with a part of himself that felt hurt and abandoned when his girlfriend had a number of conversations with other men at a party. As he was working with this part of himself, he got an image of a brick wall. He said he was stuck and couldn't get any more responses from the hurt part. We welcomed the brick wall image, and treated it as an expression of another part. When he asked the brick wall, "What do you want?", the answer he got was "Control." When he asked what the purpose of control was, he got "To be loved." After finishing the process with this part of himself, he returned to the part that initially felt hurt and abandoned. This time, no interference or objection came up, and he transformed his response of feeling hurt and abandoned into a feeling of security, caring, and alertness. Rather than negotiating with resistance, reframing it, or finessing it, Core Transformation results in the resistance's "melting" away.

COMMENTS IN CLOSING

How Does Core Transformation Create Such Deep Healing?

The often profound shift in experience that happens through this process comes primarily through the core states we discover within. As we have watched many people go through the process, and have gone through it ourselves many times, we have come to the sense that many (if not most) of our human difficulties out of a sense of separation between ourselves and others, or arise out of a separation within ourselves. Since the process inevitably takes us to something like wholeness (reintegration within ourselves as individuals) or oneness (reintegration of ourselves with the universal whole), this is what enables seemingly unresolvable difficulties and pain to be finally healed and resolved. For example, if we are afraid of others, when we tap into a universal sense of oneness with others, it no longer makes sense to be afraid of them. We *are* them. Similarly, if we are angry with others and blame them, when we go to a level of oneness with all, there is nothing separate from us to judge and blame.

In addition, the more we come to an experience of wholeness within ourselves, we embody a degree of vitality, strength, and empowerment that often spontaneously leads to resourceful, effective action in the world, and to a meeting of others without sacrificing ourselves. The combination of wholeness and oneness leads naturally to inner clarity, as well as to appropriate boundary setting that is relaxed rather than tense or defensive. The result of this kind of inner work is that we attain an experience of wholeness and integration, in contrast to further developing an "act" that looks good and is successful, but is another way of being split.

An Evolutionary Process

People who have worked with this process in a regular way over time have reported that their core states evolve over time: They become more intense and full, and cycle to more transcendent domains of experience. For example, the "oneness" we experience after doing this process periodically for quite a few years is significantly enriched from the one we experience at the beginning. It's as if there is a gradual awakening at the level of our inner essence. People often report that their whole lives tend to move in greater harmony with this deep inner nature.

How to Get the Best Results

We and those we have trained have experienced surprisingly dramatic and long-lasting changes in even quite difficult "problems" when we use Core Transformation as a complete transformation process. This involves the following:

1. *Using all the steps.* In this chapter, we have presented the primary exercise—the core state exercise. To increase the percentage of success, the remaining five steps are extremely enriching and important.
2. *Using the process with the entire system of parts involved.* Usually in a major issue or major life change, a system of parts is involved, rather than only one part.
3. *In our experience, it is possible to gain the most from this process through using it over time, in an almost meditative fashion.* Some people experience dramatic results the first time. For others, the dramatic results happen in a more cumulative fashion, through use over time. For everyone, whatever is gained from the process paves the way to even greater gains the next time.

It is also important to realize that our using Core Transformation successfully does not mean that all life's difficulties are now magically gone. It is more that we have moved to a new set of challenges from which to learn. We experience personal development as an ongoing process. The gains we and many others have made through this process are enduring; people have permanently resolved such difficult habits as smoking. The increases in self-confidence remain. Yet as we attain a new level of consciousness, we can become aware of new desires and goals for ourselves.

This shift of consciousness is to us a very important aspect of this process. It is not just resolving difficulties and making life okay. It is not just getting over smoking or a drug habit, or overcoming shyness. It shifts the nature of our being—our sense of ourselves and the world. It leads to the dissolution of self-righteous judgments. This shifting of consciousness is clearly what we as a world culture need to meet the challenges and hurdles of our times.

REFERENCES

Andreas, C., & Andreas, S. (1989). *Heart of the Mind.* Moab, UT: Real People Press.

Andreas, C., & Andreas, T. (1994). *Core Transformation: Reaching the Wellspring Within.* Moab, UT: Real People Press.

Andreas, S. (1991). *Virginia Satir: Patterns of Her Magic.* Palo Alto, CA: Science & Behavior Books.

Andreas, S., & Andreas, C. (1987). *Change Your Mind–and Keep the Change.* Moab, UT: Real People Press.

Andreas, S., & Andreas, C. (1992). Neurolinguistic programming. In S. H. Budman, M. F. Hoyt, & S. Friedman (Eds.), *The First Session in Brief Therapy* (pp. 14–35). New York: Guilford Press.

Bandler, R. (1985). *Using Your Brain–for a Change.* Moab, UT: Real People Press.

Bandler, R., & Grinder, J. (1975). *The Structure of Magic* (Vol. 1). Palo Alto, CA: Science & Behavior Books.

Bandler, R., & Grinder, J. (1979). *Frogs into Princes.* Moab, UT: Real People Press.

Bandler, R., & Grinder, J. (1982). *Reframing.* Moab, UT: Real People Press.

Budman, S. H., Hoyt, M. F., & Friedman, S. (Eds.). (1992). *The First Session in Brief Therapy.* New York: Guilford Press.

Grinder, J., & Bandler, R. (1976). *The Structure of Magic* (Vol. 2). Palo Alto, CA: Science & Behavior Books.

Hoyt, M. F. (Ed.). (1994). *Constructive Therapies.* New York: Guilford.

Jung, C. G. (1966). The practice of psychotherapy. In *The Collected Works of C. G. Jung* (Vol. 16, complete). Princeton, NJ: Princeton University Press. (Original work published 1954)

Satir, V. (1989). *Forgiving Parents.* [Videotape]. Boulder, CO: NLP Comprehensive.

CHAPTER 13

A Golfer's Guide to Brief Therapy (with Footnotes for Baseball Fans)

MICHAEL F. HOYT

It's not what the teacher says, but what the student hears that matters.
> —HARVEY PENICK, *And If You Play Golf, You're My Friend* (Penick with Shrake, 1993, p. 27)

In the Name of Jack, Arnie, and the Australian Shark. Amen.
> —FRANK & MIKE in the Morning, KNBR Radio, San Francisco

While Aristotle said, "The greatest thing by far is to have command of metaphor," Korzybski (1933) also cautioned that "The map is not the territory." I recognize that psychotherapy (or life) may not be an adequate symbol to capture the richness of golf (or baseball), but I hope that my remarks will at least suggest a few helpful resemblances. As golfers and ballplayers know, many a useful principle has been revealed on various fields of dreams.

THE FRONT NINE

1. When I was a teenager I attended the Los Angeles Open back in the early 1960s. I followed Arnold Palmer around the course, and actually got to talk with him a number of times. On one hole he drove deep into the rough. As he surveyed his next shot, there was a big tree and a long way between his ball and the hole. He walked down the fairway to check the location of the distant flag, and then came back. I was standing maybe 10 feet away from him and asked, "Mr. Palmer, where are you going to hit it?" He looked back and forth several times, and then replied, "In the hole." The ball didn't go in on that shot, but it did wind up on the green, and I learned a useful lesson: *It's a long day on the course if you don't know where the hole is. Have a specific goal and be purposeful on every stroke.*

2. "Play it where it lies" is a basic rule (Watson with Hannigan, 1984). This is it, and the craft and art come when one appreciates the wind, the downhill lie, and the bunkers. "Setting up is 90% of shotmaking," says Jack Nicklaus in *Golf My Way* (Nicklaus with Bowden, 1974). He also advises a high tee, since the sky offers less resistance than the ground. The grip is where inner meets outer, where we and the world connect (Pressfield, 1995). This gets at the importance of *alliance and utilization,* with the key being to meet the patient in his or her world and to use whatever is available to achieve therapeutic purpose. Blaming "resistance" is like cursing the ball or throwing your clubs.

3. Another basic rule is to take as few shots as necessary, since the winner is the one who plays the stipulated round (or hole) in the fewest strokes. This requires that we keep score to learn what works, lest the game devolve, as Mark Twain (quoted in Feinstein, 1995) rued, into "a good walk spoiled." Fortunately, successful single-session therapy (Hoyt, 1994a; Talmon, 1990) is not as uncommon as a hole in one. *Making the most of each session—efficiency—defines brief therapy.*

4. A related point is to play in a timely manner. Being ready and being decisive are important, since slow play breaks tempo and results in frustrating delays for others who are ready to go forward.[1] Although the old joke has it that players who dawdle and take innumerable strokes are "getting their money's worth," the truth is that courses with long backups

---

[1]This raises the issue of cultural factors, such as the role of authority, the value of emotional expression, various senses of self, time construction, and so on. Yapko (1990) notes three factors that determine whether a patient will benefit from brief therapy interventions: (1) the person's primary temporal orientation (toward past, present, or future); (2) the general value given to "change"—whether he or she is more invested in maintaining tradition or seeking change; and (3) the patient's belief system about what constitutes a complete therapeutic experience. In his fascinating account of Japanese baseball, *You Gotta Have Wa,* Whiting (1990, p. 50) notes: "Perhaps another reason for baseball's attraction for the Japanese is its relatively slow pace. As any Western business-man familiar with Japan will agree, the Japanese are extremely careful. They like to fully discuss and analyze a problem before reaching a decision. On a baseball field the natural break between pitches and innings allows ample time for verbose and dilatory strategy sessions, since the game is never over until the last man is out. Japanese pro games—like Japanese business meetings—can seem interminable. . . . Most games last well over three hours."

and clinics with long waiting lists are not serving their members well.[2] *Don't rush, but don't tarry, either.*

5. The venerable golf instructor Harvey Penick (Penick & Shrake, 1993) suggested that one can build a fair game around two or three clubs; and Lee Trevino once counseled the great woman golfer Nancy Lopez (Lopez with Schwed, 1979, p. 24), "You can't argue with success. If you swing badly but still score well and win, don't change a thing." Bobby Jones (1960, p. 17) advised, "Learn by playing," and said that his favorite swing key was "Whatever worked best, last" (quoted in Snead with Wade, 1989, p. 34). These solution-oriented ideas appreciate existing abilities.[3] One should also study and expand skills, of course, instead of simply relying on early training or natural talent. Passion and discipline are both required (Wallach, 1995). As Ben Hogan (quoted in Davis, 1994, p. 68) said when asked about the role of luck, "The more I practice, the luckier I get." *Brief therapists use strengths and hone skills.*

6. "Play the game one shot at a time" is basic advice. As Nancy Lopez (Lopez with Schwed, 1979, p. 127) says, "If a wasted shot or a poor round keeps gnawing away at your mind and spirit, it's going to affect your next shot or your next round. If you don't let it, it won't." Sam Snead (Snead with Wade, 1989, p. 77) similarly recommends: "The key to concentrating properly is to play in the present tense. Don't spend all your energies on something that just happened—either good or bad—and avoid thinking about what lies ahead. . . . I've always told people, you can't do anything about the past, and you've got to play your way into the

---

[2]The design of certain mental health care delivery systems may include incentives to keep patients in treatment as long as possible. As Haley (1990, pp. 14–15) has noted: "When we look at the history of therapy, the most important decision ever made was to charge for therapy by the hour. Historians will someday reveal who thought of this idea. The ideology and practice of therapy was largely determined when therapists chose to sit with a client and be paid for durations of time rather than by results." Those of us who suffered through the U.S. baseball strike of 1994–1995 know the impact money can have on the game. That economics can have a pernicious influence is not new, of course. As the great Buck O'Neil, whose playing was restricted to the old Negro Leagues because of racial segregation, said about Jackie Robinson's integration of the major leagues: "For Jackie to play in the major leagues, that meant that one white boy wasn't going to play. We had played against these fellas and they knew we could play. And they knew if we were *allowed* to play, a lot of them wouldn't play. See?" (quoted in Ward & Burns, 1994, p. 230). Whom do our policies include and exclude?

[3]The value of focusing on what works instead of what doesn't work was illustrated when the great Henry Aaron went into a rare slump. One day, the story has it, his manager found Aaron reviewing tapes of himself smashing line drives and hitting home runs. "Why aren't you watching tapes of strike-outs and pop-ups, to see what you're doing wrong?" he asked. Aaron replied, "Why would I do that? It wouldn't show me what I need to do!" This also suggests the therapeutic usefulness of *solution-focused body awareness*, having patients recall times when they were in a desired state (e.g., strong and competent) and having them increase verbal/nonverbal congruence by evoking the posture and intonation of these preferred times.

future."[4] It is interesting to note that Bernard Darwin, the famous golf writer and grandson of evolutionist Charles Darwin, wrote an article in 1925 entitled "To Think or Not to Think: Speculation on Just How Much Mental Activity is Good for a Golf Shot" (discussed in Rubenstein, 1991, p. 41). Watching Jack Nicklaus or Ben Hogan set up over a shot is a lesson in single-pointed concentration. There is no time but the present, and recognizing this, *brief therapy usually has a here-and-now(-and-next) orientation.*

7. *Keep it in the fairway and seek progress, not perfection.* As another golf adage has it, "It's not how well you hit it; it's how well you mis-hit it" (see Lardner, 1960).[5] More advanced and strategic players sometimes try to "play the course backward"; that is, they plot backward from where they want to wind up, calculating the best way to get there—sort of like de Shazer's (1988) Miracle Question and its progenitor, Erickson's (1954) Crystal Ball Technique. In *Harvey Penick's Little Red Book* Penick reminds us that "a good follow-through position . . . is important because [it] is a reflection of what has gone on before it" (Penick with Shrake, 1992, p. 156).

8. Tom Watson (Watson with Hannigan, 1984), in *The New Rules of Golf,* reminds us that golf may be the only game in which the playing arena must be maintained, in part, by the players. In *Golf in the Kingdom,* Michael Murphy (1972) tells us that you can tell a lot about people by whether they replace their divots. Mark McCormick (1984), the chief executive officer of a major sports management group, recounts receiving in the mail an unexpected envelope containing some cash from golf pro Doug Sanders (who had made a promise that could easily have been overlooked) to illustrate the importance of honesty and building trusting relationships. Players like Bobby Jones (who once called a penalty on himself that cost him a tournament) and Tom Watson are known for the elegance of their

---

[4] Beware "analysis paralysis." One can prepare, but in the moment the enactment is mostly spontaneous. The story has it that when Yogi Berra was asked what he thought about while batting, he replied, "I'm not thinking. I'm batting!" Everyone has favorite Yogi-isms, including "When you come to a fork in the road, take it!", "It ain't over 'til it's over," "It's *déjà vu* all over again!", and "Ninety percent of the game is half mental!" Once, when asked for the correct time, Yogi replied, "Do you mean now?" It should also be noted that when asked about the veracity of statements attributed to him, he responded, "I really didn't say everything I said" (Pepe, 1988; Ward & Burns, 1994).

[5] The importance of keeping it in the fairway, of avoiding iatrogenesis by not unnecessarily aggravating a bad situation, was nicely underscored by Sam Snead (Snead with Wade, 1989, p. 3): "By now, I expect most people have heard the story about my debate with Ted Williams, the Red Sox Hall of Famer who was the last major leaguer to hit over .400 for a season. . . . One day we got talking about whether it was harder to hit a baseball or a golf ball. Ted said that hitting a baseball was the toughest act in sports because you were trying to hit a round ball with a round bat and the ball was traveling around 90 miles an hour. 'That may be true, Ted,' I told him. 'But in golf we have to play our foul balls.' "

ethics and etiquette as well as for their scores.[6] Among the lessons here are these: *Be respectful, keep your agreements, pass through lightly, and avoid doing harm.*

9. There are these old guys at my home course in Mill Valley, California, who don't hit it very hard but always seem to know which side of the fairway gets more roll and which side of the green will trickle down to the hole. The message I get is *use local knowledge* (a term that refers to the wisdom of exploiting vernacular circumstances).[7] There is the "psychotherapy of everyday life" (Bergin & Strupp, 1970) as well as the "rub of the green" (Hallberg, 1988)—that is, appreciating and taking advantage of fortuitous events—and it is wise to look for natural helpers, ethnic angles, and family resources. It may be helpful for therapists to have a few organizing "swing keys." Collaborative competency-based therapists may like the thought: "I'm the caddy, not the pro—my job is often to hand them one of *their* clubs, offer encouragement, and maybe give some advice about traps and strange winds."

MAKING THE TURN

The Basic Rule of Golf, Number 1:1 (Watson with Hannigan, 1984), states that "The Game of Golf consists in playing a ball from the teeing ground into the hole by a stroke or successive strokes in accordance with

---

[6]Joltin' Joe, the Yankee Clipper—the epitome of talent, grace, and discipline—also had something to say about impeccability. As George Will tells it in *Men at Work* (1990, p. 325), "When DiMaggio was asked why he placed such a high value on excellence he said, 'There is always some kid who may be seeing me for the first or last time. I owe him my best.' "

[7]Golfers used the term *local knowledge* long before Geertz (1983) applied it in anthropology and therapists like Anderson and Goolishian (1992), White and Epston (1990), and others (see Hoyt, 1994b; O'Hanlon, 1994) took it to mean respecting clients' own expertise. Geertz (1983, p. 69) uses a baseball analogy to illustrate the contextual importance of prior knowledge: "In order to follow a baseball game one must understand what a bat, a hit, an inning, a left fielder, a squeeze play, a hanging curve, and a tightening infield are, and what the game in which these 'things' are elements is all about." de Shazer (1993, pp. 114–115) extends the baseball analogy to practice as a psychotherapist: "As we watch a performer, whether it is a sax player or a center fielder, we are watching the culmination of a long practice. That is, in order for a performer to perform, she must master the basic techniques and have absolute control over her horn. This is true in the classical music world and, perhaps more so, in the jazz world and it is certainly true in center field. Without a mastery of the basic skills, the 'how' of performance is a mystery. To some extent, the doing of therapy, and the doing of jazz and baseball are very similar. At each point along the way, the performer (therapist and/or the musician and/or center fielder) 'spontaneously' decides which of his skills are germane within the context of the endeavor." Perhaps some of Milton Erickson's long and legendary success was based on the complexity and power of his knowledge; like an old baseball player who has lost a step or two, Erickson knew where to "stand" and used more subtle language to achieve his results.

the Rules." Or, as John Weakland (quoted in Hoyt, 1994c, p. 25) was wont to say, "It's one damn thing after another."

THE BACK NINE

10. In his humorous collection of golf stories, *Fore!*, P. G. Wode-house (Bensen, 1983) tells of a fellow who, before he knew otherwise, always shot par because he thought that was all the strokes one was allowed![8] An article in *Sports Illustrated* (Horn, 1994) reports that a 430-year-old Zen temple in Annaka, Japan, now has a special shrine replete with a statue of the Buddhist goddess of mercy, Kannon, holding a putter and surrounded by 13 drivers displayed in the traditional lotus fan shape. (Fourteen is the maximum number of clubs the rules allow.) Above these, in Japanese, are the words "Hole in One." Given the power of self-fulfilling prophecies,[9] brief therapists know that they should *foster hope and expect change*.

11. Although I am normally a "bogey" golfer (i.e., one who typically shoots around 90), I have had a few (alas, brief) visits to what is sometimes called "The Zone," that space/place where everything "clicks" and one can do no wrong: a few 5-woods here and there, a several-hour taste of Nirvana early one morning on a course near Lake Tahoe. Remarkably, shortly after studying *The Inner Game of Golf* (Gallway, 1981), I scattered balls on a green at the little course in San Francisco's Golden Gate Park and, barely hesitating to line up the putts, made eight of nine varying from 10 to 30 feet! (Since then I have missed many long and short ones on the same hole.) Another time (at the Banff Springs course in Alberta, Canada), I just knew I was going to make a monster 60-footer . . . and did! Another time, having to get down in two, on the 18th at Dartmouth

---

[8]We sometimes have to stretch our thinking or break out of our "frame" or expectation, as I did when I was listening a few years ago to an interview with the great Mickey Mantle. He was asked, "How much do you think you'd make playing nowadays?" and answered "Oh, maybe $700,000 a year." The interviewer was incredulous: "How could that be, with your stats?" Mickey replied: "Well, you've got to remember, I'm 61 years old!" Milton Erickson (as told to me by Jeffrey Zeig, personal communication) used to provide students with a learning experience in the form of a quiz, asking how many ways could they get into the rooms of a house that he would describe. After the students would exhaust the conventional, pedestrian ways, he would point out options such as driving to the airport, taking a plane to another city, returning via a different route, and then entering through various windows. Baseball fans may enjoy answering the following: What are five ways to get to first base without hitting the ball?

[9]A number of wonderful baseball movies illustrate, in different ways, the power of faith: *Damn Yankees, Field of Dreams, Angels in the Outfield.* In *Bull Durham,* Susan Sarandon's character, Annie Savoy, decides to give baseball a chance after discovering that there are 108 beads in a rosary and 108 stitches on a baseball (Ward & Burns, 1994, p. 101). My favorite remains the elegiac *Bang the Drum Slowly* (with Robert DeNiro in his first major screen role), in which lessons in T.E.G.W.A.R. (The Exciting Game Without Any Rules) teach friendship and creative living.

I somehow "zoned in" on a 50- or 60-footer with multiple breaks; the ball miraculously followed the exact line I had envisioned, stopping one-half turn from falling into the cup—a putt that allowed me to halve the round and thus avoid being the sole purchaser of the beverages our group was soon to enjoy.

How does one find "The Zone"? We all have been there—that sense of being especially "on," seemingly able to do magic and make anything happen. (Sometimes the opposite is true, too, and we're "off" and nothing seems to work.) Golf writer Lorne Rubenstein (1991, p. 59) quotes philosopher/psychologist William James: "An athlete sometimes wakens suddenly to an understanding of the fine points of the game and to a real enjoyment of it. . . . If he keeps on engaging in the sport, there may come a day when all at once the game plays itself through him—when he loses himself in some great contest." In the wonderful tale *Golf in the Kingdom* (Murphy, 1972, p. 64; see also Murphy & White, 1978), Scottish golf pro Shivas Irons (a kindred spirit of Castaneda's Don Juan) advises, "Ye'll come away from the links with a new hold on life, that is certain if ye play the game with all your heart." He then takes author Michael Murphy out for a midnight round (employing whiskey and wielding an old shillelagh as culturally appropriate teaching tools) and instructs him in such vital esoteric mysteries as "True Gravity."[10] Brief therapists may find that *staying loose, tuning in, trusting the unconscious* ("no mind"), and *recalling and modeling earlier successes*—the concepts underlying solution-focused (de Shazer, 1985) and solution-oriented (O'Hanlon & Weiner-Davis, 1989) therapy and neurolinguistic programming (Mackenzie with Denlinger, 1990)—may help jiggle the keys to the kingdom within. How much sweeter could it be than the story about Ben Crenshaw winning the 1995 Masters golf tournament? Only a few days earlier, Crenshaw had been a pallbearer at the funeral of his long-time teacher, Harvey Penick. As a last lesson, on his deathbed Penick "checked Crenshaw's grip the same way he had been checking it since Ben was a child. Then he said, 'Just trust yourself' " (Reilly, 1995, p. 18).

12. *Individualize treatment to suit the particular person.* As golfer and clinical psychologist Harry (Bud) Gunn says in his multileveled book, *How to Play Golf with Your Wife—and Survive* (1976, p. 32), "It is also an axiom that what works for Jack Nicklaus or Arnold Palmer may not work for you or your wife. I don't know about your wife, but mine is not built anything like either of these two gentlemen." This is what Milton Erickson also seemed to be saying in his oft-quoted statement: "Each person is a unique individual. Hence, psychotherapy should be formu-

---

[10]Perhaps this is part of the magic behind Satchel Paige's (1962) sage and natural "Stay loose," as well as Malamud's (1952/1993) *The Natural.* Similarly, the Japanese slugger Sadaharu Oh (1985, p. 108), who intensely studied aikido to improve his hitting, advises: "If your body is not at one with your mind, you are lost."

lated to meet the uniqueness of the individual's needs, rather than tailoring the person to fit the Procrustean bed of a hypothetical theory of human behavior" (quoted in Zeig & Gilligan, 1990, frontispiece).[11] Gunn also displays a systemic/strategic therapist's eye when he reports the case of a couple who

> had complaints about their love life, which the wife said was too frequent and the husband said was too sparse. Seeing the enjoyment that I derived from golf, they decided to try it themselves. I cautioned them repeatedly about the dangers, but they went right ahead. To my surprise, they claimed a few months later that golf and not my counseling had provided the answer. It was not so much that my wallet hurt when they informed me they were discontinuing marital counseling, but my curiosity was aroused. With a certain tone of doubt I asked, "You mean that golf has improved your love life?" "Oh, yes," the husband replied, "now I find that while the frequency of love making has dropped I don't complain because I am too tired to care. I get angry just as often, but it's at my golf game and not my wife." (1976, pp. 16–17).

13. Sounding like a narrative constructivist, Rubenstein (1991, p. xiv) has said: "To be part of golf is to come upon stories, to become a story, to tell stories." As effective therapists know, *it is important to speak the client's language.* For many people, golf and baseball evoke rich memories, oftentimes rooted in childhood experiences.[12] Sports lan-

---

[11]Generalities have their limits; the "action" is in the details. As Keith Hernandez (1994, p. viii) comments in *Pure Baseball: Pitch by Pitch for the Advanced Fan,* "When we go to the park or turn on the local television or radio broadcast, we don't watch generic 'pitching,' 'hitting,' and 'fielding.' We watch this pitcher throw to this batter with this glove work and this base running as a result. I can't think about baseball other than in such specifics." He also goes on to say: "My motto: Pay attention." (For ways to sharpen attention, see Dorfman & Kuehl, 1989.) The importance of case study is also emphasized by Gustafson (1992, p. viii): "What is very distressing to me is the disappearance of individual patients. Presenters tag one big noun to another like 'resistance' and 'therapeutic alliance' and never tell you about the actual work with a person, or they tell you a success in which the person is a typical case of 'passivity' or whatever. No individual beings loom before us at all."

[12]Childhood sports heroes may model "exceptions" and "sparkling moments" with far-reaching consequences. Consider Archbishop Desmond Tutu's report: "I must have been nine years of age, and I was in one of our ghetto townships . . . in South Africa. It must have been in winter but I still don't know who bought the tattered copy of *Ebony* magazine that I was paging through. It was the issue describing how Jackie Robinson broke into Major League Baseball. He was going to play for a team called the Brooklyn Dodgers, and what was important to me, I still recall, is how I shot up in stature because although I didn't know what baseball was, what was significant for me was that here was a Black guy, admittedly several thousand miles away, but he was Black and even in that stage of my life I knew that we had a commonality and solidarity in our Blackness and that his achievement was somehow my achievement. These guys had been telling us there was a ceiling beyond which we couldn't go, and here was a guy who had broken through that ceiling, overcome obstacles, and therefore, he did something for me—and I think it must have been the case that it would have affected other people—but for me *(continued)*

guage has come into common parlance, as we hear someone say about a success that they "hit a home run" or "got a hole in one" and describe something untoward as "striking out" or being "subpar." (This use of "below par" to signify something bad is actually a reversal of the golf meaning, where a low score is good; this appropriation is an example of languages crossing groups and distinguishing different communities. See Rubenstein, 1991, pp. 152–153.) A husband I knew was spending a great deal of time playing golf. He complained of his wife's social and emotional distance but made only weak efforts to engage her more until, after a particularly feeble overture during a counseling session, I dryly commented, "You're still away." (The uninitiated may not have heard the golfer's postflub refrain: "The saddest words they'll ever say, hit again, you're still away.") A colleague (Jeff Goldman, personal communication) told me about a brief therapy success with an avid golfer who sought treatment because of erectile dysfunction. The client may have been learning something he already knew as he described the details of successful putting: the importance of being simultaneously keenly alert and totally relaxed, "visualizing the ball rolling toward the hole." At the third session he reported that he was back to "enjoying the game, the walk in the early morning," and "letting the score take care of itself."

14. In *Mind over Golf,* R. H. Coop (Coop with Fields, 1993) discusses the importance of timing in teaching golf to youngsters—matters that could also be applied by therapists who want to work briefly and avoid unnecessary "resistance." He says (on p. 150): "The concept of readiness to learn must be understood. One time I asked Jack Nicklaus, the father of five children, how soon kids should be encouraged to play golf. His answer: 'You should start them as soon as they are as interested in golf as they are in chasing bullfrogs.' " (At the time, Nicklaus's youngest son would join the family for a round of golf, hit a few shots, then turn his attention to a pond where a number of frogs made their home.) In addition to *the importance of knowing when,* Coop goes on to suggest a number of useful teaching and therapy pointers: creating positive experiences and associations, stopping a practice session at a good point that will leave the learner wanting more, and starting with high-success experiences.

15. Recently I joined some fellows and was hacking my way around the Prince Course on Kauai, Hawaii. On one hole on the back nine, Robert Trent Jones, Jr., has laid out a particularly formidable arrangement: A large tree guards the right side and awaited our drives. One of my foursome looked at the tree and laughed with a tickle. "My wife hit six shots into that tree. Damn, that woman could swear!" He looked down

---

(*continued from p. 313*) it was an incredible sort of fresh air, a breaking of at least one of the shackles that racism had bound us with" (1995, p. 35).

the fairway and laughed again. "Are you still married to her?" I asked, noticing something about the "could" in his sentence. "No, she's passed away," he said, pausing—and then looked at the tree and the spot before it and laughed joyously again. Brief therapy involves choosing a "viewing and doing" (O'Hanlon & Weiner-Davis, 1989), *constructing a story that provides a useful meaning.*[13]

16. When I'm feeling frazzled or overwhelmed, and ready to start calling the patient names like "borderline" or "resistant" (see Vaillant, 1992), I try not to lose my grip or throw my clubs. In what some people call the greatest golf match in history, the 1977 British Open at Turnberry, Tom Watson and Jack Nicklaus played the last two rounds in 65–65 and 65–66, respectively. Their shots were extraordinary and repeatedly and reciprocatedly heroic. Even when Watson had all but cinched the match with a great shot dead to the pin on the 18th hole—after making a 60-foot putt a couple of holes earlier to pull even—Nicklaus answered by draining a 40-footer on the 18th green. As Nicklaus (1994, p. 62; see also Wind, 1985) tells it: "On the 14th tee that last day, Tom's eye caught mine and he said, 'This is what it's all about, isn't it, Jack?' I agreed with him then, and still do even though I lost." It sometimes helps to remember that *the challenge of tough cases can make us reach in for something extra.*

17. In 1895, Lord Wellwood (quoted in Morrison, 1994, p. 39) noted: "The game is not as easy as it seems. In the first place, the terrible inertia of the ball must be overcome." The seeming paradox is that the strategic therapist (Haley, 1977) *assumes responsibility for making something happen.* We cannot *not* influence, of course, although it requires art and craft, great power and a deft touch, to achieve good results consistently.

18. Getting the job done, finishing successfully, is what counts. In golf, they say, "You drive for show, but you putt for dough" (see Palmer & Dobereiner, 1986). In therapy, we call it "termination": knowing how and why to say when. To make treatment no longer than necessary, we have to *pay attention to ending.*

BACK AT THE CLUBHOUSE

After a round, golfers may repair to the lounge, often called "The 19th Hole," to seek refreshments, improve their lies, and enjoy fellowship and

[13]Many therapists are now situating their practice under the theoretical rubric of narrative constructivism, the essence of which may be captured in the story about the three baseball umpires disputing their acumen. The first one, who prides himself on ethicality, says, "I call 'em as I see 'em." The second ump, who believes in objective accuracy, says, "Not bad, but I call 'em the way they are." Finally, the third ump speaks: "They ain't nothing until I call 'em!" He's the narrative constructivist. (Lincoln & Guba, 1985, p. 70, attribute this statement to the National League umpire Jocko Conlan.)

support. As the famous sportswriter Grantland Rice (quoted in Nelson, 1992, p. 27) observed, "Golf is 20% mechanics and technique. The other 80% is philosophy, humor, tragedy, romance, melodrama, companionship, camaraderie, cussedness, and conversation." We therapists are in the strange but wonderful business of going into small rooms with unhappy people and trying to talk them out of it.[14] *To prevent isolation and burnout, enjoy the 19th hole!*

ACKNOWLEDGMENTS

Portions of this chapter were presented at the Sixth International Congress on Ericksonian Approaches to Psychotherapy and Hypnosis, held in Los Angeles in December 1994, and at the First Pan-Pacific Brief Therapy Conference, held in Fukuoka, Japan, in July 1995. I am grateful to many friends and colleagues for helpful suggestions.

REFERENCES

Anderson, H., & Goolishian, H. (1992). The client is the expert: A not-knowing approach to therapy. In S. McNamee & K. J. Gergen (Eds.), *Therapy as Social Construction* (pp. 25–39). Newbury Park, CA: Sage.

Bensen, D. R. (Ed.). (1983). *Fore! The Best of Wodehouse on Golf.* New York: Ticknor & Fields.

Bergin, A. E., & Strupp, H. H. (1970). New directions in psychotherapy research. *Journal of Abnormal Psychology, 76,* 13–26.

Coop, R. H., with Fields, B. (1993). *Mind over Golf.* New York: Macmillan.

Davis, M. (Ed.). (1994). *The Hogan Mystique.* Greenwich, CT: American Golfer.

de Shazer, S. (1985). *Keys to Solution in Brief Therapy.* New York: Norton.

de Shazer, S. (1988). *Clues: Investigating Solutions in Brief Therapy.* New York: Norton.

de Shazer, S. (1993). Commentary: de Shazer and White: Vive la difference. In S. G. Gilligan & R. Price (Eds.), *Therapeutic Conversations* (pp. 112–120). New York: Norton.

Dorfman, H. A., & Kuehl, K. (1989). *The Mental Game of Baseball: A Guide to Peak Performance.* South Bend, IN: Diamond Communications.

[14]I love the story my father told me (recounted in Hoyt, 1995, pp. 331–332) about the time he was at a baseball game at Wrigley Field in Chicago, and a drunken and belligerent fan in the bleachers was verbally abusing one of the ballplayers. The man let it be known that he was packing a gun, and it became alarmingly possible that he might use it. My father—who was a salesman by trade and something of a strategic therapist by nature—got involved. Dad was also a gun fancier; and he got the irate fan engaged in a discussion about the type of gun, showed some interest, and wound up bargaining for and buying the gun on the spot. (The police never came.) When I asked my father what he had done with the weapon, he said he had taken it the next day to a shop and sold it, for a profit. When I asked why he had done that, he replied, "Hey, you've got to get paid for this kind of work!"

Erickson, M. H. (1954). Pseudo-orientation in time as a hypnotic procedure. *Journal of Clinical and Experimental Hypnosis, 6,* 183–207.

Feinstein, J. (1995). *A Good Walk Spoiled: Days and Nights on the PGA Tour.* Boston: Little, Brown.

Gallway, W. T. (1981). *The Inner Game of Golf.* New York: Random House.

Geertz, C. (1983). *Local Knowledge.* New York: Basic Books.

Gunn, H. E. (1976). *How to Play Golf with Your Wife–and Survive.* Matteson, IL: Greatlakes Living Press.

Gustafson, J. P. (1992). *Self-Delight in a Harsh World: The Main Stories of Individual, Marital and Family Psychotherapy.* New York: Norton.

Haley, J. (1977). *Problem-Solving Therapy.* San Francisco: Jossey-Bass.

Haley, J. (1990). Why not long-term therapy? In J. K. Zeig & S. G. Gilligan (Eds.), *Brief Therapy: Myths, Methods, and Metaphors* (pp. 3–17). New York: Brunner/Mazel.

Hernandez, K. (1994). *Pure Baseball: Pitch by Pitch for the Advanced Fan.* New York: HarperCollins.

Hallberg, W. (1988). *The Rub of the Green.* New York: Bantam.

Horn, R. (1994, August 8). Tee ceremony. *Sports Illustrated,* no pagination.

Hoyt, M. F. (1994a). Single-session solutions. In M. F. Hoyt (Ed.), *Constructive Therapies* (pp. 140–159). New York: Guilford Press. (Reprinted in M. F. Hoyt, *Brief Therapy and Managed Care: Readings for Contemporary Practice* [pp. 141–162]. San Francisco: Jossey-Bass, 1995.)

Hoyt, M. F. (Ed.). (1994b). *Constructive Therapies.* New York: Guilford Press.

Hoyt, M. F. (1994c). On the importance of keeping it simple and taking the patient seriously: A conversation with Steve de Shazer and John Weakland. In M. F. Hoyt (Ed.), *Constructive Therapies* (pp. 11–40). New York: Guilford Press.

Hoyt, M. F. (1995). *Brief Therapy and Managed Care: Readings for Contemporary Practice.* San Francisco: Jossey-Bass.

Jones, R. T. (1960). *Golf Is My Game.* Garden City, NY: Doubleday.

Korzybski, A. (1933). *Science and Sanity.* New York: International Non-Aristotelian Library.

Lardner, R. (1960). *Out of the Bunker and into the Tress: Or, the Secret of High-Tension Golf.* Indianapolis: Bobbs-Merrill.

Lincoln, Y. S., & Guba, E. G. (1985). *Naturalistic Inquiry.* Newbury Park, CA: Sage.

Lopez, N., with Schwed, P. (1979). *The Education of a Woman Golfer.* New York: Simon & Schuster.

Mackenzie, M. M., with Denlinger, K. (1990). *Golf: The Mind Game.* New York: Dell.

Malamud, B. (1993). *The Natural.* New York: Avon. (Original work published 1952)

McCormick, M. H. (1984). *What They Don't Teach You at Harvard Business School.* New York: Bantam Books.

Morrison, A. (Ed.). (1994). *The Impossible Art of Golf.* New York: Oxford University Press.

Murphy, M. (1972). *Golf in the Kingdom.* New York: Delta/Viking.

Murphy, M., & White, P. A. (1978). *The Psychic Side of Sports.* Reading, MA: Addison-Wesley.

Nelson, K. (1992). *The Greatest Golf Shot Ever: And Other Lively and Entertaining Tales from the Lore and History of Golf.* New York: Fireside/Simon & Schuster.

Nicklaus, J. (1994, May). *Golf Magazine.*

Nicklaus, J., with Bowden, K. (1974). *Golf My Way*. New York: Fireside/Simon & Schuster.

O'Hanlon, W. H. (1994). The third wave. *Family Therapy Networker, 18*(6), 18–26, 28–29.

O'Hanlon, W. H., & Weiner-Davis, M. (1989). *In Search of Solutions: A New Direction in Psychotherapy*. New York: Norton.

Oh, S. (1985). A Zen way of baseball. In R. S. Heckler (Ed.), *Aikido and the New Warrior* (pp. 99–113). Berkeley, CA: North Atlantic Books. (Excerpted from S. Oh with D. Falkner, *Sadaharu Oh*. New York: Random House, 1984.)

Paige, L. S. (1962). *Maybe I'll Pitch Forever*. Garden City: Doubleday.

Palmer, A., & Dobereiner, P. (1986). *Arnold Palmer's Complete Book of Putting*. New York: Atheneum.

Penick, H., with Shrake, B. (1992). *Harvey Penick's Little Red Book: Lessons and Teachings from a Lifetime in Golf*. New York: Simon & Schuster.

Penick, H., with Shrake, B. (1993). *And If You Play Golf, You're My Friend: Further Reflections of a Grown Caddie*. New York: Simon & Schuster.

Pepe, P. (1988). *The Wit and Wisdom of Yogi Berra*. Westport, CT: Meekler Books.

Pressfield, S. (1995). *The Legend of Bagger Vance: Golf and the Game of Life*. New York: William Morrow.

Reilly, R. (1995, April 17). For you, Harvey. *Sports Illustrated*, pp. 16–23.

Rubenstein, L. (1991). *Links: An Exploration into the Mind, Heart, and Soul of Golf*. Rocklin, CA: Prima.

Snead, S., with Wade, D. (1989). *The Lessons I've Learned: Better Golf the Sam Snead Way*. New York: Macmillan.

Talmon, M. (1990). *Single Session Therapy*. San Francisco: Jossey-Bass.

Vaillant, G. E. (1992). The beginning of wisdom is never calling a patient a borderline: Or, the clinical management of immature defenses in the treatment of individuals with personality disorders. *Journal of Psychotherapy Practice and Research, 1*, 117–134.

Wallach, J. (1995). *Beyond the Fairway: Zen Lessons, Insights, and Inner Attitudes of Golf*. New York: Bantam.

Ward, G. C., & Burns, K. (1994). *Baseball: An Illustrated History*. New York: Knopf.

Watson, T., with Hannigan, F. (1984). *The New Rules of Golf*. New York: Random House.

White, M., & Epston, D. (1990). *Narrative Means to Therapeutic Ends*. New York: Norton.

Whiting, R. (1990). *You Gotta Have Wa*. New York: Vintage.

Will, G. F. (1990). *Men at Work: The Craft of Baseball*. New York: Macmillan.

Wind, H. W. (1985). Nicklaus and Watson at Turnberry. In *Following Through* (pp. 168–181). New York: Ticknor & Fields.

Yapko, M. D. (1990). Brief therapy tactics in longer-term psychotherapies. In J. K. Zeig & S. G. Gilligan (Eds.), *Brief Therapy: Myths, Methods, and Metaphors* (pp. 185–195). New York: Brunner/Mazel.

Zeig, J. K., & Gilligan, S. G. (Eds.). (1990). *Brief Therapy: Myths, Methods, and Metaphors*. New York: Brunner/Mazel.

CHAPTER 14

Three Styles
of Constructive Therapy

HAIM OMER

Constructive styles of therapy are based on the assumption that "language games" are central to the formation and resolution of problems. Summarily put, their unifying idea is that language not only describes events but constitutes them. This process operates mainly interpersonally: It is in the act of conversing about the world that a reality is defined that becomes true to the participants.

A strictly scientific psychotherapy should be uniform in its practices and devoid of peculiarities. Under the positivist aegis, if any stylistic variety came to exist within a single theoretical viewpoint, research—it was piously hoped—would bring everything back to homogeneity. From a constructive perspective, however, psychotherapy loses some of its affinity to science, coming closer to the lettered disciplines (Frank, 1987; Omer, 1993). In this new professional neighborhood, style becomes highly pertinent and worthy of study. Let us begin by illustrating how stylistic differences may become manifest under what is "officially" the same therapeutic approach.

Two therapists decide to treat a case of fear of heights by imaginal flooding. They accept the theoretical hypotheses underlying extinction of fear and learn the basics of the technique. The first therapist tells the patient, Mr. B., to visualize himself at the edge of a cliff, to pay attention to the sensations in his body, to look downward and steady his gaze, to experience the tension and the fear, to imagine the length of the fall, to imagine himself slipping, to imagine himself falling, and so on for about half an hour. The second therapist tells Mr. B. to visualize himself at the brink of the Grand Canyon looking downward and then slipping, slipping, slipping, hanging with his hands onto the rocks, slowly losing his grip, hanging by his fingers, fingernails, little finger, little fingernail, and then falling, falling, falling, people on the trails stunned by his flying figure swishing past the bored mules, head downward, legs upward, tie leftward, shirt ballooning, one of the trackers letting fall a cup of coffee, cup and coffee, then coffee and cup following him, but he is faster than cup, much faster than coffee, now he is approaching the bottom, closer, closer, his head enters his shoulders, his shoulders his belly, his belly his thighs, his everything his heels, he becomes a flat mush of pressed flesh except for his left eye, which rolls into the Colorado River and is eaten by a perch. The approach followed by these two therapists may go by the same name and follow the same theoretical rationale, but there the similarity ends.

Style is not only a matter of individual differences, but characterizes whole trends and schools. It is transmitted from master to pupil as the living bond of a creative community. In what follows, I describe three constructive stylistic trends: the *conversational*, the *narrative*, and the *strategic*. Although conceptually separable, these trends overlap in practice; some therapists may be pure representatives of a trend, but most show a blend of more than one.

CONVERSATIONS

The concept of "therapeutic conversation" was coined as an alternative to a view of psychotherapy as a process of unimpeded informational exchange. From a traditional perspective, patient and therapist were believed to be able to relay meanings in a dependable manner (at least when therapy was going well). This view of human communication was criticized by constructivist thinkers as "the myth of instructive interaction" (Efran, Lukens, & Lukens, 1990; Maturana & Varela, 1980): Packages of information cannot be transferred from one mind to another. In all probability, what is received is usually a highly distorted version of what the sender thought he or she was transmitting. This news, however, may not be as bad as it seems. In every dialogue there are two views of reality (at least), but there is also some common ground between the two, or there would be no dialogue. This difference *cum* congruence is precisely what makes for an enrichment of interpersonal reality. People are moved along by the differences, and their views are expanded by the attempt to go on talking. As in binocular vision, a depth bonus accrues (de Shazer, 1991). This view has inspired a therapeutic style that stresses multiperspectival conversations, absence of privileged knowing (by the therapist), and encouragement of mutual reflexivity. In different combinations, these features characterize the work of such practitioners as Luigi Boscolo, Harold Goolishian, Tom Andersen, and Lynn Hoffman. I want to argue, however, in favor of a more elusive stylistic commonality among these "conversationalists": They love *ambiguation*.

In the Milan school, for instance, ambiguation is pursued for its power to melt the family's all-too-solid assumptions and interactive patterns. The targets of ambiguation are called "openings" by the Milanese (Boscolo, Cecchin, Hoffman, & Penn, 1987). Although the term is never explicitly defined, it is lavishly illustrated, showing that openings are situations indicative of the family's sacred beliefs, obdurate rules, black-and-white distinctions, inflexible roles, and changeless interactions. The Milanese openings actually designate closedness. Ambiguation is thus directed at the rigid patterns that stabilize the family's present function. Like the later Romantic musicians who created harmonic instability by modulating farther and farther from the home key, the Milanese excel in setting the family's world view adrift through ambiguation.

The first and probably most famous type of ambiguation developed by the Milan school is embodied in the procedure of circular interviewing (Selvini Palazzoli, Boscolo, Cecchin, & Prata, 1980), in which the therapist elicits different points of view from family members on how the other family members are engaged on a given issue. Circular interviewing was first developed as a way for amassing information toward systemic hypotheses. Whereas straightforward questioning (in which each person answers only for himself or herself) usually leads to linear hypotheses, circular questioning should lead to circular ones. Soon, however, the Milanese shifted their emphasis from the informational to the deliberately interventional function of circular questions. The procedure sent ripples all over the family system—a condition the Milanese learned to value for itself.

Say, for instance, that the mother defines the problem as the father's depression. Milanese-style therapists might choose this stabilizing label as an opening and submit it to the process of circular ambiguation: Who noticed the problem first? For whom is it less of a problem? For whom is it not a problem at all? What happens to the mother and the eldest daughter when the father stays in bed? What happens to them when the father goes back to work? How do the other children react to the changes in the mother? By the end of the session, the once stable "father's depression" has been transmuted into a shifting reality that shimmered in a multiplicity of facets.

This interview style had a powerful influence in the systemic literature, issuing in a veritable avalanche of new kinds of multiperspectival conversations (e.g., Andersen, 1987; Tomm, 1987). The unsettling vision that was furthered by a doubling, trebling, and multiplying of superimposed perspectives became almost an end in itself.[1]

---

[1]"Methinks I see these things with parted eye, When every thing seems double" (Shakespeare, 1600/1974, *A Midsummer Night's Dream*, IV. i. 189–190).

A second type of ambiguation is embodied in the Milan school's concept of neutrality (Selvini Palazzoli et al., 1980). This is not merely a passive withholding of judgment, but an active process whereby the therapeutic team assiduously ambiguates its own values, attitudes, and interests. Neutrality is achieved if the family is thoroughly mixed up about what the therapists' goals, focuses, and sympathies are.

In their pursuit of neutrality, the Milanese have developed some peculiar guidelines for team discussion (Boscolo et al., 1987). For instance, they forbid expressions of agreement between team members, for such expressions would tend to crystallize the team in one direction, which would then be transmitted to the family. They also proscribe solutions, at least in the early stages of discussion. At times they assign each team member a different causal perspective on the family—for instance, by deciding that one member will blame it all on the mother, one on the father, and one on the daughter. If even then the threat of agreement persists, team members are required to respond to each other in nonsequiturs. For example:

A: "I feel the mother cannot bear the idea of separation."
B: "I think the father controls by the pocket."
C: "I think the daughters say a lot by silence."

A team striving for neutrality may thus sound not unlike a Samuel Beckett play.

The Milanese version of neutrality is in many respects similar to the Galveston group's cultivation of the attitude of "not knowing" (Anderson & Goolishian, 1988). This therapeutic stance consists of approaching the client the way an ethnographer encounters a new culture: with total openness and a sense of absolute ignorance. If the client talks about demons, the therapist should want to learn about the demons. If the client complains of having a sexual disease that is transmitted by phone, the therapist should wipe out all previous ideas about sexual diseases and their ways of transmission. This is no mere strategic ploy for humoring the client. The therapist's activity is actually more inner- than outer-directed. It is an attempt to develop an empty mind so as to open up dialogic space for the unfolding of the client's narrative. Untrammeled by the therapist's "knowing" or "expert" stance, the client's story will grow and change. Problems loosen up when steeped in this totally elastic conversational medium. They can thus be said not to be solved, but dis-solved. The solvent of ambiguity and of not knowing blurs their contours and melts their solid core.

A third kind of ambiguation is produced by role equivocation: The therapists refuse to act as bona fide therapists. Their behavior is intentionally puzzling. They not only won't supply information and guidance;

they may even change their minds from session to session, within the same session, or even the selfsame utterance. At times they deliberately declare themselves not to be therapists. On one occasion, Boscolo and Cecchin (Boscolo et al., 1987) told the members of a family that they had many things to tell them. They could not do so, however, for doing so would be doing therapy, which they could not do, for they were not the family's therapists. To their readers, they added that the family reacted excellently to the message. I wonder whether the family members were as dumbfounded as I was.

A family's assumptions concerning appropriate role behaviors are treated with no more reverence: The youngest child is to comment on the parents' sex life; the daughter is to pronounce judgment on the mother; the identified patient is proclaimed family prophet. Invariably the "wrong" person is asked the "right" questions. Therapy becomes a carnival of roles.

Other procedures for achieving role diffusion have been developed by other conversationalists, focusing mainly on the traditional therapeutic roles of observer and commentator. In this respect, Andersen's (1987) reversal of the one-way screen signaled the rise of a brave new world of reflecting games. In one dazzling variation (Madigan, 1993), the family is interviewed by a therapist, watched by another observing therapist, watched in turn by a team. After the interview has proceeded in this fashion for awhile, the observing therapist interviews the interviewer in front of the family. Some of the questions are quite personal and are designated to further erode the boundary between professional and client. Still later in the session, the team behind the screen takes the forefront and the family members, together with the interviewer and the observer, listen to the team's discussion of the whole session. Everyone is then invited together to comment on the team's commentaries. And we thought Lewis Carroll's Wonderland peculiar!

The process of role diffusion is abetted by a further type of ambiguation, which focuses upon the implicit rules that underlie interactional stability. Usually, personal utterances not only express content but also limit the viable responses of others. Thus, if a family member starts to cry, a therapist might express sympathy, ask the person why he or she is crying/ or at times keep silent. Similarly, if two siblings are having a laugh, the therapist might ask them what they are laughing about, laugh together with them ("join the tea party," in Boscolo and Cecchin's felicitous expression), or ask the parents whether they are willing to take charge. If two members of the family indicate that they share a secret, the therapist might try to crack the secret or decide to respect it and pass it by. All of these responses show an expected fit to the clients' acts. They confirm the implicit rules of the interaction. Crying elicits sympathy or silent deference; laughter induces mirth or irritation; secrets arouse curiosity or respect. The contours of the original acts are steadied by the expected responses.

A blurring ensues, however, if the response is unfitting. The Milanese assiduously opt for such an unfitting course. Thus, with crying or laughing clients, the therapists may ask *other* members why they think these people are crying or laughing, whether they often do this at home, whether there are other people in the family who cry or laugh in similar circumstances, and so forth. When a secret is indicated, the therapist may tell the family members to keep the secret, but to answer a series of questions concerning the secret without revealing it. The questions are such as to nibble at the secret's boundaries until its interactional function gets quite muddled up. We are back at circular interviewing, but with a difference. In circular questioning, the purpose is to elicit different perspectives; here, it is to undermine interactional rules. The first type of ambiguation is focused on content, the present one on process.

A fifth kind of ambiguation is embodied in the Milanese end-of-session interventions. Originally, the typical intervention would include a systemic rationale followed by the prescription of a paradox or ritual. When the technique of circular interviewing was developed, however, question arose as to whether the end-of-session intervention might not be superfluous or even counterproductive by shortcutting the ambiguity evoked by the interview. I think that an answer could be given in terms of stylistic balance between the interview and the intervention. Let me explain.

The Milan school's prescriptions—and not only the paradoxical ones—are actually concentrated packages of ambiguity. For example, conflicting parents are directed to follow contrary policies on odd and even days of the week, and then to act "spontaneously" on Sundays; family members are praised for their willingness to separate, but are also told that they have gone too far; spouses or partners are enjoined to go out together every other day, but are also told that they may actually spend the time apart. The ambiguity persists in the follow-up session: Whatever the family reports counts as fulfillment of the injunction. The very concept of prescription is thus thoroughly muddled up: Therapists tell clients to do something, the clients do the opposite, and the therapists endorse what they did as the clients' own way of cooperating. Interestingly, this very attitude toward prescriptions has also been adopted by de Shazer (1985), whose style is in other respects quite different from that of the Milanese. de Shazer at times compounds the ambiguity by prescribing two contrary tasks, each ambiguous in its own way, and suggesting that the clients should determine when to perform which by tossing a coin. Needless to say, a double nonperformance is also accepted as a valid response.

With this in mind, we can understand the relationship between the interview and the prescription as dialectical: The prescription synthesizes, without resolving, the many strands that the interview has left hanging. All communicational interchanges oscillate between a centrifugal tendency toward multiplicity and a centripetal one toward unity. This interplay creates a balance between discordance and consensus, movement and repose. The Russian philosopher and literary critic Mikhail Bakhtin (1981) has given a cogent description of this tension as the chief constituent of the novel. His term for the chorus of multiply interacting voices is *heteroglossia*. The novel's achievement is precisely that of manifesting heteroglossia within a unifying artistic context. Bakhtin's analysis, however, reaches beyond the confines of the novel to the vital tension inherent in all discourse. The combination of intervention and interview by the Milanese might be understood in terms of this tension. The two limit and complement each other: What the interview fragments, the intervention brings together. Heterogeneity, however, is not eliminated; on the contrary, the multiple voices of the interview are preserved in the intervention. As in a Hegelian synthesis, the opposing elements are raised onto a new integrative plane without losing their difference. Multiplicity and unity, separateness and togetherness, are thus harmonized.

NARRATIVES

Narrative concepts have had a stupendous career in psychotherapy. Since they rose to the forefront of the field with Spence's (1982) epoch-making book *Narrative Truth and Historical Truth: Meaning and Interpretation in Psychoanalysis*, they have extended their reach not only among psychoanalytically inspired approaches (Strupp & Binder, 1984), but also to systemic (Parry, 1991; Sluzki, 1992; White & Epston, 1990), cognitive (Russell & Van den Broek, 1992), humanistic (Polster, 1987), and integrative ones (Omer & Strenger, 1992).[2] The assumptions of the narrativists are similar to those of the conversationalists; the chief differences are stylistic. Succinctly, narrativists stress thematic unity, conflict, characterization, drama, and plot. They stand for coherence where the conversationalists favor ambiguation.

Take, for instance, the work of Michael White (1989, 1995; White & Epston, 1990). His procedure of narrative reconstruction starts with the villain. Singularly, the villain is not a human being at all, but a personal-

---

[2]See *Critical Interventions in Psychotherapy* (Omer, 1994), and also Omer (1991, 1995), for an extended discussion of some of the ways impasses in the therapeutic narrative, strategy, and alliance can be resolved.

ized version of the client's problem.[3] The naming of the problem is highly pertinent in this respect: Sneaky Poo, Sneaky Wee, The Voices, The Monsters, Misery, and Dependence are some of the denizens in White's bestiary. This portrayal of the problem leads to a new portrayal of the client, for in the world of narrative there is no dragon without a knight. Given such a powerful antagonist, we might ask, who is the protagonist? White trusts the client's narrative propinquities to guarantee that as the villain begins to fill the stage, the hero must be buckling on armor in the wings.

The portrayal of the client/hero is thus the next therapeutic task. Consider the following questions: "How did you ready yourself for this step?" "What preparations led up to it?" "What can you tell me about your history that would help me to understand how you managed to do this?" "What did you do when younger that could provide some clue that this development was on the horizon of your life?" "What does this tell you about yourself as a person?" "How will this new picture of yourself change what you plan to do in the near future?" These questions establish narrative continuity. In heroic tales, past actions foretell future ones. Hercules throttled snakes in his crib, and young King Arthur pulled swords from rocks. Clients, families, and therapists grow in their conviction of the hero's destiny as the heroic plot is spun between past and future.

There are other ways to construct character and create narrative continuity. Hans Strupp and Jeffrey Binder (1984), for instance, portray character by searching for recurrent interpersonal themes. In their narrative scheme, a full-fledged interpersonal episode is built out of four elements: acts of self, expectations of others, acts of others, and internalized acts of self. These elements are woven together in stories that begin with the client's attempt to act in the world, continue with others' response to this attempt, and end with the client's taking stock of the whole episode. Therapy is the process of unfolding, filling in, and piecing together these interpersonal accounts.

Of particular interest is the way Strupp and Binder explain what, in this process, is therapeutic. The narratives of patients, they argue, are punctured throughout by lacks and leaps. The story may proceed from acts of self to acts of others, overlooking the expectations of others; or it may jump from acts of self directly to internalized acts of self, missing altogether the contribution of others; or it may broadly elaborate on the acts of others, while barely sketching those of the self. Such persons experience life as chaotic and as refractory to prediction and control.

---

[3]As O'Hanlon (1994) says, "Externalization basically entails a linguistic separation of the problem from the personal identity of the patient. . . . The hallmark of the narrative approach is the credo, 'The person is never the problem; the problem is the problem' " (pp. 21–23).

The therapeutic process may then be viewed as a cooperative editorial enterprise by means of which the gaps are gradually filled in, making the narrative continuous and coherent.

In James Mann's (1973) style of characterization, the smoothness and continuity stressed by Strupp and Binder give way to dramatic polarity: The central issue that summarizes the client's stance in life is framed as a clash between a boundless dominant striving and a limiting and frustrating reality. Take the following life sketches, for instance: "You have always wanted to be special and authentic, but you feel inadequate and phony instead." "Your major goal in life was to feel personal closeness; more than ever, however, you now feel a deep sense of alienation and loneliness." Or "You have always striven for a sense of security, but the more you tried the farther away it seemed to lie." Such a description is offered to the client as the central issue for a therapy that is to last for exactly 12 sessions. Clients and clinicians alike are often deeply impressed by these blitz characterizations. It seems unbelievable that by the end of one session a therapist may succeed in expressing so succinctly the central drama of a client's life. Mann has assured the would-be skeptics that the task is easier than it seems, for people's major strivings are not so diverse, after all: One person puts love first, another work, and a third security. This candid reply shows how far Mann's life sketch stands from the positivist ideal of perfect correspondence between description and reality. We are clearly within the realm of sympathetic narrative caricature. In my view (see Omer, 1993b), this places Mann very close to the narrative tradition.

Mann has argued that the fixed number of sessions in the therapy intensifies the client's inordinate longings and adds urgency to the encounters. There is nothing like an approaching end to make a person wish for more. In this manner, the 12-session format reinforces the polarity of the central issue: Therapy, personhood, and life are all about the tragedy and the pity of boundless striving in a world that is ruled by time, separation, and death.

Mann's dramatic polarity brings us back to White. Both types of narratives are built on polarity, but they could hardly differ more: Mann's drama is conducive to compromise and resignation, White's to insurrection. A different rhetoric and ethos pervade these two kinds of therapeutic dialogue. If we think of Mann and White as two narrators,[4] we could say that White identifies with the client in the fight against the problem, whereas Mann identifies with inexorable fate (for instance, Mann determines the 12-session limit, thus making therapy mimic destiny). The semantic and metaphoric preferences of the two illustrate their respective rhetorics: Mann talks of "approaching sepa-

---

[4]"Co-narrators" would be the usual phrasing. Here, however, I am mainly interested in outlining the contribution of the therapist's style to the narrative.

ration," "the limit of time," and "our doomed yearning for infinity"; White talks of "oppression," "recruitment," and "liberation." Mann evokes a sense of fatefulness, of resigned separation, of a mellow readiness to depart; White, a sense of indignation and of the dawning consciousness of possible freedom. On Mann's mantelpiece we should expect to find a *memento mori*, on White's a copy of the *Declaration of the Rights of Man*.

STRATEGIES

Conversationalists search for the ambiguity inherent in multiple views and voices; narrativists, for the continuity of character and plot; and strategists, for a sense of unimpeded action and movement.

Some constructivist manifestos have been rather unkind to strategic styles of therapy (Hoffman, 1985, 1992), describing them as hierarchical and controlling. On this view, to be a real constructivist, one should give up all presumption of controlling the therapeutic process. This view, however, has not gone unchallenged. Some strategists have voiced cogent reminders that one cannot *not* communicate, *not* influence, or *not* attempt to control (Efran & Clarfield, 1992; Weakland, 1993). Maybe one possible way out of this tangle is to allow that the relationship between constructivism and therapeutic control is orthogonal. Some therapists feel just as comfortable issuing prescriptions within an invented as within an objective reality.

Early strategic approaches to psychotherapy (Haley, 1963; Watzlawick, Weakland, & Fisch, 1974) were developed in tandem with the antipositivist critique. What is perhaps the chief assumption of strategic approaches—to wit, that therapeutic goals are constructed and negotiated—would make little sense within a positivist perspective. Equally constructivist is the attitude of most strategic therapists to so-called "resistance," which is viewed neither as a characteristic of clients nor as a necessary therapeutic event. Resistance actually reflects a mismatch between the therapist's and the client's constructions of goals and means. Better-fitting constructs would lead to nothing like it. Strategic therapists have also emptied the concepts of "motivation for therapy" and "motivation for change" of an objective ground: Motivation is not a quantum of energy residing within the client, but evolves from the formulation of goals. Similarly, putative entities such as "therapeutic relationship" or "alliance" should be best viewed not as endowed with independent ontological status, but as resulting from the give and take between the two constructed realities: To the extent that these match, there will be an alliance; when they do not, there will be none.

Steve de Shazer (1982, 1985, 1988, 1991) is my chosen representative of strategic style.[5] In his writings, as in those of other strategists (e.g., O'Hanlon & Weiner-Davis, 1989; Omer & Alon, 1989), goal construction rules over the therapeutic dialogue. de Shazer follows two stylistic guidelines in formulating goals: Keep them small, and make them concrete. This tangible minimalism is essential for inducing a sense of immediate and ubiquitous change. Large, abstract, or fuzzy goals would stifle the sense of change: How much could one experience progress toward self-actualization, contact with the inner self, or separation–individuation, say, between this morning and the coming Wednesday at 7:00 P.M.?

Passive change, however, does not count with strategists. Consider the following interchange:

CLIENT: For a while, I completely lost interest in exposing myself.

THERAPIST: How did you do that?

CLIENT: I just wasn't interested. I just don't have the urge anymore.

THERAPIST: How did you do that?

CLIENT: It almost came natural to me. The more I paid attention to the job, the less I paid attention to the urge.

THERAPIST: Good. (de Shazer, 1991, p. 100)

We might almost say that unless an experience can be translated into action language, it has no right of entrance into the strategist's reality. The therapist in the excerpt reacts as if something is missing from the client's report until the change is tagged as resulting from some kind of activity.

de Shazer's preoccupation with movement underlies his avoidance of a problem focus, which, in his view, clutters the way with impediments. The best way to avoid obstacles is to focus on the free areas in between, like skiers on a slope who manage not to look at the tree with which they would surely collide if it were to capture their attention.

de Shazer's love of movement has led to what may well be the swiftest opening to therapy ever devised. New clients are asked: "Many times in between the call for an appointment for therapy and the first session people notice that already things seem different. What have you noticed about your situation?" (Weiner-Davis, de Shazer, & Gingerich, 1987). As the client finds examples of already occurring new behaviors (which most do), the next questions are these: "What do you need to do to keep

---

[5]In an interview with Michael Hoyt presented in Chapter 3 of this volume, de Shazer stresses that his approach has veered away from its early strategic emphasis. I am using the term *strategic*, however, not to designate the use of "strategic maneuvers," but as a characteristic of a style that is goal- and movement-oriented. In this sense, de Shazer has perhaps become more rather than less strategic.

these changes going?" and "Are additional changes necessary or do you simply need more time to assure yourself that these changes will stick?" (Weiner-Davis et al., 1987). Therapy is no more than five minutes old and it has already reached the follow-up stage!

Many of de Shazer's technical innovations make sense once we capture his guiding stylistic vision. Take, for instance, what he calls the "miracle question" (de Shazer, 1985): Clients are enjoined to imagine that they wake up one morning to find out that their problem has been completely and miraculously solved. This may appear to be a strange question for de Shazer. Has he forgotten about the desirability of minute partial and concrete goals? For a moment we might think that de Shazer has relinquished his minimalism. If we think, however, of de Shazer's drive for unflagging movement and of his systematic avoidance of obstacles, the miracle question makes supreme strategic sense: It works like parachuting behind the enemy's lines. It lands the therapeutic dialogue, at one stroke, in a world of pure solution.

Change is to be experienced as all-pervasive, as a daily matter, as something with which the client is so familiar as even to fail to perceive it. To this end, the most hallowed ideas of the strategic/systemic movement may be sacrificed. This was the case, for instance, with the concept of second-order as opposed to first-order change. de Shazer (1991) jettisons this distinction for turning change into something precious and rare.

In de Shazer's world, one can then truly be said never to step twice into the same river. His style is a swift run, which avoids clashes, eschews drama, and abhors the statuesque. This may explain his critical pronouncements against White (de Shazer, 1993), which have caused no little perplexity among admirers of the two (see Chang & Phillips, 1993). de Shazer holds against White that by personalizing the problem he reifies it, establishing a problem focus that bogs therapy down. The therapy cannot but be shadowed by the towering figure it has erected. Instead of the fluidity of change, we get gigantized, arresting dichotomies. This difference in style is clearly shown in de Shazer's contraposition of his "exceptions" against White's "unique outcomes." *Prima facie,* the two concepts look similar. de Shazer, however, points to the uniqueness of White's outcomes. The word *unique* carries the connotation of something rare and special. de Shazer's exceptions are, on the contrary, meant to sound almost trivial. White's unique outcome is the gateway to or the incipient core of the new identity. It defines the new self who has shaken off the problem's yoke. de Shazer's exceptions are just so many different ways of perceiving and acting—mere pointers to other new perceptions and acts. White's unique outcome is carved to serve as the centerpiece of an arresting drama. de Shazer's exceptions are quick stepping-stones on the way to the treatment's vanishing point.

CONCLUSION

In the present chapter, instead of looking at practice from the viewpoint of theoretical premises, I have chosen to focus on style. I believe that this perspective captures much that is missed when we follow a theoretical one. Indeed, if we are to take seriously the decline of positivism in psychotherapy, questions of style must rise in importance relative to questions of theory. Theory ruled supreme in a scientifically inspired world view. Once we begin to view therapy as a craft of language games, style should be given pride of place.

The danger, however, is that a recourse to style as an explanatory concept may bog the profession down in a morass of fuzziness and encourage lazy habits of arbitrary justification. To the question "Why did the therapist say that?", one might pithily answer "Well, that's his style!" We might soon have our heads full with "Milanese style," "Milwaukee style," "Adelaide style," "exceptionism," and "unique-outcomism." I believe, however, that we can do better than that. An understanding of the "elements of style" (Strunk & White, 1979) has been developed in the lettered disciplines, and many of the relevant concepts are eminently applicable to psychotherapy. A systematic analysis of a given therapeutic style might include, for instance, a description of its peculiar semantics, syntax, imagery, characterization, plots, forms, thematics, rhetoric devices, and hermeneutic practices (Omer, 1993a). The potential gains of such an approach for psychotherapy go well beyond mere description. We would enrich our teaching and training. Finding ways to analyze, characterize, and transmit therapeutic style would help turn psychotherapy into a responsible constructive craft.

REFERENCES

Andersen, T. (1987). The reflecting team: Dialogue and meta-dialogue in clinical work. *Family Process, 26,* 415–428.

Anderson, H., & Goolishian, H. A. (1988). Human systems as linguistic systems: Preliminary and evolving ideas about the implications for clinical theory. *Family Process, 27,* 371–393.

Bakhtin, M. M. (1981). *The Dialogic Imagination* (C. Emerson & M. Holquist, Trans.). Austin: University of Texas Press.

Boscolo, L., Cecchin, G., Hoffman, L., & Penn, P. (1987). *Milan Systemic Family Therapy.* New York: Basic Books.

Chang, J., & Phillips, M. (1993). Michael White and Steve de Shazer: New directions in family therapy. In S. G. Gilligan & R. Price (Eds.), *Therapeutic Conversations* (pp. 95–111). New York: Norton.

de Shazer, S. (1982). *Patterns of Brief Family Therapy.* New York: Guilford Press.

de Shazer, S. (1985). *Keys to Solution in Brief Therapy.* New York: Norton.

de Shazer, S. (1988). *Clues: Investigating Solutions in Brief Therapy*. New York: Norton.

de Shazer, S. (1991). *Putting Difference to Work*. New York: Norton.

de Shazer, S. (1993). Commentary: de Shazer and White: Vive la difference. In S. G. Gilligan & R. Price (Eds.), *Therapeutic Conversations* (pp. 112–120). New York: Norton.

Efran, J. S., & Clarfield, L. E. (1992). Constructionist therapy: Sense and nonsense. In K. Gergen & S. McNamee (Eds.), *Therapy as Social Construction* (pp. 200–217). Newbury Park, CA: Sage.

Efran, J. S., Lukens, M. D., & Lukens, R. J. (1990). *Language Structure and Change*. New York: Norton.

Frank, J. D. (1987). Psychotherapy, rhetoric, and hermeneutics: Implications for practice and research. *Psychotherapy, 24*, 292–302.

Haley, J. (1963). *Strategies of Psychotherapy*. New York: Grune & Stratton.

Hoffman, L. (1985). Beyond power and control: Towards a "second-order" family systems therapy. *Family Systems Medicine, 3*, 381–396.

Hoffman, L. (1992). A reflexive stance for family therapy. In K. Gergen & S. McNamee (Eds.), *Therapy as Social Construction* (pp. 7–24). Newbury Park, CA: Sage.

Hoyt, M. F. (1994). On the importance of keeping it simple and taking the patient seriously: A conversation with Steve de Shazer and John Weakland. In M. F. Hoyt (Ed.), *Constructive Therapies* (pp. 11–40). New York: Guilford Press.

Madigan, S. P. (1993). Questions about questions: Situating the therapist's curiosity in front of the family. In S. G. Gilligan & R. Price (Eds.), *Therapeutic Conversations* (pp. 219–236). New York: Norton.

Mann, J. (1973). *Time-Limited Psychotherapy*. Cambridge, MA: Harvard University Press.

Maturana, H. R., & Varela, F. J. (1980). *Autopoiesis and Cognition*. Dordrecht, The Netherlands: Reidel.

O'Hanlon, W. H. (1994). The third wave. *Family Therapy Networker, 18*(6), 18–26, 28–29.

O'Hanlon, W. H., & Weiner-Davis, M. (1989). *In Search of Solutions: A New Direction in Psychotherapy*. New York: Norton.

Omer, H. (1991). Writing a post-scriptum to a badly ended therapy. *Psychotherapy, 28*, 484–492.

Omer, H. (1993a). Quasi-literary elements in psychotherapy. *Psychotherapy, 30*, 59–66.

Omer, H. (1993b). Short-term psychotherapy and the rise of the life-sketch. *Psychotherapy, 30*, 668–673.

Omer, H. (1994). *Critical Interventions in Psychotherapy*. New York: Norton.

Omer, H. (1995). Troubles in the therapeutic relationship: A pluralist perspective. *In Session: Psychotherapy in Practice, 1*, 47–57.

Omer, H., & Alon, N. (1989). Principles of therapeutic strategy. *Psychotherapy, 26*, 282–289.

Omer, H., & Strenger, C. (1992). The pluralist revolution: From the one true meaning to an infinity of constructed ones. *Psychotherapy, 29*, 253–261.

Parry, A. (1991). A universe of stories. *Family Process, 30*, 37–54.

Polster, E. (1987). *Every Person's Life Is Worth a Novel*. New York: Norton.

Russell, R. L., & Van den Broek, P. (1992). Changing narrative schemas in psychotherapy. *Psychotherapy, 29,* 344–354.

Selvini Palazzoli, M., Boscolo, L., Cecchin, G., & Prata, G. (1980). Hypothesizing, circularity, neutrality: three guidelines for the conductor of the session. *Family Process, 26,* 3–13.

Shakespeare, W. (1974). A midsummer night's dream. In G. B. Evans (Ed.), *The Riverside Shakespeare* (pp. 217–249). Boston: Houghton Mifflin. (Original work published 1600)

Sluzki, L. (1992). Transformations: A blueprint for narrative changes in therapy. *Family Process, 31,* 217–230.

Spence, D. (1982). *Narrative Truth and Historical Truth: Meaning and Interpretation in Psychoanalysis.* New York: Norton.

Strunk, W., Jr., & White, E. B. (1979). *The Elements of Style* (3rd ed.). New York: Macmillan.

Strupp, H. H., & Binder, J. (1984). *Psychotherapy in a New Key.* New York: Basic Books.

Tomm, K. (1987). Interventive interviewing: Part II. Reflexive questioning as a means to enable self-healing. *Family Process, 26,* 167–183.

Watzlawick, P., Weakland, J., & Fisch, R. (1974). *Change: Principles of Problem Formation and Problem Resolution.* New York: Norton.

Weakland, J. (1993). Conversation—but what kind? In S. G. Gilligan & R. Price (Eds.), *Therapeutic Conversations* (pp. 136–145). New York: Norton.

Weiner-Davis, M., de Shazer, S., & Gingerich, W. (1987). Constructing the therapeutic solution by building on pretreatment change: An exploratory study. *Journal of Marital and Family Therapy, 13,* 35–363.

White, M. (1989). *Selected papers.* Adelaide: Dulwich Centre Publications.

White, M. (1995). *Re-authoring lives: Interviews and essays.* Adelaide: Dulwich Centre Publications.

White, M., & Epston, D. (1990). *Narrative Means to Therapeutic Ends.* New York: Norton.

CHAPTER 15

Resource-Focused Therapy

BRADFORD P. KEENEY
WENDEL A. RAY

WHAT IS RESOURCE-FOCUSED THERAPY?

Resource-focused therapy (RFT) is a practical approach to working with people who complain of difficulties, dilemmas, and impasses. By paying the least amount of attention to pathologizing problems, RFT focuses strictly on bringing forth the natural resources of both clients and therapists. By resource, we mean any experience, belief, understanding, attitudes, event, conduct, or interpersonal habit that contributes to the positive contextualization of one's experience in living. In its ideal form, RFT does not even appear as therapy (Ray & Keeney, 1993).

RFT differs from most therapies in that it discounts *both* the metaphor of "therapist" *and* that of "client." We prefer seeing both parties as caught in the same dilemma: How can each be resourceful to the other? What must the "client" say or perform to evoke a response from the "therapist" that will be resourceful to the "client"? What must the "therapist" say that evokes the "client" to evoke the "therapist"? What must take place in order for the participants to have conversation that is resourceful to both? Until the client says something that brings forth the creative imagination and positive contributions of the therapist, the therapist is in the situation of being treated by the client. From our perspective, both therapist and client are problems until each is transformed, with the help of the other, into being resourceful, therapeutic, and healing to the situation.

Portions of this chapter are adapted by permission of the publisher from the introduction of *Resource Focused Therapy* (Ray & Keeney, 1993).

334

Our focus is specifically on *resourceful contexts*. Whether an action, spoken word, or experience is resourceful is determined by the context embodying it. *Resourceful* does not refer to particular events, but to the context of events. For example, praise from a mother to her child is not resourceful on the basis of the words spoken *in vitro;* praise is resourceful only when uttered in a resourceful context.

Most of the knots clients and therapists get themselves into stem from the confusion they generate by confounding the difference between context and the events being contextualized. A major contribution of Gregory Bateson (1972) was his noting over and over again how different levels of abstraction or understandings are often mixed up, breeding problematic configurations. Therapy is not the name of a single action; it is the name of a context of actions. When the idea that therapy is a context and not a simple action is fully realized, a major shift in understanding takes place for the therapist. It then becomes clear that there are no particular right words, actions, or interventions that will necessarily work for a specific situation. What is called for is the movement of a problematic context into a resourceful context. In a resourceful context, all uttered lines and enacted conduct are contextualized, experienced, and realized as therapeutic.

Without a commitment to recognizing the meaning of context, therapists can become confused by doing the right thing in the wrong context ("It doesn't work, but it should") or by doing the wrong thing in the right context ("It works, but it shouldn't"). From this perspective, the paradigm of therapy is conceptually quite simple. It involves the transformation of the context within which client and therapist converse.

In the beginning of the theatrical play called "therapy," the opening context is often named "the problem." Act One, "the problem," finds a client stuck in a situation where his or her experience is contextualized as "problematic." When a therapist enters the client's problem context, the therapist participates in maintaining it. No matter what is said to the client—whether it be inquiring about the behavioral specifics of the problem, descriptions of attempted solutions, hypotheses about its origin, or professional categorizing and stigmatizing—if it contributes to the theme of the problem, then the therapist is potentially helping the client stay stuck in a problem context.

In RFT, the goal of Act One is to get out of it and move into the next act, Act Two. In most plays, the middle act is the transformational hinge, linking the beginning to the end. The final act, Act Three, is (for plays with resourceful endings), a situation of resolution and generativity. In schematic terms, we have the following:

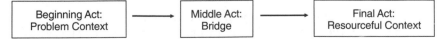

This diagram, the paradigm of a play (whether therapy or otherwise), is a simple map for understanding the structure of therapy.

With this map, therapy involves doing whatever is necessary to get out of the problem context. Again, anything said or done in the problem context, even if it seems the "right thing," is always a potential problem by virtue of its being contextualized as a member of the problematic context. *How* one gets out of this context is less important than getting out of it. Talking about the World Series or fishing or cooking is usually more resourceful than discussing anxiety or depression. The trick, however, is eventually getting into a context where all that is discussed can be contextualized as a resource. Here what was formerly called the "presenting problem" may now be discussed as a resource.

What is never to be forgotten is that therapy does not address problem particulars, but problem contexts. Problem behaviors are not the whole of the problem. The contextualization of any behavior as a problem is the whole that embraces the problem. This orientation to therapy, previously presented in *Improvisational Therapy: A Practical Guide for Creative Clinical Strategies* (Keeney, 1991), is rooted entirely in keeping track of the context of one's performance.

In theatrical terms, the name of the scene in which one's lines are spoken must always be kept in mind. Offering "help" in a problematic or impoverished scene is often not helpful. Creating an opening that helps get both therapist and client out of impoverished contexts is the first step toward being therapeutic. Getting into and maintaining presence in a resourceful context is the final act of therapy.

RFT is concerned with getting clients and therapists into a resourceful context as quickly and efficiently as possible. If it is possible to ignore the problem completely, this may be done. If the problem must be exaggerated to break into another scene, this may be encouraged. Focusing on getting into and staying in a resourceful context requires minimizing other actions and understandings previously associated with the profession of therapy.

In RFT, therapy ideally ends up being outside of therapy. Therapy ends in a context of resourceful conduct—action that by its very definition does not require therapy. At the final stage, both the client and therapist may be embarrassed to find themselves in therapy. As may be seen in the case studies presented later in the chapter, clients and therapists participate in bringing forth the breath of life and imagination within each other.

HISTORICAL BACKGROUND

Historically speaking, RFT is rooted to the genre of therapy called "brief therapy." Brief therapy as we know it today emerged out of Harry Stack

Sullivan's (1953) interpersonal theory, and was expanded after his death by one of his students, Don D. Jackson. Sullivan was one of the first to insist that it makes no sense to talk of a self and its strivings apart from the interpersonal relations nexus of which it is a part (Mullahy, 1967). Jackson and his colleagues—first as members of the Bateson research projects on paradox in communication (Bateson, Jackson, Haley, & Weakland, 1956; Jackson & Weakland, 1961; Jackson, 1967a, 1967b; Ray, 1995), and later in the conjoint family therapy model pioneered at the Mental Research Institute (MRI), which Jackson founded in 1958—laid the foundations for brief therapy. These pioneers did not work in isolation. They studied and were influenced by many of the leading therapists of their time, particularly the prodigious hypnotherapist Milton Erickson.

The birth of the most influential form of brief therapy was associated with the classic text *Change: Principles of Problem Formation and Resolution,* written by three of Jackson's colleagues at the MRI, Paul Watzlawick, John Weakland, and Richard Fisch (1974). They abandoned much of the excessive weight of theoretical psychotherapy baggage, to focus on problem definitions and descriptions of attempted solutions. As a therapeutic Occam's razor, this orientation helped free many therapists to focus on designing imaginative interventions that aim at disrupting the interactional patterns embodying problem conduct.

In a similar vein, Jay Haley (another former member of Bateson's distinguished research team), in his classic contribution *Problem-Solving Therapy* (1976), took specific aim at busting problems. Less parsimonious than Watzlawick, Weakland, and Fisch, Haley preferred a more elaborated mythology to account for explaining the occurrence and persistence of symptoms. Influenced by his colleagues Salvador Minuchin and Bruno Montalvo, he developed a sociological map for contextualizing symptoms in terms of coalitions, hierarchy, and social power. To Haley's credit, he never constructed a formal theory. Instead, his text drew loosely on simple heuristics and generalizations that aid the therapist in focusing in a specific way on alleviating problems in social sequences.

However, a potential weakness of both the Weakland, Fisch, and Watzlawick team's and Haley's approaches is their focus on the problem as the theme of therapy. Although their intention is to free the social system from being organized by a problem, their focus on the problem carries the risk that the therapist may contribute to maintaining presence in the problem context.

The work of de Shazer (1982, 1988), a student of Weakland, emphasizes solutions—the necessarily implied and complementary side of all problems. Here less emphasis is placed on problems per se, and an effort is made to search for solutional conduct. Nevertheless, a potential difficulty with de Shazer's approach is that a focus on solutions does not necessarily remove one from the problems they are supposed to solve.

To focus on either problems *or* solutions is to remain contextualized within the complementary whole of problems ↔ solutions. The two are inseparable, and one side brings forth the other. As Fisch, Weakland, and Segal (1982) demonstrate, problems bring forth attempted solutions. Blocking the type or class of attempted solution is for them the efficient way of alleviating the problem. For de Shazer and other solution-focused therapists, a focus on solutions brings forth problems, whether these are spoken about or not. Thus, a potential disadvantage for both problem-focused and solution-focused therapies is that each risks keeping the theme of therapy in Act One—the context called "problem." That is, whether solutions are "right" or "wrong," they risk remaining ways of preserving the problem context. Some therapists who attempt to learn problem- or solution-focused therapies have too readily overlooked the context within which problems and solutions are discussed. As a result, these orientations sometimes tend to have a behavioristic feel to them that easily seduces the therapist into looking at bits of action or sequences of action, without regard to the context of rhetoric that gives the action meaning.

The contribution of the Milan approach to systemic family therapy, particularly the work of Cecchin and Boscolo (Boscolo, Cecchin, Hoffman & Penn, 1987; Cecchin, Lane, & Ray, 1992, 1993, 1994a, 1994b), has helped to correct this deficiency in contextual vision. Their approach radically emphasizes the contexts of meaning (see Keeney & Ross, 1985; Keeney, 1982). At the same time, being influenced by the theoretical ideas of coalitions, paradox, and so forth, this orientation also potentially falls into the trap of maintaining a focus on the problem ↔ solution distinction, particularly with its focus on "The problem is the solution." This reversal of the Watzlawick et al. (1974) slogan, "The solution is the problem," is half of the whole distinction ("The solution is the problem/the problem is the solution"). Either side implies the other and maintains the whole theory of being in a universe of problems, solutions, problem solutions, and solution problems.

As part of this historical tradition of brief therapies, our work has developed naturally out of our understanding and practice of the contributions of Bateson, Sullivan, Jackson, Erickson, Weakland, Fisch, Haley, Cecchin, and Boscolo, among others. What we bring to the theoretical table is an identification of what all these approaches seem to be after, in spite of the very different metaphors they use to discuss their understanding. Specifically, the goal of RFT is to get clients and therapists out of problem–solution contexts and get them into a resourceful context. In a resourceful context the problem can be seen as a solution and solutions as problems. Here, however, the new understanding takes place outside of a problem–solution context.

THE CLINICAL PROCEDURE

Act One: The Setup

As noted earlier, RFT regards a session as the creation of a theatrical play. In this therapeutic play, three different acts take place. Act One, the setup, is the occasion for hearing the presenting lines of the client(s). The therapist may evoke these lines in any fashion. What is more important concerns the therapist or team of observers identifying any lines that provide a hint or direction toward a more resourceful contextualization of therapist–client talk. Act One simply creates the building blocks, the setting of the stage, the props, and the characters that will make up the play; the following acts move the conversation toward a more resourceful context.

Act Two: Creating a Resourceful Context

As soon as the therapist or therapy team begins to have a hunch about how the conversation may be moved forward, a question will be designed and delivered to the client(s). Typically, in a team situation, the discussion and construction of this question take place behind the observing mirror. Often several lines given by a client in the setup are tied together in a way that creates a more general theme concerning how they are linked. This linkage and the proposed theme (which may be from another client line) form the basis for the question.

The resourceful theme, idea, explanation, suggestion, or hunch is then dropped on the client or clients, with instructions for them to think and talk about it for a few minutes. The therapist or team may then leave and watch the response from the observing room. If the idea is accepted, the therapy moves forward. If it is rejected or partially rejected, then the process is repeated, and a discussion of the idea is listened to as if it were another Act One.

This approach does not create hypotheses—that is, possible understandings of a situation. We prefer to create what Gerald Rademeyer (personal communication, 1992) calls a "diathesis," defined as a disposition for organizing things in a certain way. Questions are ways of setting forth these diatheses or dispositions toward a more resourceful theme.

Act Three: Enacting the Resourceful Context

Whereas Act Two sets the stage for change by introducing the name of a therapeutic theme or context, Act Three aims at stabilizing this change through prescribing action that only makes sense when performed in the redefined situation. As the assignment is discussed, the client's or clients' lines are carefully woven into justifying, legitimizing, and fine-tuning the new understanding(s) brought about by the change in context of conversation.

All subsequent sessions begin with this same format—eliciting lines (usually from a follow-up to the previous assignment), further constructing the resourceful context, and calling for additional enactments in the new reality. To summarize, Act One is where the client or clients bring the opening lines, typically understood as derived from an impoverished, often painful context. Act Two is the creation of new themes and understandings that are resourceful to both client(s) and therapist(s). And finally, Act Three is the prescription of action based on that resourceful understanding. Act Two and Three embody the two sides of therapeutic change—change in understanding and change in action—both based on the offerings given by the client(s) in Act One. In the case studies that follow, the structure of each case in terms of Acts One, Two, and Three is identified.

A CASE STUDY[1]

Act One: The Setup

A Hispanic woman left a message with a university clinic's answering service, saying she was calling because her children insisted she seek help. "They" were worried about her "depression."

When a therapist returned the woman's call, she explained that during the preceding several months she had not been her "usual happy self." She complained of being preoccupied with worry, and described herself as moping around the house and depressed. Her children had been unable to cheer her up. She was not sure whether anything could be done for her, but wanted to come in for an appointment because her children thought she needed to.

Maria came to the interview alone. She seemed unsure of herself, laughing nervously. This 52-year-old Hispanic woman explained that she had been married for 35 years and had raised 10 children. She began by describing the pride she felt in having been a good parent and grand-parent, having taken most of the care of her grandchildren. In addition, she had provided a home for several foster children over the years. Seven months ago, her husband had been accused by their ex-daughter-in-law of molesting two of their granddaughters, ages 10 and 8. He was babysitting with them at home one day when he allegedly fondled them

---

[1]In this case study, Bradford Keeney was the consultant and Wendel Ray the therapist.

and exposed himself to them. The ex-daughter-in-law reported the incident to the police and child care officials, but not to Maria, and Maria's husband was arrested. He then moved out of the house to another town. He continued to provide some financial support to Maria, but she had seen him infrequently since "all this began."

Maria had first found out about the accusations when she read about them in the local newspaper. She was shocked and shaken. "I've read about these sort of things, but never imagined it could happen in my family."

Maria maintained that "life has to go on," but since "this thing happened" her family was shattered. She described herself as constantly being worried and preoccupied with what this would mean to her family's future. She felt that with time she would be able to accept the situation, because "Life goes on," but her children were concerned about her moping around the house and being depressed all the time. When asked how she thought the therapist could be helpful, Maria stated that she saw the problem not so much as depression over the situation with her husband, but more as worry and anxiousness over her lack of formal education (she had dropped out of school in the seventh grade), very little work experience outside the home, loss of confidence in herself, and fear that she would not be able to find a job and make a living as a result of all this. Her identity as a competent, experienced parent and grandparent appeared threatened by the situation with her husband.

Act Two: Creating a Resourceful Context

The consultant suggested that the therapist go into the session and display uncertainty and nervousness about the case. He was to tell Maria that he had recently moved to town and was just starting the family therapy doctoral program. (These were accurate descriptions.) He was to stress how important it was for him to be successful with Maria, because she was one of his first clients and he needed to make a good impression on the director of the program, who would be observing from behind the one-way mirror.

This message was preceded with the comment that the consulting team had been called away on an emergency, and while alone, the therapist thought he would take advantage of the opportunity to ask for her help. The more unsure and nervous the therapist betrayed himself as being, the more competent Maria became. After delivering this message, the therapist kept leaving the room, under the pretext of checking to see whether the team had returned. In this context, Maria turned to her maternal resources and began adopting a posture that could help the therapist.

Act Three: Enacting the Resourceful Context

The therapist began asking Maria for some advice on another case he was working with. He described a family with an uncontrollable adolescent boy. The parents had no idea how to control the boy, and the therapist wondered, in light of Maria's many years of experience in raising children, whether she could give him some advice. He explained that he was new at this and did not really know what to do.

Maria provided detailed and specific suggestions and expert advice on how to coach the parents to be in charge and take control of their adolescent. She gave solid structural advice of putting the parents in control, using and withholding rewards, and so forth. She went on to advise the therapist that the child might not be the problem, but that the misbehaving might be a result of the parents' strained relationship.

As Maria continued to provide sound advice, the therapist continued to solicit her help. Maria became visibly more in control and sure of herself. By the end of the session she was calm and exuded confidence. She was told that the team members were not going to be able to return and continue the session because of the emergency that had called them away, and she would not be charged for the session; after all, she really had helped the therapist and not the other way around. The therapist thanked Maria for the advice, and she left beaming.

Later during the week, the therapist called her and related that since he had started using her advice with the members of the other family, satisfactory changes had occurred with them. She was quite pleased.

Maria did not show up for the next two scheduled sessions. When she did return three weeks later, she presented herself as being much more in control of and confident in herself than in the earlier session. She expressed pleasure at being told how well the family she had provided advice on was doing. She was told that the case had turned around so fast and with such profound changes that the program director wanted to know how it had been done. The therapist had explained to him the advice she had provided. Maria was then told that the director had been so impressed by her advice that he wanted to know whether she would be willing to provide consultation on cases involving child-focused problems.

Maria was delighted and said she would be very willing to provide consultation on such cases. She was also told that the therapist and the director would be willing to write letters of reference for her in regard to her family counseling expertise.

The therapist and Maria never returned to the presenting context of worrying about her problems. Maria had found a way of moving into a future with hope, confidence, and acknowledged skills.

Follow-Up

In a follow-up interview conducted several months later, Maria told us that she had been hired to work at a local children's home. Showing none of the signs of depression present in the first session, Maria said that she felt capable of handling the situation on her own, and therapy was discontinued.

A SECOND CASE STUDY[2]

Act One: The Setup

A therapist trainee was seeing a family during live supervision. The family came to therapy because the 16 year old adolescent son was described as being "polyaddicted." He had been thrown out of three treatment programs because the treatment staff feared his violence. Part of the story was that he had killed a dog with a baseball bat and had blown up a truck. He was living with a maternal aunt and uncle, who were giving him "one last chance to straighten up."

His mother was described as being sexually "loose," being a "drunk," and living with a boyfriend who was also a "drunk." The mother had divorced the father when the son was an infant, and the father had been out of the picture for years.

The therapist was a self-described "recovering alcoholic" enrolled in a two-year marriage and family therapy program. In the supervised session, a fascinating family secret was revealed: Many years earlier the maternal grandfather, who had died in prison, had been a severe alcoholic who was very violent. On several occasions he had nearly killed the grandmother by beating her severely, stabbing her, and shooting her with a shotgun.

The aunt, grandmother, and mother had never told the children about the grandfather, but regularly said to the 16-year-old boy that he was "just like your grandpa" (meaning dangerously violent and addicted). In turn, the grandmother was revered by family members for her "saintly" behavior. Everyone was very protective toward her. It was also reported that the 16-year-old's mother, now seen as the black sheep of the family, used to take up for her siblings and protect them from the grandfather when he became violent.

The boy was furious with his mother for not being more available to him. He also said that he tended to get nervous and subsequently

---

[2]In this case study, Wendel Ray was the team leader, and Bradford Keeney provided consultation by telephone.

drink, smoke pot, or use "crank" (synthetic amphetamine) whenever the aunt, mother, or grandmother began to worry out loud that he would relapse. When the alleged violence of the son was explored, it turned out that the stories had been greatly exaggerated. He had not blown up a truck, but rather had blown up the engine while driving too fast; he *had* killed a dog with a baseball bat, but in self-defense after having been attacked by the dog.

Act Two: Creating a Resourceful Context

The team took a break to discuss the family's situation. At first there was a long period of silence, because the entire team felt overwhelmed by the family story. Slowly, team members began to discuss the kind of hypotheses that therapists often formulate: The boy's behavior was irresponsible; the family was only coming to therapy to help the boy avoid going to jail; the boy was dangerous and possibly a hopeless psychopath who came to therapy to avoid justice; the mother was irresponsible and promiscuous; there was very little space in this family for a male to gain a position of dignity and worth, in the shadow of the grandfather's history of violence and drunkenness, and the father's history of abandonment; the grandmother was exploiting the grandson in order to punish her daughter for being loyal to the grandfather; and the grandmother had invalidated the dignity of the grandson by keeping the secret about the grandfather's violence for so many years and then revealing it to the therapist, an outsider, without first discussing it privately with him. All of these ideas—ideas of the sort that often tempt therapists—were regarded as nonresourceful and were subsequently neglected.

The team and clients began moving toward the creation of a story of family loyalty, which contextualized the boy's behavior as being a manifestation of the desire of the entire family to keep the grandfather's memory alive. This recontextualization brought the mother to be empowered by her recalling, in front of the whole family, stories of how she took care of her siblings during the grandfather's drunken tirades. The mother's feelings of sorrow and grief about how the family had tried to push the memory of the grandfather out of existence were played out. This resourceful contextualization revealed how the grandson had become the living embodiment of stories about the grandfather as a way of keeping his memory alive. The stories carefully kept in place the protected image of the grandmother as a pillar of the family who had managed to keep them together under very difficult circumstances.

Act Three: Enacting the Resourceful Context

In further work the family began to recall other characteristics of the grandfather that were worthy of remembering. For example, he had been a carpenter who was very talented at making things with his hands, just like his grandson. Movement toward carpentry was now encouraged as a more resourceful way of keeping the grandfather's memory alive.

One consequence of this telling of the resourceful family story was that the grandson suggested a method for helping his aunt, mother, and grandmother handle their worries about him: Any time he (the grandson) noticed them becoming nervous about the possibility of a relapse, he would reassure them by suggesting they take him for a urinalysis checkup to confirm that he had not resumed substance use.

The resourceful family story was maintained in subsequent sessions and was used to encourage more productive conduct in the everyday life of the family.

Follow-Up

Two years after therapy ended, the adolescent was continuing to stay out of trouble. He was a senior in high school; his grades had improved; he was a star of the football team; and his use of drugs and alcohol was minimal. His relationship with his mother was greatly improved, as was the rapport among the mother, grandmother, and aunt.

CONCLUSION

RFT requires an abandonment of building therapeutic Towers of Babel and practicing one-upmanship games of political expertise over the client. It is an invitation for the therapist to learn to be more imaginative, more playful, more resourceful, and more human. As the therapist's humanity evolves, the appearance of "therapy" will diminish. What is left is a rebirth of occasions free from the straitjacket of prescribed templates, simplistic moralisms, and power games. Here the therapist abandons being a "therapist" in order to be more genuinely helpful. The absence of the "therapeutic" and the presence of resourceful creation are the goals of RFT. In its most complete form, RFT abandons its own ideals about being a school or orientation of therapy, and instead moves into the territory of human beings joined together in the healing dance played out in the experience of living collaboratively with one another—one of the greatest mysteries that can ever be known.

REFERENCES

Bateson, G. (1972). *Steps to an Ecology of Mind*. New York: Jason Aronson.
Bateson, G., Jackson, D., Haley, J., & Weakland, J. (1956). Toward a theory of schizophrenia. *Behavioral Science, 1*(4), 251–264.

Boscolo, L., Cecchin, G., Hoffman, L., & Penn, P. (1987). *Milan Systemic Family Therapy*. New York: Basic Books.

Cecchin, G., Lane, G., & Ray, W. A. (1992). *Irreverence: A Strategy for Therapists' Survival*. London: Karnac Books. (Distributed in the United States by Brunner/Mazel)

Cecchin, G., Lane, G., & Ray, W. A. (1993). From strategizing to non-intervention: Toward irreverence in systemic practice. *Journal of Marital and Family Therapy*, *19*(2), 125–136.

Cecchin, G., Lane, G., & Ray, W. A. (1994a). *The Cybernetics of Prejudices in the Practice of Psychotherapy*. London: Karnac Books. (Distributed in the United States by Brunner/Mazel)

Cecchin, G., Lane, G., & Ray, W. A. (1994b). Influence, effect, and emerging systems. *Journal of Systemic Therapies, 13*(4), 13–21.

de Shazer, S. (1982). *Patterns of Brief Family Therapy: An Ecosystemic Approach*. New York: Guilford Press.

de Shazer, S. (1988). *Clues: Investigating Solutions in Brief Therapy*. New York: Norton.

Fisch, R., Weakland, J., & Segal, L. (1982). *The Tactics of Change: Doing Therapy Briefly*. San Francisco: Jossey-Bass.

Haley, J. (1976). *Problem-Solving Therapy*. San Francisco: Jossey-Bass.

Jackson, D. (1967a). Schizophrenia: The nosological nexus. In P. Watzlawick & J. Weakland (Eds.), *The Interactional View* (pp. 193–208). New York: Norton.

Jackson, D. (1967b). The myth of normality. *Medical Opinion and Review, 3*(5), 28–33.

Jackson, D., & Weakland, J. (1961). Conjoint family therapy: Some considerations on theory, technique, and results. *Psychiatry, 24(Suppl. 2), 30–45.*

Keeney, B. P. (1982). *Aesthetics of Change*. New York: Guilford Press.

Keeney, B. P. (1991). *Improvisational Therapy: A Practical Guide for Creative Clinical Strategies*. New York: Guilford Press.

Keeney, B. P., & Ross, J. (1985). *Mind in Therapy: Constructing Systemic Family Therapies*. New York: Basic Books.

Mullahy, P. (1967). *A Study of Interpersonal Relations*. New York: Science House.

Ray, W. A. (1995). The interactional therapy of Don D. Jackson. In J. Weakland & W. Ray (Eds.), *Propagations: Thirty Years of Influence from the Mental Research Institute*. New York: Haworth Press.

Ray, W. A., & Keeney, B. P., (1993). *Resource Focused Therapy*. London: Karnac Press. (Distributed in the United States by Brunner/Mazel)

Sullivan H. S. (1953). *The Collected Works of Harry Stack Sullivan*. New York: Norton.

Watzlawick, P., Weakland, J., & Fisch, R. (1974). *Change: Principles of Problem Formation and Problem Resolution*. New York: Norton.

CHAPTER 16

Postmodernism, the Relational Self, Constructive Therapies, and Beyond

A Conversation with Kenneth Gergen

MICHAEL F. HOYT

A long-time proponent of a social constructionist perspective, Kenneth Gergen is Professor of Psychology at Swarthmore College in Swarthmore, Pennsylvania. His wide-ranging interests, along with those of his colleague and wife, Mary Gergen, bridge intellectual traditions and popular culture. His edited volumes include *The Self in Social Interaction* (Gordon & Gergen, 1968), *Historical Social Psychology* (K. J. Gergen & Gergen, 1984), *The Social Construction of the Person* (Gergen & Davis, 1985), *Texts of Identity* (Shotter & Gergen, 1989), *Everyday Understanding: Social and Scientific Implications* (Semin & Gergen, 1990), *Therapy as Social Construction* (McNamee & Gergen, 1992), and *Historical Dimensions of Psychological Discourse* (Graumann & Gergen, 1993). His authored books include *Toward Transformation in Social Knowledge* (1985b), the much-acclaimed *The Saturated Self: Dilemmas of Identity in Contemporary Life* (1991), and his recent *Realities and Relationships: Soundings in Social Construction* (1995a).

Perhaps especially apropos of the postmodern sensibility discussed herein, the following interview was not conducted in one time, place, or state of mind. Rather, questions were asked, answered, adumbrated, and amplified over many months, from airplanes, trains, offices, hotels, and homes. The conversation commenced in June 1994. When Gergen graciously telephoned in response to my letter of invitation, I quickly asked, "Why did you call your *Networker* speech [Gergen, 1992] 'The Polymorphous *Per*versity of the Postmodern Era' rather than 'The

Polymorphous *Diversity*'? I know the reference to Freud [1905/1953],[1] but 'perversity' implies a deviance from a 'normal' or 'right' way." Gergen responded, "Let's talk." Our conversation, constructed over time, follows.

HOYT: How do you conceptualize the *self*, and how does this change moving from a modern to a postmodern perspective?

GERGEN: For purposes of contrast, let's start with the tradition we inherit in the West, one which posits some form of inner essence. Whether we are speaking of Christian religion and its belief in a soul; Romanticists of the past century, with their championing of passion, inspiration, or *élan vital*; recent existentialist thinkers and their emphasis on conscious choice; or the belief of modernists in reason or cognition—all begin with the assumption of an essential core of the self. It is this essence that constitutes one's being and without which one would be something less than human.

  As a social constructionist, I view all these perspectives as culturally and historically situated. It is not that they are mistaken, somehow failing to see the self as it truly is. The mistake is perhaps in presuming that we can determine "what truly is." The words we use to describe our being are not simply pictures of what exists, not maps of a territory. Rather, they construct us as this or that, and in doing so serve as logics for action. I think it is this de-essentializing that is the major ingredient of the move from the modern to postmodern conception of self. Within the spectrum of postmodern thought, it is the social constructionist who will treat the self as a manifestation of human interchange.

HOYT: If the self is socially constructed, is there something essential that may be shaped or influenced, but is not created *sui generis*? I'm thinking, for example, of Stern's [1985] studies of infant development and Margaret Mahler's [Mahler, Bergman, & Pine, 1975] ideas about the "psychological birth of the infant." Other writers, such as Singer and Salovcy [1993], have suggested that one's sense of self is "remembered"—organized or influenced by cognitive–affective processes.

GERGEN: Again, the challenge for the constructionist is to avoid pronouncements about what is essential. This is not to say that the constructionist doesn't participate in culture, and would not use words like *soul, intentional choice, cognition,* and the like. Rather, it is to recognize that when we use these utterances we are participating

---

[1]In *Three Essays on the Theory of Sexuality*, Freud (1905/1953) used the phrase "polymorphous perversity" to describe the undetermined potential pansexuality of children.

in a particular set of cultural traditions, and not pronouncing truth beyond culture and history. To say "I love you" is not then a description of a mental state; it is active participation in a deeply valued form of relationship.

To deal with your question more directly, I don't want to say either one way or the other that there is or is not something essential to be shaped or influenced. Rather, let's ask what hangs on the question for different social or cultural practices. What will follow if I take one route in a conversation as opposed to another? As I mentioned previously, we have a substantial tradition of essentialism, giving an affirmative answer to your question. So for me as a scholar, I scarcely succeed in pressing our ideas forward if I simply say, yet once again, "We are emotional beings," or "cognitive beings," or "intentional beings."

One of my central interests has been to generate a new sense of what it is to be a person, a sense of what I call a "relational self." The hope is to transform the meaning of what it is to be a self—to have an identity, emotion, memory, motivation, and the like— so that we can understand it as constituted within relationship. Vygotsky [1986] and Bakhtin [1981] are useful as first steps in this direction, as are Mead [1934] and Bruner [1986]. However, in each of these cases there remains a strong commitment to an individual subjectivity that precedes relatedness. My hope (and I must say that there are many scholars and therapists who are engaged in these dialogues) is to go beyond this work by positing relatedness as the essential matrix, out of which a conception of self (or identity, emotion, etc.) is born, objectified, and embedded within action. On this account, for example, emotion is a constructed category, and emotional performance is culturally prescribed. However, such performances are never cut away from a relational dance or scenario. We participate in the dance together, and without the dance there would be no occasion for the performance. In this sense, it is *we* who possess the emotion. Much of this is spelled out in my new book, *Realities and Relationships* [1995a].

HOYT: This is very consistent with the interactionalist notion that "the basic unit of analysis is at least two people," as I recently heard Jay Haley express it, as well as the idea that "the mind is not in the head" [Maturana & Varela, 1987]. In your view, where is the *unconscious*? Is the term useful? Is there a *self* outside (beyond, below) narrative?

GERGEN: As you can see, whether we posit an unconscious mind is optional. There is nothing about whatever we are that makes this kind of description necessary. Our beliefs in the unconscious as a reality are also culturally and historically situated, growing most recently from the soil of 19th-century Romanticism.[2] However, whether the term is *useful* or not is a very interesting one. It is not useful if what we mean by the term is that the concept gives us an accurate description—"real" insight into human functioning. However, if what we mean by "useful" is viewed in terms of social functioning—where does it get us in our relations to speak of the unconscious?—then the answer would be very multifaceted.

HOYT: How so?

GERGEN: For example, the concept has been very useful in augmenting our tendency to place moral judgment on the deviant in society. Rather than simply placing moral blame on the rapist, child molester, or murderer—leading unequivocally to punishment—the concept of the unconscious adds to our cultural repertoire by enabling us to see the deviant as in some sense "ill." We think increasingly, then, about ways to restore the individual to full functioning (as opposed to forms of punishment that will virtually ensure their remaining deviant). There is much more that could be said on behalf of the concept of the unconscious. However, there is also a very strong down side, and I guess I find it more compelling than the positive account. Here I am speaking of the many critiques of the assumption of the unconscious, for example, for its reducing all problems to the intrapsychic level, its blindness to cultural and economic conditions, its championing of the authority of the all-knowing doctor (in contrast to the ignorant patient), its alliance with the medical model of illness, and its providing the individual excuses for all forms of brutishness.[3]

HOYT: How do you define *therapy*? Is that the right word? What might be an alternative?

GERGEN: I would prefer not to define it. Rather, let's say that we find ourselves at this time in cultural history engaged in a range of interrelated conversations in which the concept of therapy plays a very significant role. The precise meaning of the term is contested, and it should ideally remain so. To legislate in this case would be to stop the conversation, oppress the many voices, and arbitrarily and misleadingly freeze history.

HOYT: How do you currently see the therapeutic endeavor?

GERGEN: My preference in this conversation is to view therapy as a process of constructing meaning. To be sure, we exist in what we

[2]See de Shazer's comments regarding Freud and Wittgenstein in Chapter 3. For an extended discussion of the history of the idea of the unconscious, see Ellenberger (1970).

[3]See also Michael White's discussion in Chapter 2 of how even altruistic acts can be destructively made suspect, pathologized, and invalidated.

commonly call "real-world" conditions—"biological," "material," "economic," and the like. However, in the main what we take to be the successes and failures in our lives, the worthwhile and the worthless, the satisfying as opposed to the frustrating, are byproducts of human meaning. It is not so much "how things are" as how we interpret them that will typically bring us into therapy. A physical touch may itself be unremarkable; however, in different frames of meaning it may spark a sense of friendly support, move one to ecstasy, or incite litigation for harassment. A blow to the chin will send a family member in search of a therapist, but will move a boxer to change his tactics. With this emphasis in place, we are invited to see effective therapy as a transformation in meaning. However, as you can see from the preceding remarks, I don't see this transformation principally as a cognitive event. Rather, it is an alteration in actions—relying importantly on language but not at all limited to language.

HOYT: As therapy moves more into postmodern context, what are the continuities from past tradition and practice, and what "new directions" should we consider? It would be perhaps premature and too specific to propose a curriculum, but what do you see as the major issues and challenges?

GERGEN: These are very complicated issues and we could talk at length. For now, however, let me focus on just one aspect of what many see as the postmodern condition, and its particular implications for therapeutic practice. As I tried to describe in *The Saturated Self* [1991], the communication technologies of this century bring us into confrontation with a vastly expanded range of others—both in terms of physical presence and vicarious figures of the media. Our otherwise parochial worlds become shattered by the intrusion of a multiplicity of opinions, values, attitudes, personalities, visions, and ways of life. At the same time, there has been an increasing tendency for various groups to generate common consciousness. Again, the technologies allow otherwise voiceless people to organize, develop common goals, consider entitlements, and so on.

  Under these conditions of increasing pluralism, it is very difficult for any therapeutic school to claim—as was long the tendency—ubiquitous authority. To reduce all problems, for example, to early family conditions, conditioned responses, or deficits in self-regard not only seems excessively parochial, but in a certain sense tyrannical.

HOYT: The death of an orthodoxy makes it difficult to organize a counterorthodoxy.

GERGEN: How then does therapeutic practice respond to these conditions? Of course, the most common practice among therapists is simply to "go eclectic." Rather than continuing in the school favored in their training, they continue to explore, learn, adapt, and eventually develop multilayered approaches. In my view, a constructionist orientation favors just this kind of practice, but as well furnishes such practice with a needed sense of integration and purpose.

HOYT: I prefer the term *multilayered* or *multitheoretical* rather than *eclectic*. Being multiply informed is important, but to me *eclectic* sometimes seems like a cross between *electric* and *chaotic*, a directionless hodgepodge of techniques.[4]

GERGEN: We could also use the term *polyvocal*, which better fits the metaphor of conversation. In any case, the greater the range of "vocabularies" available to the therapist, the greater his or her efficacy within wide-ranging relationships. At the same time, the constructionist therapist is drawn to the use-value of these various vocabularies (words and actions) as they are developed in the therapeutic relationship, and extended to further relationships outside. How well do the vocabularies travel, and what do they do to and for people's lives as they are pressed into action?

HOYT: Holy hermeneutics! If modernism gave us "ontological insecurity," postmodernism could produce a panic attack! As Sheila McNamee and you [1992, p. 2] have commented, "Little confidence now remains in the optimistic program of scientifically grounded progress toward identifying 'problems' and providing 'cures.'" With conventional standards of "what's right" no longer valid compasses, what suggestions do you have for therapists as we search for (and co-create) therapeutic realities with our clients? Any guides for the perplexed?

GERGEN: At the outset, I think we must all remain humble and interdependent in the face of the problem. This is not the time to look to a new guru who can remove our perplexities; we must together work toward new visions. With this said, my own preference is for a therapeutic approach that appreciates the force of local realities, but within an expanded context of connection. By this, I mean that the therapist would not begin with a single set of criteria as to what constitutes an effective intervention or a cure. Rather, he or she would be maximally sensitive to how such matters are defined within the local communities. What are the standards for judging satisfaction or dissatisfaction within the most immediate relationships at

---

[4]Like Pirandello's *Six Characters in Search of an Author*, the practice of therapy has sometimes seemed like "100 Techniques in Search of a Theory." Surveying the psychotherapy field, Hoyt and Ordover (1988) called for a "unified field theory" to coordinate the various "strong forces" that theorists and practitioners have evolved. A constructionist perspective provides this meta-potential.

hand? At the same time, the therapist must remain concerned with the fuller range of relationships in which the immediate case is embedded. Meaning within the local condition is ultimately dependent upon broader cultural context. Again, this won't lead to a single standard. But the point is to allow the mix of standards into the therapeutic conversation.

HOYT: This gets at one of the challenges of a multicultural society, where different groups have different mores and standards. How do we steer between the Scylla of a Balkanized, "anything goes" separatism and the Charybdis of a colonization by the dominant culture?

GERGEN: It is in the mix of voices, it seems to me, that we find the answer—in the blending, appropriation, and paradox. Yet, a therapist could find a family in which a certain degree of incestual activity or physical abuse was tolerated—simply "not part of the problem" as they see it. In this sense, it wouldn't be the therapist's immediate task to deconstruct the family's system of beliefs (legal issues notwithstanding). However, given the ultimate interdependence of this family on the broader array of cultural meanings, in the longer run therapy might usefully be directed to coordinating family meanings (and actions) with those of the dominant society.

HOYT: In the last chapter of *Therapy as Social Construction* [McNamee & Gergen, 1992], Efran and Clarfield [1992] review what they consider to be "sense and nonsense" in constructionist therapy. They evoke Coyne's [1982] term "epistobabble" and note, to use their words [p. 200], that some critics dismiss such therapies as "little more than recombinations of familiar 'reframing' and team observation techniques already in use. They question whether constructionist lingo will prove any more substantive or long-lived than a dozen earlier infatuations." What do you see as truly different and likely to endure?

GERGEN: It's difficult to understand why Efran and Clarfield were so hostile—to almost everyone unfortunate enough to draw their gaze. I think disagreements can be useful and wonderful means toward new visions, but it seems primitive to me to abuse your colleagues in the ways they selected.

HOYT: Beyond the mean-spiritedness of their critique, what is added?

GERGEN: In my view, the importance of social constructionism to current therapeutic theory and practice is that it enables many practitioners to articulate emerging beliefs and practices in such a way that they can more clearly see (1) how they truly differ from the "modernist" tradition; (2) the similarities between what they are doing and what many others are doing in the field; and (3) how their orientation is related to a vast range of cultural changes, including major intellectual transformations in the academy and changes in societal life

patterns. I don't see constructionism as offering just another model
of therapy, another "silver bullet" cure, a specialized vocabulary, or
a new set of "musts." Rather, I see constructionism as inherent in a
vast array of conversations taking place around the world—conversations that bring people together over pressing issues of common
concern. To be sure, there are a circumscribed array of topics in these
conversations, and in this sense constructionist discussions cannot
do everything one might wish. However, they do raise fundamental
questions about long-cherished traditions in Western culture. Given
the rapid changes taking place in meanings, values, and practices,
and the enormous conflicts among meaning systems around the
world, they are likely to remain focal for some time.

HOYT: Raising consciousness via the question, as Watzlawick [1976] put
it, "How real is real?", recognizing that we are "constructive" [Hoyt,
1994a] and that reality is "invented" [Watzlawick, 1984], could have,
if not a humbling effect, at least suggest some pause and respect. It
could open dialogic space, one would hope. In this regard, let me
note that in your foreword [Gergen, 1993] to Friedman's *The New
Language of Change,* you comment that this shift entails a "formidable
change of seas" in which there is "the suspicion of all reality posits
. . . coupled with a related distrust of the authoritative voice" [p. x].
Given that we cannot stand outside the equation, how can we
practice therapy without imposing our values or ethics?

GERGEN: There is no therapy that stands outside values or ethics; even
the most politically neutral therapist is acting for good or ill by some
standard. Given this fact, many therapists are drawn to the conclusion that therapy should thereby operate as advocacy. If we are
bound to be advocates in any case, it is reasoned, then why not be
clear and open about what it is we stand for and what we are against,
and use therapy to build a better society? In certain ways I am drawn
to this kind of thinking; it is surely an improvement over the old
modernist attempt to step outside the conversation by declaring
value neutrality. However, I also worry about the implications of the
advocacy orientation if it is fully extended. Can you imagine the
results for the profession if we split into hundreds of political
encampments—the gay, the gray, the lesbian, the black, the Chicano,
the Asian, and so on—each with suspicion or antipathy toward the
other? This would be multiculturalism gone mad. If we separate
along moral–political lines, not only do we diminish the possibility
for dialogue and communality, but we also generate a therapeutic
world of all against all. Perhaps you can see again why I favor forms
of therapy that enable people to speak in many voices, to compre-
hend the paradoxes in their own values, to appreciate the positive

force of many local intelligibilities. The challenge here would not be to locate the one right position, ethic, or political ideal; nor would it be to suppress informed political action. Rather, it is to enable people to move with greater fluidity in the world, with a greater potential perhaps for coordinating the disparate as opposed to eradicating the opposition.[5]

HOYT: You have written eloquently [Gergen, 1995b] about ways that the therapeutic professions have developed and disseminated a language of mental deficit—a language that creates hierarchies, dependencies, and endless ways of constructing the self as deficient. We now seem to have a flood of new self disorders, such as multiple personality disorder, narcissistic disorder, borderline disorder, codependency, and the like. How can we redress this situation? Can we reeducate the profession, the media, and the public?[6]

GERGEN: I do think the therapeutic community has provided an invaluable resource to people over the years, and particularly as the traditional social bonds have eroded. As families, committed friendships, and communities disappear into the past, therapists continue to "be there" for support, insight, renewal, and the like. And given our technologies of saturation, this trend is only likely to continue. However, if there is one marked failure of the therapeutic communities, it is not in terms of outcome evaluation. (Personally, I think outcome evaluations are no more than window dressing for a given school of therapy, and the entire concept is misleading.) Rather, there has been a profound disservice in generating an enormous set of concepts through which people can see themselves as deficient. Worse, these vocabularies are self-serving; when people come to

[5]"Being transparent," laying our cards on the table, can help reduce subtle or duplicitous manipulation; but we may also need to embrace, not erase, inevitable tensions. Writing within the context of race relations, West (1994, pp. 150–151) suggests jazz as a useful metaphor: "I use the term 'jazz' here not so much as a term for a musical art form, as for a mode of being in the world, an improvisational mode of protean, fluid, and flexible dispositions toward reality suspicious of 'either/or' viewpoints, dogmatic pronouncements, or supremacist ideologies. . . . The interplay of individuality and unity is not one of uniformity and unanimity imposed from above but rather a conflict among diverse groupings that reach a dynamic consensus subject to questioning and criticism. As with a soloist in a jazz quartet, quintet, or band, individuality is promoted in order to sustain and increase the *creative* tension with the group—a tension that yields higher levels of performance to achieve the aim of the collective project."

[6]See the discussion by de Shazer and Weakland (Hoyt, 1994b), "On the Importance of Keeping It Simple and Taking the Patient Seriously," including their discussion of whether one functions as a mental *health* professional or a mental *illness* professional; see also Gergen's (1994a) remarks, "On Taking *Ourselves* Seriously." Some commentators, such as Masson (1994), seem to have gone so far as to conclude that the whole idea of professional psychotherapy is inherently wrong, and have suggested that it be abandoned and replaced with self-help groups.

believe they possess these "diseases" or "failings," a therapist is required for "cure."

Yes, to be sure, education can be an important means of redress. However, this first means a major change within the therapeutic community. That is, it is first necessary to get our own house in order. Family therapists have been in the vanguard of criticism of diagnosis; however, there is simultaneously a move within the family arena to develop an entirely new range of deficit categories—namely, relational diagnostics. And there are still the clinical psychology and psychiatric professions for whom these deficit categories are no less than maps of the real world.

Coupled with this self-critical effort, and perhaps more realistic, is the decoupling of diagnosis and third-party billing procedures.[7] So long as diagnostic categories are necessary for insurance payments, the professions will knuckle under. This procedure can and should be reversed. After all, we have learned to live with "no-fault" divorce processes. Why can the same logic not apply in the case of difficulties in living? The day is also soon coming when an activist ex-mental patient will bring lawsuits against therapists for such unjustifiable and injurious classification. Perhaps such litigation can speed the process of change.

HOYT: Some cultures, such as the traditional Balinese (Suryani & Jensen, 1993], create or construct "selves" that in some ways resemble the condition we call "multiple personality disorder" [MPD]. Other writers, such as Glass [1993] in *Shattered Selves: Multiple Personality in a Postmodern World,* are very critical of postmodern conceptions of the self, arguing that true MPD[8] is a fragmentation of self resulting from horrible childhood abuse and that such individuals suffer greatly for having to live without a firm identity. How do you see the relationship between a postmodern view of "self" and "multiple personality disorder"?

GERGEN: First, the assumptions embraced by Glass—that there simply are "MPD" persons in the world, and that they chiefly suffer from the lack of a firm identity—are exactly the kind of mentality I view as detrimental to the culture. Such presumptions not only serve to objectify the "illness," and to suggest that others may also possess

---

[7]See Wylie's trenchant (1995) article, "Diagnosing for Dollars?", in the *Family Therapy Networker* issue "The Power of DSM-IV." See also Blum (1978) and Tomm (1990). Long ago Ambrose Bierce (1906/1957) offered this definition from *The Devil's Dictionary:* "*Diagnosis,* n, A physician's forecast of disease by the patient's pulse and purse" (1957, p. 36).

[8]MPD is now called "dissociative identity disorder" in the DSM-IV (American Psychiatric Association, 1994). A good pros and cons summary of issues is available in Spiegel and McHugh (1995).

this particular infirmity, but as well imply that there is something privileged in a state of "unified and coherent" being. In a certain sense, then, this kind of analysis is part of the problem.

Now this is not to doubt that Glass confronts clients who are in deep pain, and that they can understand themselves in just the way he describes. But there are many other ways in which one's personality can be rendered meaningful—many alternative conceptions that can be generated of what he is authoritatively classifying as "MPD." And many of these alternatives would, in my view, be far more promising for the client (and society) as they move from therapeutic relations into daily life.[9]

There is also a certain genre of postmodern writing that provides just such a promise. If one feels split among selves, torn between competing tendencies, capable of multiple personalities, this literature suggests that such a condition may be the newly emerging cultural form. And it is not to be lamented—but explored for its potential riches. Contributions to this genre would include the work of Jim Wertsch [1985, 1991] in psychology, and Peggy Penn [1982, 1985; Penn & Frankfurt, 1994] in family therapy.

HOYT: Reading through some of the chapters in *The Saturated Self* in the rapid way you recommend [Gergen, 1991, p. 49] did produce the existentially dizzying, almost disorienting "multiphrenic"[10] effect

---

[9]As Grove and Haley (1993, p. 183) report: "[Milton] Erickson did not approach the phenomenon of having more than one personality as a form of psychopathology. Instead, Erickson would treat the problem as the client actually possessing two or more personalities which happened to occupy the same body. . . . In Erickson's approach, the goal was not to try to merge the personalities or to search for additional personalities. The goal was to persuade the personalities to communicate directly with each other and to learn to collaborate while sharing the same body. . . . Additional personalities are not thought of as dissociated states to be merged. Instead they are seen as helpers who can collaborate and make a positive contribution to the life of the total person." In an extended case report, Grove (1993, pp. 16–17) elaborates: "There are several advantages to this orientation. By approaching secondary personalities as real individuals with their own independent needs and motivations, the therapist can more easily win the trust and cooperation of the secondary personalities. Resistance by the secondary personalities over the idea that the therapist wants to 'kill' them by having them merge is reduced. Resistance by the dominant personality over the idea that they possess multiple personalities can be lessened by focusing on what the client is most motivated to change, such as eliminating amnesia and undesirable behaviors conducted by the secondary personalities. Because the client's presentation of having multiple personalities is not viewed as a psychopathology, the therapist can approach all personalities with a more positive view. Personalities can be framed as having special abilities and motivated to help each other." For a related perspective, see O'Hanlon's discussion in Chapter 4 of treating a patient with "MPD."

[10]Gergen (1991, p. 16) describes "the fragmenting and populating of self-experience, a condition I call 'multiphrenia.' Critical to my argument is the proposal that social saturation brings with it a general loss of our assumption of true and knowable selves. As we absorb multiple voices, we find that each 'truth' is relativized by our (*continued*)

that, by parallel process, was the subject. The medium became the message, as Marshall McLuhan [1964] said. Writers such as Kegan [1994] have suggested that we're "in over our heads," that the complexity of (post)modern life exceeds our cognitive grasp. In "multiphrenia," what will provide a sense of stability/identity/self?[11]

GERGEN: As you might guess from what I just said, we might ask, "What is necessarily wrong with 'instability' and 'fragmentation'?" These are, after all, negative labels for conditions that might also be described as "fascinating," "exciting," and "transformative," on the one hand, and "multi-faceted" or "richly complex" on the other. The opposite of instability could be viewed as a boring and oppressive status quo, while the opposite of fragmentation might be seen as rigidity and narrow-mindedness.

This is not to say that I wish to abandon the quest for stability and simplicity. There are days and hours in which I long for it. But I can also understand these wishes in terms of my immersion in a cultural history in which these conditions are valued, and understand that these yearnings are not for something fundamental, deeply ingrained in nature. They are simply one of the facets or desires of self within the vast multiplicity. That idea in itself I find helpful.

HOYT: What will *character* mean in a postmodern world? How do we understand *ethics* and *integrity* (acting consistent with one's values) if we are "saturated" and "polymorphous"?

GERGEN: I do feel that postmodern writers have been unfairly criticized for their inability to support firm moral values and their exploration of relativism.[12] For who in this century, outside the highly parochial and fanatic, are willing to declare what is good and right for all people for all time? The postmodern writers are too frequently scapegoated for the incapacities of those who criticize.

(continued from p. 357) simultaneous consciousness of compelling alternatives. We come to be aware that each truth about ourselves is a construction of the moment true only for a given time and within certain relationships."

[11]Tom Hanks, the actor who played the title role in the film *Forrest Gump*, described preparing for the part: "I went to a school for mentally challenged kids who are now adults. But Forrest wasn't quite like that. It was more like creating an alien. What are the rules of his world? It was like creating a whole new take on the universe" (Morrison, 1994, p. 49). His intellectual limitations and resultant literalism seemed to render Forrest a kind of "master of deconstruction." Is part of Forrest's wide appeal that he is today's Everyman (and Everywoman) looking for simple truths amidst the multiphrenia? Everyone is not as sweet and open-minded as Forrest, however. Might there be the peril that too much complexity, especially if coupled with economic hard times, could generate a backlash "escape from freedom" (Fromm, 1976) of reactionary fundamentalism?

[12]See the exchange between Gergen (1994b; also 1985a) and Smith (1994), plus Comment (1995), for their (and others') responses to the dialogue.

I also feel that in their explorations of relativism, multiple selves, and constructed realities, postmodern writings open important new vistas in our comprehension of morality and for practices more fully suited to living together in a world of differences. They suggest, for one, that we should cease looking to a slate of ideals, ethical foundations, a code of justice, or canons of morality in order to create "good persons" or "the just society." High-sounding words and phrases themselves require nothing in the way of subsequent action, and may be interpreted in so many ways that even the most violent persecution can be justified on the basis of the most glowing ideals. I believe we should turn away from abstract justifications and look to *ourselves*, to our relationships. For it is out of these relationships that we generate the hells for ourselves that we term *unjust, oppressive, immoral,* and so on.

HOYT: I take what you're saying as suggesting a higher moral challenge. If we give up the notion of an "ultimate truth," then we have to take full responsibility for all of our constructions and actions, *and* realize that others are just as entitled to theirs.

GERGEN: Almost. Faced now with ourselves, we may then *together* ask about the kinds of practices that bring about these conditions, and the ways in which these practices might be altered. This kind of thinking has also inspired some work I am doing with Sheila McNamee [McNamee & Gergen, 1995], on what we are calling "relational responsibility." Here we are raising criticisms with the traditional view of holding individuals morally responsible for problematic actions, and trying to develop some conversational resources that might enable people to explore the forms of relatedness in which the problematic action takes place.

HOYT: I expect that this may be related to the experience you wrote about [Gergen, 1994c, pp. 76–77] in "The Limits of Pure Critique." Let me quote at length:

At the beginning of a three-day conference, the organizers arranged a confrontation pitting radical constructivism (as represented by Ernst von Glazerfeld) against social constructionism (which I was to profess). The subsequent critiques were unsparing, the defenses unyielding, and as the audience was drawn into the debate polarization rapidly took place. Voices became agitated, critique turned ad hominem, anger and alienation mounted. As the moderator called a halt to the proceedings, I began to see the three days before me as an eternity. . . . Here [Karl] Tomm asked if von Glazerfeld and I would be willing to be publicly interviewed. Most important, would we be willing to do so *as the other*? Uneasily, we agreed. . . . Our exposure to each other did allow each of us to absorb aspects of the other—intellectual views, attitudes, values—which we now carried with us as potentials. The initial question was whether we were willing and able to give these potentials credible voice. Through an extended series of questions, carefully and sensitively addressed, Tomm was able to elicit 'the other within.' Playing the other's identity, we discussed issues of theory, views of the other, self-doubts, fears, personal relationships, feelings about the conference and so on.

The results of the procedure were striking. As both we and the audience learned, we could communicate intelligibly and sympathetically from within the other's framework. Each could give voice to the rationality of the other. Further, the binary was successfully broken. Rather than a showdown between competing epistemologies, the debate could be understood within the context of a long interpersonal history, imbricated friendships, private aspirations and doubts, the demands of public debate and so on. A new level of discussion ensued. The conference was thereafter marked by its civility of interchange; there was expression without domination, careful listening and sensitive reply. No, this did not mean a resolution of differences; the lines of difference remained clear. However, it did allow the exploration to move forward, and with the resulting emergency of new complexities, the old yearnings for victory and defeat—heroes and villains—receded from view.

When I recently asked David Epston what he would like to ask you, he called my attention to this passage and said he would ask, "Where do you think you will take such developments both in the realm of ideas and everyday life from here?" Pray tell?

GERGEN: On the theoretical side, you might imagine from my earlier comments that my major concern is with expanding consciousness of relatedness. I call this "relational theory," a project that begins with *Realities and Relationships*, but has since expanded in several directions. Given the quotation you just cited, you can imagine that such theorizing is directed toward more practical domains—including therapy, education, organizational management, and politics. The challenge is to bring about metaphors, stories, distinctions, images, and so on that don't so much reflect what is, but create what can be. I also work with various therapists, organizational consultants, global businesses, and the like to develop practices that embody a relational perspective. With some friends, we created The Taos Institute, an institute centered in New Mexico that brings theorists and practitioners together to work on cutting-edge issues in relational process. Perhaps the most wonderful thing about this kind of work is that you never feel you are alone—fully responsible for all the ideas, plans, practices, outcomes, and so on. The work becomes lighter, more joyous, and more optimistic. Also, I find the creative potential of dialogue is just enormous.

HOYT: The work of Michel Foucault [e.g., 1975, 1978, 1980], especially his views on the relationship of power and knowledge, has influenced many therapists working within narrative constructive frameworks. Not everyone is so impressed, however. Camille Paglia [1992, p. 174] has written: "Foucault's biggest fans are not among the majority of philosophers, historians, and sociologists, who usually perceive his glaring inadequacies of knowledge and argument, but among well-meaning but foggy humanists, who virtually never have the intellectual and scholarly preparation to critique Foucault competently. The more you know, the less you are impressed by Foucault." What do you think of Foucault's contribution, and what do you think of Paglia's dismissal?

GERGEN: To pick up on an earlier theme, I don't look to Foucault or any other writer now for "the truth," nor for a perfect and well-defended logic, new set of guides, ideals, or premises for a new life. Rather, from my constructionist background, I am inclined to ask whether a given piece of writing can offer resources for the kinds of conversations in which I now find myself. If I borrow from the words, the metaphors, the logics within the writing, what happens now to my various relationships? In this sense I have found certain Foucaultian concepts very useful—as have many others. They seem to help us do things in conversations that we could less easily or not possibly do before. No, I don't find all of Foucault so useful; by contemporary American standards the writing is often opaque, incoherent, and mystifying, and his major analyses of history unjustifiable. However, in his critiques of earlier views of power, and in his emphasis on the relationship of language to power and on the effect of various professional discourses on society, for example, he has been enormously useful.

HOYT: How about Paglia?

GERGEN: Along these same lines, I don't find Paglia so very helpful. If I put her discourse into action, I am more likely to find myself in a set of conflictual and aggressive relationships. To borrow her discourse too often leads to an argumentative form of relationship in which mutual annihilation is the implicit end. Do we need more of this in our current cultural condition?

HOYT: In "The Social Construction of Narrative Accounts," you and Mary Gergen [M. M. Gergen & Gergen, 1984; see also K. J. Gergen & Gergen, 1986, 1988; M. M. Gergen & Gergen, 1993] discuss *progressive*, *stabilizing*, and *regressive* narratives. You also comment [1984, p. 177] that what might look "regressive" could be a part of a forward movement ("unless the crisis is viewed as a critical integer in a progressive narrative") or a larger homeostasis. As the French say, to make an omelette you have first to break the eggs. With multiphrenia and such a complexity of competing goals, how is primacy established? What dialectic, what values guide complex, competing choices?

GERGEN: Perhaps I can answer this in a way that will clarify what I was trying to say regarding value positions. It seems to me that in the Western tradition we are supposed to possess some personal logic, set of values, or well-considered aim in life that should guide us through such complex situations. Yet, it is just such a view that social constructionism calls into question. From this perspective logic, values, aims, and the like are positions in language. As language they do not require any particular form of action; they are action in themselves. And if they occur privately (what we have traditionally considered "in the mind"), nothing necessarily follows in terms of "choices" (another term heavily weighted by our psychologistic and individualistic tradition).

Further, as I have tried to stress, we might usefully see intelligible action in terms of its place within a set of relationships. In this context, rather than trying to work out a fully developed set of priorities abstracted from concrete conditions of relationship, it seems more promising from the constructionist standpoint to immerse oneself more fully within ongoing relationships. This does not mean acting only within the present moment, for one is also a participant in numerous other relationships. These relationships, too, should ideally be made salient to the ongoing process. I rather like as an illustration the actions of the unmarried pregnant adolescents interviewed in Gilligan's [1982] In a Different Voice. When confronted with the difficult question of abortion, they didn't resort to abstract principles, but primarily engaged in an array of conversations—with friends, parents, the potential father, and so on.[13] From the process of relating, decisions emerged—decisions which were presumably lodged within the array of existing coordinations.[14]

---

[13]In fairness to Camille Paglia, in light of the earlier discussion it should be noted that in a recent interview (Paglia, 1995, p. 58), she too advocates—without abandoning her in-your-face style—that recognition be given to the legitimacy of competing views in the abortion controversy: "The people who are pro-abortion—I hate the cowardly euphemism of pro-choice—must face what they are opposing. The left constantly identifies the pro-life advocates as misogynists and fanatics, but that doesn't represent most of those people. They are deeply religious and they truly believe that taking a life is wrong. If the left were to show respect for that position and acknowledge the moral conundrum of unwanted pregnancy, the opposition to abortion would lessen. We must acknowledge that people should be a little troubled by abortion. Not to acknowledge that this is a difficult decision is wrong. . . . You have a stronger case if you give due respect to the other side."

[14]As the well-known business negotiator Chester Karrass (1992, p. 11) observes, "The children of tomorrow must be good negotiators. They must be prepared to resolve differences in a civilized way; to listen; to be responsible; and to be unafraid to (continued)

HOYT: There seem to be two opposite trends occurring simultaneously. One involves the emergence of the "relational self," the other a tendency toward greater isolation and loneliness. Do you agree? How do you understand the "relational self" and what's happening?

GERGEN: There are a number of ways to go with this question; let me try only one. There is a sense in which I want to argue that all selves are relational, and always have been. (This position is part of my own attempt to create a sense of the reality of relatedness.) Unless a feral child or severely cerebrally damaged, even the isolated individual (for example, the elderly shut-in or the derelict) is immersed in otherness. At the same time, I think you are absolutely correct in your surmise that people are more physically isolated than ever before. This is part of the irony of *The Saturated Self*. The very technologies that bring the teeming array of images, voices, dramas, logics, and so on into our lives (e.g., television, radio, mass print, telephone, VCRs, personal computers), are also the same technologies that allow us to exist without others' physical presence. So we are more multiply related but more physically alone. I worry a great deal about this trend; the consequences for society are profound. A major interest for me now is whether we might use some of these same technologies (and especially computer networks) to generate new forms of community.

HOYT: The information and networking possibilities are thrilling, but I hope "virtual reality" and "cybersex" won't replace older forms! In *We've Had a Hundred Years of Psychotherapy and the World's Getting Worse*, James Hillman and Michael Ventura [1992] argue that the pendulum has swung too far toward the individual self, producing a narcissistic preoccupation, and call for a greater identification with society. Some religious and spiritual practices also advocate connection to humanity or nature as part of a larger sense of self. How does this fit with your idea of the relational self?

GERGEN: I entirely agree with the thesis that the pendulum has swung too far toward the individual self. A narcissistic preoccupation is only one of the problematic consequences. I'm less positive about a solution which requires a greater identification with society, as it suggests that I exist separate from society. In the same way I can resonate with some spiritual, religious, and ecological movements which generate a sense of our greater relatedness. A great deal of my recent work explores the ways in which we are always already constituted by relationship. As I mentioned earlier, I try to focus on

---

(*continued from p. 362*) adjust conflicting values. The alternative in an age of rising expectations is violence." He goes on (p. 215) to give some sage marital advice: "Love, honor, and negotiate."

various ways in which to be a self, to have an idea, to possess an emotion is to be acting out of and into relatedness. And as in the case of the work with McNamee [McNamee & Gergen, 1995], we try to generate practices of relationship (as opposed to individual) responsibility. I am also working with therapists and organizational consultants to bring these kinds of ideas into practice, and with an artist and a filmmaker in trying to give this consciousness a visual dimension.

HOYT: In an earlier discussion with Michael White and Gene Combs [see Chapter 2], I promised to ask you about your remarks at the end of your keynote speech at the Therapeutic Conversations 2 conference in Washington, D.C., when you commented that "We don't live in narratives, we live with them," and spoke of moving "beyond stories to relatedness itself."[15] It's hard to talk about what is beyond words. At the risk of asking an oxymoronic question, would you expound on the ineffable lightness of being?

GERGEN: My major aim in that conclusion was to "put language in its place."[16] That is, as we move in this constructionist and narrational direction, we sometimes fix on the words as ends in themselves. We try as therapists to generate new sense of meaning, new narratives, new constructions, as if a new set of words would "do the trick." In fact, I tend to talk that way myself at times. However, this is to miss

[15]Gergen's (1994d) words: "So is it right that we live in narratives? Well, the communicational view, this relational view that I'm trying to develop here would say, 'No, we don't live in them, we live *with* them. They are what we *do* with people. . . .' Well, if that's the case—and this is the part that interests me—is it possible that we could imagine therapy or relationships themselves as moving to the point where pure relatedness is honored before the meaning? When you move, let's say, with a client not to the point where they've got a good or better story, but *beyond* stories to relatedness itself. I tried at one place to call this a kind of 'relational sublime,' beyond reason. A sublime state where one is simply in an inarticulable sense of relatedness with others, with the world—not like swimming in an ocean, but more like being in the ocean and moving with all the waves, not like having a direction but moving in synchrony. A kind of inarticulable state beyond meaning where one is simply *embedded with*: that intrigues me."

[16]As Gergen (1991, p. 157) explained in *The Saturated Self*: "The case is clarified by focusing on the languages of self-construction—the words and phrases one uses to characterize the self. . . . It is impossible to sustain the traditional view of language as an outer expression of an inner reality. If language truly served as the public expression of one's private world, there would be no means by which we could understand each other. Rather, language is inherently a form of relatedness. Sense is derived only from coordinated effort among persons. One's words remain nonsense (mere sounds or markings) until supplemented by another's assent (or appropriate action). And this assent, too, remains dumb until another (or others) lend it a sense of meaning. . . . In this way, meaning is born of interdependence. And because there is no self outside a system of meaning, it may be said that relations precede and are more fundamental than self. Without relationship there is no language with which to conceptualize the emotions, thoughts, or intentions of the self."

the ultimate concern, which is relatedness itself—out of which meanings are generated. In effect, relations precede meaning.

However, in trying to speak about moving "beyond stories to relatedness itself" I find myself resisting clarity, wanting rather to move by intimation. This is because in the struggle to articulate a state of relatedness out of which articulation springs, you rather place walls around that state; you construct it as "this as opposed to that."[17] And in doing so relations themselves are delimited. So I look to metaphors, ambiguous concepts, or parables. In the concept of a *relational sublime*, I borrowed heavily from the Romanticist idea of a mental condition which transcends the capacity of rational comprehension [Gergen, in press]. The Romanticists often used the term to depict a condition in which one sensed the incomprehensible scope and power of nature (and by implication, God). I rather like these images, and feel that we might develop a sense of ourselves as fully immersed in relatedness—with all humanity, all that is given—and that we might conceive of this awesome sensibility of pure relatedness (itself born of relationship) as approaching what we might mean by the domain of the spiritual.

HOYT: We're all in this together. Thank you.

REFERENCES

American Psychiatric Association (1994). *Diagnostic and Statistical Manual of Mental Disorders* (4th ed.). Washington, DC: Author.

Bakhtin, M. (1981). *The Dialogic Imagination.* Austin: University of Texas Press.

Bierce, A. (1957). *The Devil's Dictionary.* New York: Sagamore Press. (Original work published 1906)

Blum, J. D. (1978). On changes in psychiatric diagnosis over time. *American Psychologist, 33,* 1017–1031.

Bruner, J. (1989). *Actual Minds, Possible Worlds.* Cambridge, MA: Harvard University Press.

Comment (1995). *American Psychologist, 50*(5), 389–394.

Coyne, J. C. (1982). A brief introduction to epistobabble. *Family Therapy Networker, 6*(4), 27–28.

Efran, J. S., & Clarfield, L. E. (1992). Constructionist therapy: Sense and nonsense. In S. McNamee & K. J. Gergen (Eds.), *Therapy as Social Construction* (pp. 200–217). Newbury Park, CA: Sage.

Ellenberger, H. F. (1970). *The Discovery of the Unconscious.* New York: Basic Books.

Foucault, M. (1975). *The Birth of the Clinic.* New York: Vintage.

---

[17]See Rosenbaum and Dyckman's discussion in Chapter 11 about how we delimit ourselves by constructing what we will *not* include within our identities; related ideas are also discussed by O'Hanlon in Chapter 4 and Gilligan in Chapter 10.

Foucault, M. (1977). *Discipline and Punish: The Birth of the Prison.* New York: Pantheon.

Foucault, M. (1980). *Power/Knowledge: Selected Interviews and Other Writings, 1972–1977.* New York: Pantheon.

Freud, S. (1953). Three essays on the theory of sexuality. In J. Strachey (Ed. and Trans.), *The Standard Edition of the Complete Psychological Works of Sigmund Freud* (Vol. 7, pp. 125–243). London: Hogarth Press. (Original work published 1905)

Fromm, E. (1976). *Escape from Freedom.* New York: Avon.

Gergen, K. J. (1985a). The social constructionist movement in modern psychology. *American Psychologist, 40,* 266–275.

Gergen, K. J. (1985). *Toward Transformation in Social Knowledge* (2nd ed.). Beverly Hills, CA: Sage.

Gergen, K. J. (1991). *The Saturated Self: Dilemmas of Identity in Contemporary Life.* New York: Basic Books.

Gergen, K. J. (1992). *The Polymorphous Perversity of the Postmodern Era.* Keynote speech, Family Therapy Networker Conference, Washington, DC.

Gergen, K. J. (1993). Foreword. In S. Friedman (Ed.), *The New Language of Change: Constructive Collaboration in Psychotherapy* (pp. ix–xi). New York: Guilford Press.

Gergen, K. J. (1994a). On taking *ourselves* seriously. *Journal of Systemic Therapies, 13*(4), 10–12.

Gergen, K. J. (1994b). Exploring the postmodern: Perils or potentials? *American Psychologist, 49,* 412–416.

Gergen, K. J. (1994c). The limits of pure critique. In H. A. Simons & M. Billig (Eds.), *After Postmodernism: Reconstructing Ideology* (pp. 58–78). Newbury Park, CA: Sage.

Gergen, K. J. (1994d). *Between Alienation and Deconstruction: Re-Envisioning Therapeutic Communication.* Keynote speech, Therapeutic Conversations 2 Conference, Washington, DC.

Gergen, K. J. (1995a). *Realities and Relationships: Soundings in Social Construction.* Cambridge, MA: Harvard University Press.

Gergen, K. J. (1995b). Therapeutic professions and the diffusion of deficit. In K. J. Gergen, *Realities and Relationships: Soundings in Social Construction.* Cambridge, MA: Harvard University Press. (An abbreviated version appeared in *Journal of Mind and Behavior,* 1990, *11,* 353–368.)

Gergen, K. J. (in press). Technology and the self: From the essential to the sublime. In D. Grodin & T. Lindlof (Eds.), *Constructing the Self in a Mediated Age.* Thousand Oaks, CA: Sage.

Gergen, K.J., & Davis, K.E. (Eds.). (1985). *The Social Construction of the Person.* New York: Springer-Verlag.

Gergen, K. J., & Gergen, M. M. (Eds.). (1984). *Historical Social Psychology.* Hillsdale, NJ: Erlbaum.

Gergen, K. J., & Gergen, M. M. (1986). Narrative form and the construction of psychological science. In T. R. Sarbin (Ed.), *Narrative Psychology: The Storied Nature of Human Conduct.* New York: Praeger.

Gergen, K. J., & Gergen, M. M. (1988). Narrative and the self as relationship. In L. Berkowitz (Ed.), *Advances in Experimental Social Psychology* (Vol. 21, pp. 17–56). New York: Academic Press.

Gergen, M. M., & Gergen, K. J. (1984). The social construction of narrative accounts.

In K. J. Gergen & M. M. Gergen (Eds.), *Historical Social Psychology* (pp. 173–189). Hillsdale, NJ: Erlbaum.

Gergen, M. M., & Gergen, K. J. (1993). Narratives of the gendered body in popular autobiography. In R. Josselson & A. Lieblich (Eds.), *The Narrative Study of Lives* (pp. 191–218). Newbury Park, CA: Sage.

Gilligan, C. (1982). *In a Different Voice.* Cambridge, MA: Harvard University Press.

Glass, J. M. (1993). *Shattered Selves: Multiple Personality in a Postmodern World.* Ithaca, NY: Cornell University Press.

Gordon, C. & Gergen, K. J. (Eds.). (1968). *The Self in Social Interaction.* New York: Wiley.

Graumann, C. F., & Gergen, K. J. (Eds.). (1993). *Historical Dimensions of Psychological Discourse.* New York: Cambridge University Press.

Grove, D. R. (1993). Ericksonian therapy with multiple personality clients. *Journal of Family Psychotherapy, 4*(2), 13–18.

Grove, D. R., & Haley, J. (1993). *Conversations on Therapy: Popular Problems and Uncommon Solutions.* New York: Norton.

Hillman, J., & Ventura, M. (1992). *We've Had a Hundred Years of Psychotherapy and the World's Getting Worse.* New York: HarperCollins.

Hoyt, M. F. (1994a). Introduction: Competency-based future-oriented therapy. In M. F. Hoyt (Ed.), *Constructive Therapies* (pp. 1–10). New York: Guilford Press.

Hoyt, M. F. (1994b). On the importance of keeping it simple and taking the patient seriously: A conversation with Steve de Shazer and John Weakland. In M. F. Hoyt (Ed.), *Constructive Therapies* (pp. 11–40). New York: Guilford Press.

Hoyt, M. F., & Ordover, J. (1988). Book review of J. K. Zeig (Ed.), *The Evolution of Psychotherapy. Imagination, Cognition, and Personality, 8*(2), 181–186.

Karrass, C. L. (1992). *The Negotiating Game* (rev. ed.). New York: HarperCollins.

Kegan, R. (1994). *In Over Our Heads: The Mental Demands of Modern Life.* Cambridge, MA: Harvard University Press.

Mahler, M., Bergman, A., & Pine, F. (1975). *The Psychological Birth of the Human Infant.* New York: Basic Books.

Masson, J. M. (1994). *Against Therapy* (rev. ed.). Monroe, ME: Common Courage Press.

Maturana, H. R., & Varela, F. J. (1987). *The Tree of Knowledge.* Boston: New Science Library.

McLuhan, M. (1964). *Understanding Media: The Extension of Man.* New York: Signet.

McNamee, S., & Gergen, K. J. (Eds.). (1992). *Therapy as Social Construction.* Newbury Park, CA: Sage.

McNamee, S., & Gergen, K. E. (1995). *Relational responsibility.* Unpublished manuscript, University of New Hampshire.

Mead, G. H. (1934). *Mind, Self and Society.* Chicago: University of Chicago Press.

Morrison, M. (1994, August). The evolution of Tom Hanks. *Us: The Entertainment Magazine,* pp. 46–52.

Paglia, C. (1992). Junk bonds and corporate raiders: Academe in the hour of the wolf. In C. Paglia, *Sex, Art, and American Culture: Essays* (pp. 170–248). New York: Vintage.

Paglia, C. (1995, May). Interview. *Playboy,* pp. 51–64.

Penn, P. (1982). Circular questioning. *Family Process, 21*(3), 267–280.

Penn, P. (1985). Feed-forward: Future questions, future maps. *Family Process, 24*(3), 299–310.

Penn, P., & Frankfurt, M. (1994). Creating a participant text: Writing, multiple voices, narrative multiplicity. *Family Process, 33*(3), 217–231.

Semin, G., & Gergen, K. J. (Eds.). (1990). *Everyday Understanding: Social and Scientific Implications.* Newbury Park, CA: Sage.

Shotter, J., & Gergen, K. J. (Eds.). (1989). *Texts of Identity.* Newbury Park, CA: Sage.

Singer, J. A., & Salovey, P. (1993). *The Remembered Self: Emotion and Memory in Personality.* New York: Free Press.

Smith, M. B. (1994). Selfhood at risk: Postmodern perils and the perils of postmodernism. *American Psychologist, 49,* 405–411.

Spiegel, D., & McHugh, P. (1995). The pros and cons of dissociative identity (multiple personality) disorder. *Journal of Practical Psychiatry and Behavioral Health, 1*(13), 158–166.

Stern, D. N. (1985). *The Interpersonal World of the Infant.* New York: Basic Books.

Suryani, L. K., & Jensen, G. D. (1993). *Trance and Possession in Bali: A Window on Western Multiple Personality Disorder, Possession, and Suicide.* Oxford: Oxford University Press.

Tomm, K. (1990). A critique of the DSM. *Dulwich Centre Newsletter, 2*(3), 5–8.

Vygotsky, L. S. (1986). *Thought and Language* (rev. ed.). Cambridge, MA: MIT Press.

Watzlawick, P. (1976). *How Real Is Real?* New York: Random House.

Watzlawick, P. (Ed.). (1984). *The Invented Reality: How Do We Know What We Believe We Know?* New York: Norton.

Wertsch, J. V. (Ed.). (1985). *Vygotsky and the Social Formation of Mind.* Cambridge, MA: Harvard University Press.

Wertsch, J. V. (1991). *Voices of the Mind: A Sociocultural Approach to Mediated Action.* Cambridge, MA: Harvard University Press.

West, C. (1994). *Race Matters.* New York: Vintage.

Wylie, M. S. (1995). Diagnosing for dollars? *Family Therapy Networker, 19*(3), 22–33.

Songs for
Constructive Therapists

TRANCEPLANTS

Bill O'Hanlon

I worked in your garden
I really grew a lot
Most of the things you taught me
I'm sure that I forgot
So I had to start all over
With a garden of my own
And wish that you could see it
And the ways that I have grown

> *Chorus:*
> You plant a seed and you don't know what will grow
> But you'll get what you need, something inside will know
> You gave me room and now that you are gone
> My garden is in bloom and your seeds will carry on

When winter breezes blow
You might think they'll never end
But every gardener knows
That spring brings growth again

> *Chorus:*
> You plant a seed and you don't know what will grow
> But you'll get what you need, something inside you knows
> You gave me room and now that you are gone
> My garden is in bloom and it's time to carry on

Note. Written in Mesa, Arizona, April 19, 1982, for Milton H. Erickson, MD. Copyright 1995 by Bill O'Hanlon. Reprinted by permission of the author.

RAPNOTIC INDUCTION NO. 1

(Courtesy of Discfunctional Records)

Joseph A. Goldfield

Word up to you all, it's fresh that you're here
To honor John Weakland's illustrious career
My style's indirect, but my message ain't oblique
You're in a win–win situation with my hip-hop technique
Forty years ago his ideas sounded criminal
Now today we know he's the master of the minimal
I'm paying my respects, Yo! I'm meta-rapping
Let's go back in time and see how it all happened:

It started in the '50s in unconnected places
Studying schizophrenic families and their homeostasis
There was some bloods ahead of their time
Mapping out the injunctions of the double bind
Circular epistemology of the feedback loop
These were early contributions of the Palo Alto group
But when it came to therapy change was slow
Pointing out the marital quid pro quo?!
They continued to describe cybernetics of psychosis
And got mesmerized by Ericksonian hypnosis

They all got excited, went their separate ways
Haley started going through a structural phase
Bateson went off studying dolphins and Zen
Weakland, Fisch, and Segal started doing it in ten
They were the first to promulgate the notion of Brief
Which went against the tenets of all mental health beliefs
Analysts and others were freaking and annoyed
'Cause they thought he was dissing on their main man, Freud!

But things are different today due to third-party payers
If you can't work briefly b-b-better say your prayers!
Insurance demands, "Treatment must be shorter"
There's a major change of the second order!

*   *   *

Therapy's an art 'cause it ain't just a science
What's the best stance when you're with your clients
Avoid the role of utopian savior
Pursue you clients' goals in concrete behavior!
Don't criticize! Don't be insistent!
When people lose face they become resistant!
Make overt what before was tacit
Have 'em utilize their symptom as an asset!

Note. Reprinted from the *Journal of Systemic Therapies*, 1993, *12*(2), 89–91. Copyright 1993 by Joseph A. Goldfield. Reprinted by permission of the author.

Don't use a lot of jargon! Don't show your technique!
Be guided by the language that your clients speak!
Act one down like Lieutenant Columbo
If your client catches on act like a dumbo!
Retain maneuverability, be sly like a fox
Your Achilles heel will be to sell the paradox

*   *   *

Strategic therapy, it ain't a big mystery
Check it out, here's my case history:

A chronic, obsessive–compulsive, depressive
Her list of stymied therapists was totally impressive
She's home all day, bored with TV
Her entire social life was coming to see me
I told her, "Let's go slow, might be risky being normal"
In a week she had a job! For her wedding I dressed formal

Rebellious adolescent flaunting individuation
His parents couldn't wait until his graduation
He wouldn't do his chores, not even the garbage
I end those wars with benign sabotage
He keeps his room clean now and his parents feel respected
My relapse prescription they all rejected!

A man was impotent, couldn't get pleasure
He tried even harder but that made more pressure
His wife thought her body had become boring
"Maybe there's other babes he's already scoring?"
I cured them in one session, pointing out the fact
He's overwhelmed by her beauty and can't perform the act!

It ain't that complex: problem resolution
When you address the attempted solution
When you do that change will happen fast
There'll be no need to analyze what happened in the past

*   *   *

John Weakland is our mentor, that ain't no lie
Working on his moves at the MRI
He's trained a lot of people, helped with their careers
Never cops an attitude when they mess with his ideas
Even wrote prefaces to their magnum opus
Like de Shazer's books on solution focus

We all wish him well, his contributions have no measure
Being here today has been a real pleasure
I could sing his praise for days, you know that's a fact
But I gotta stop rapping, 'cause I made a devil's pact!
I ain't reframing if that was your impression
No more of the same-ing, let's terminate this session!

MODERN MAJOR THERAPISTS

(Sung to the tune of Gilbert & Sullivan's "Modern Major General")
Robert Rosenbaum

1

I am a model psychoanalytical psychologist
Of matters mental mythical I am the chief apologist
Projective identification's not for me a terrorist
For I've introjected both my parents and of course my therapist.

So I flit from ego, id, to superego's trenchant grumble-ings
I use these to interpret all my patient's awful mumble-ings
When I submit my bill don't disagree with bold persistency . . .
Or I'll lay the trouble at your door and call it your resistancy.

Chorus:
He'll lay the trouble at your door and call it your resistancy
He'll lay the trouble at your door and call it your resistancy
He'll lay the trouble at your door and call it your resistance-istancy.

And don't bother me with facts because I'm awfully good avoiding 'em
My information's absolutely, resolutely Freudian
Of matters mental mythical I am the chief apologist
I am a model psychoanalytical psychologist.

2

I am the very model of a cognitive behaviorist
Empirical and rational, a paragon positivist
If feelings, affects, impulses or drives are making you distraught
Bring them to me, I'll exorcise them with the primacy of thought.

I've got rating scales and questionnaires applied with fine inanity
I use these to erase all trace of my patients' humanity
My therapeutic intervention's eminently practical . . .
Eschewing empathy I just rely on modes didactical.

Chorus:
Eschewing empathy he just relies on modes didactical
Eschewing empathy he just relies on modes didactical
Eschewing empathy he just relies on modes didacti-actical.

So don't bother me with hopes and dreams since I've got nothing
    to discuss
I'm terrified of anything that might come from my unconscious
Empirical and rational, a paragon positivist
I am the very model of a cognitive behaviorist.

3

I identify myself as an experiential humanist
Rogerian Gestaltist flavored with an existential twist
If your Inner Child is suffering a phase of life transitional
I'll give it positive regard in manner unconditional.

If you're symptomatic, hurt and seeking validation or repair
Attending to each moment I can treat you with an empty chair
While it's true all this is lacking diagnostic specificity . . .
I substitute intuitive holistic authenticity.

    Chorus:
    He substitutes intuitive holistic authenticity
    He substitutes intuitive holistic authenticity
    He substitutes intuitive holistic authentici-ticity.

And I'm sure my therapeutic work's tremendously effectual
I'm certain since I do avoid all aspects intellectual
Rogerian Gestaltist flavored with an existential twist
I identify myself as an experiential humanist.

4

A family therapist, I seek solutions quite systemically
I posit miracles to find resources hid endemically
If clients find my interventions less than inspirational
I re-con-text-u-a-lize complaints multi-generational.

I structure boundaries and paradox patients identified
If these techniques don't work I look for kids who've been parentified
Though interventions may seem rigid, lacking elasticity . . .
They function to restore systemic homeo-stasticity.

    Chorus:
    They function to restore systemic homeo-stasticity
    They function to restore systemic homeo-stasticity
    They function to restore systemic homeo-stastici-ticity.

Though I'm steeped in cybernetics I have one mild flaw residual
When *I* have problems, *I* want therapy that's individual.
I posit miracles to find resources hid endemically
A family therapist, I seek solutions quite systemically.

5

I am a bold upholder of constructivist psychology
I preach the special virtue of my own epistemology
If you say you've got symptoms in a naive voice declarative
Externalize the problem! Catechize that truth is narrative!
I help clients eschew the norm and cross their story's Rubicon
Landscapes of consciousness provide a place free from Panopticon
I even tackle tough ones, like the self-recursive sodomist . . .
I say it's just expressive of a credo quite postmodernist.

   Chorus:
   He'll say it's just expressive of a credo quite postmodernist
   He'll say it's just expressive of a credo quite postmodernist
   He'll say it's just expressive of a credo quite postmodern-modernist.

If you find this obfuscating, quite nonsensical, confusing, I'm
Afraid you'll never understand until you shift your paradigm.
I preach the special virtue of my own epistemology
I am a bold upholder of constructivist psychology.

HAIKU

Michael F. Hoyt

Solution focus
Find exception and increase
Otherwise stay the same

More of same, no change
More of difference, not same
When will you notice?

Single session now
Kill it, make it sing, or wait
The cage is open

Note. Written July 1995 in Kyoto at 4 A.M. after being awakened by a small earthquake. Legend has it that three Japanese lords of old revealed their very different characters when asked what they would do with a nightingale that did not sing.

Index